Physical Activity for Psychological and Cognitive Development

Physical Activity for Psychological and Cognitive Development

Guest Editors

Josune Rodríguez-Negro
Víctor Arufe-Giráldez

MDPI

Basel • Beijing • Wuhan • Barcelona • Belgrade • Novi Sad • Cluj • Manchester

Guest Editors
Josune Rodríguez-Negro
Faculty of Education and Sport
University of the Basque Country
Vitoria-Gasteiz
Spain

Víctor Arufe-Giráldez
Faculty of Education
University of A Coruña
A Coruña
Spain

Editorial Office
MDPI AG
Grosspeteranlage 5
4052 Basel, Switzerland

This is a reprint of the Special Issue, published open access by the journal *Behavioral Sciences* (ISSN 2076-328X), freely accessible at: https://www.mdpi.com/journal/behavsci/special_issues/I8DM31HIFN.

For citation purposes, cite each article independently as indicated on the article page online and as indicated below:

Lastname, A.A.; Lastname, B.B. Article Title. *Journal Name* **Year**, *Volume Number*, Page Range.

ISBN 978-3-7258-5469-1 (Hbk)
ISBN 978-3-7258-5470-7 (PDF)
https://doi.org/10.3390/books978-3-7258-5470-7

Contents

Contents

About the Editors

Josune Rodríguez Negro

Josune Rodríguez Negro holds an International Doctorate in Education and Sports. She currently works at the Physical Education and Sports department of the University of the Basque Country (UPV/EHU). Her research activities are focused on education, physical education, methodology and innovation. As a researcher, she has published more than 70 publications, including books, articles and book chapters in national and international journals of high impact. She has given several talks and courses on innovation and teaching in international congresses and seminars. She is a reviewer for international scientific journals and has participated in various international congresses as a member of the scientific committee. She has also participated in several research projects.

Víctor Arufe Giráldez

Víctor Arufe Giráldez at the Faculty of Education of the University of A Coruña. His research interests focus on physical education didactics, psychomotricity, school sport, active learning methodologies and how affective pedagogies influence students' engagement. He has published over 200 scientific works, including journal articles, book chapters and educational guides. He is the editor-in-chief of two scientific journals. He has been awarded recognition for his excellence in teaching and educational innovation.

behavioral sciences

MDPI

Article

Is It Possible to Improve the Perceived Quality of Life of Overweight or Obese Older People through a Multicomponent Physical Exercise Program?

Yazmina Pleticosic-Ramírez [1,2], Víctor Arufe-Giráldez [3], Josune Rodríguez-Negro [4,5], Marcos Mecías-Calvo [6,*] and Rubén Navarro-Patón [6]

1 Departamento de Salud, Universidad Internacional Iberoamericana, Campeche 24560, Mexico; yazmina.pleticosic@doctorado.unini.edu.mx
2 Facultad de Educación, Pedagogía en Educación Física, Universidad San Sebastián, Lientur 1457, Concepción 4080871, Chile
3 Facultad de Ciencias de la Educación, Universidad de A Coruña, 15008 A Coruña, Spain; v.arufe@udc.es
4 Department of Didactics of Musical, Plastic and Corporal Expression, Faculty of Education, University of the Basque Country (UPV/EHU), 48940 Leioa, Spain; josune.rodriguez@ehu.eus
5 Research Unit of School Sport, Physical Education and Psychomotricity, University of A Coruña, 15008 A Coruña, Spain
6 Facultade de Formación do Profesorado, Universidade de Santiago de Compostela, 27001 Lugo, Spain; ruben.navarro.paton@usc.es
* Correspondence: marcos.mecias@usc.es

Abstract: Multicomponent exercise is a physical exercise modality in which various physical qualities (strength, cardiorespiratory endurance, flexibility, and balance) are developed with an equal distribution of volume in the same session (approximately 60 min) and that has been little explored in improving the quality of life of older adults. The aim of this study was to verify the effect of multicomponent training on self-perceived quality of life in Chilean overweight or obese older people. To this end, a quasi-experimental study with a control group was designed to evaluate self-perceived Quality of Life using the World Health Organization Quality of Life, brief version [Overall Quality of Life (OQOL); Overall Health (OH); Physical Health (PH); Psychological Health (PsH); Social Relations (SR); Environment (E)]. Seventy overweight or obese people aged between 60 and 86 years participated (M = 73.15; SD = 5.94) and were randomized into a control group (CG, n = 35) and an experimental group (EG, n = 35). The results in the EG (pre vs. post-intervention) indicated that there were statistically significant differences in OQOL ($p = 0.005$), OH ($p = 0.014$), PH ($p < 0.001$), PsH ($p < 0.001$), E ($p = 0.015$), and SR ($p < 0.001$) which were not found in the CG in any of the variables ($p > 0.050$) except in SR ($p < 0.001$). Regarding sex, post-intervention differences were only found between CG and EG in women in OQOL ($p = 0.002$), PH ($p < 0.001$), PsH ($p = 0.003$), and SR ($p < 0.001$), but not in OH or E ($p > 0.050$). These differences were not found among men in any of the variables ($p > 0.050$). As a conclusion, we can say that a multicomponent physical exercise program applied for 6 months significantly improves the perception of OQOL, OH, PH, PsH, SR, and E in overweight or obese older people. This perception is greater in men than in women.

Keywords: quality of life; elderly; ageing; perception; WHOQOL-BREF physical activity

1. Introduction

Nowadays, in developed countries, reaching an advanced age is no longer exceptional [1]. The demographic transformation towards an aging society is perceived as a sociodemographic change that has been increasing in recent decades [2]. Ageing brings with it physical limitations or chronic diseases that cause a lack of full well-being in this sector of the population [3,4]. However, well-being can be improved through the practice of physical exercise (PE) [5], which consequently causes an increase in the self-perceived quality of life in older adults [6]. Quality of life refers to an individual's perception of his or her position in life in the context of the culture and value system in which he or she lives and in relation to his or her goals, expectations, standards, and concerns [7,8].

Relating PE to quality of life, Vázquez et al. [5] found a positive association between quality of life and higher levels of physical activity, as well as lower levels of depression and dependence. Bouaziz et al. [9] mention that regular exercise has been shown to have many health benefits, positively impacting quality of life.

Health-related quality of life has been studied through the SF-36 questionnaire in previous research, where significant effects were obtained on physical performance and quality of life [10]; in the mental component and mental health subscale with the practice of HITT [11]; pain reduction, social and vitality improvements with the practice of moderate intensity aquatic training; improving vitality and health status with HIIT aquatic training [12]; improvement in general health, physical functioning, mental health, and vitality with resistance training [13]; and improvement in health status, vitality, and social aspects with multicomponent aquatic training [14]. Previous studies related to improvements through multicomponent exercise have analyzed improvements in BMI [15], functional capacity, or physical capacity [16], among others. Finally, the scientific evidence to date, including the WHOQOL-BREF questionnaire and multicomponent physical exercise, to evaluate quality of life in older adults is scarce or has been carried out only in women [17,18] or only to evaluate cognitive functions [19].

Multicomponent exercise is a PE modality in which various physical qualities (strength, cardiorespiratory endurance, flexibility, and balance) are developed with an equal distribution of volume in the same session (approximately 60 min) [20] and that has been little explored in improving the quality of life of older adults.

For all of the above, and given the lack of evidence on the effect of multicomponent PE on quality of life in older adults, the objective of this study was to verify the effect of multicomponent training on self-perceived quality of life in older Chilean overweight or obese people and whether these effects are the same in men and women.

2. Materials and Methods

2.1. Study Design

For this study with a quasi-experimental design with pre- and post-test measures, with a control group [21], the World Health Organization questionnaire (WHOQOL-BREF) [22] was used to evaluate quality of life, adapted to the Chilean adult population [23] (i.e., Overall Quality of Life (OQOL); Overall Health (OH); Physical Health (PH); Psychological Health (PsH); Environment (E); Social Relations (SR)) according to the group (control vs. experimental), and this was stratified according to gender (man vs. woman).

2.2. Participants

A total of 153 individuals who were overweight or obese and were 60 years of age or older—59 men and 94 women—were invited to take part in this study. A convenience sample was provided of members of clubs affiliated with the Regional Federation of Community Unions of the Elderly in the Biobío area of Concepción, Chile. The following criteria had to be met in order to be considered for inclusion: (a) being 60 years of age or older; (b) being overweight or obese people according to WHO criteria [24]; (c) not having a medical condition that would prevent them from taking part in the tests or intervention program; (d) being physically independent; (e) signing an informed consent form.

After fulfilling all the requirements for admission, 70 participants were randomly assigned to one of two groups: the experimental group (EG, n = 35; 28 women/7 men) or the control group (CG, n = 35; 33 women/2 men).

2.3. Instruments

2.3.1. Sociodemographic Data

The data on the variables age (years) and sex (male/female) were self-reported.

2.3.2. Anthropometric and Body Composition Measurements

For anthropometric and body composition measurements, the protocol of the International Society for the Advancement of Kinanthropometry (ISAK) [25] was used for both body mass and height. These two allowed us to determine the degree of obesity through the body mass index (BMI) with the formula [weight kg/height m^2], following the WHO measurements [24].

The height measurement was performed with the portable SECA 206 stadiometer in the maximum extension position, placing the square firmly on the Vertex, compressing the hair as much as possible, and asking the person to inhale deeply and hold their breath before the subject evaluated exhaled [25].

Body mass was calculated using the Omrom HBF-514C equipment. Weight was evaluated with minimal clothing, checking that the scale was at zero. These measurements were routinely performed in the morning, twelve hours after the last meal [25].

2.3.3. Adapted World Health Organization Quality of Life Questionnaire (WHOQOL-BREF)

The self-administered questionnaire of the World Health Organization (WHOQOL-BREF) [22] was used to evaluate the quality of life adapted to the Chilean older people population [23]. This self-administered questionnaire is composed of a general question on quality of life ("How would you rate your quality of life?"), a question on satisfaction with your health status ("Are you satisfied with your health?"), and 24 items grouped into four dimensions: Physical Health (e.g., "To what extent do you think that physical pain prevents you from doing what you need?"), Psychological Health (e.g., "To what extent do you feel that Does your life have meaning?"), Social Relationships (e.g., "To what extent are you satisfied with your interpersonal relationships?"), and Environment (e.g., "To what extent are you satisfied with the conditions of the place where you live?"). The items are scored on a five-point Likert 1 scale with five different formats (1 = "very bad" to 5 = "very good", 1 = "very dissatisfied" to 5 = "quite satisfied", 1 =not at all to 5= "a lot", 1= "very little" to 5= "very good", 1= "never" to 5= "always").

2.3.4. Intervention Program

The EG participated in a multicomponent physical exercise program. This is defined as a type of training that incorporates different elements, such as cardiovascular training, coordination, strength, balance, and flexibility, in a single exercise session [26] which was taught by the main researcher, who has 15 years of experience in the field of Physical Education. The program lasted 6 months, with 2 sessions per week, each lasting 60 min. Each session was organized as can be seen in Figure 1. The CG participants continued with their daily lives without modifying their habits or participating in any physical exercise program.

2.4. Procedure

Contact was made first with the management of the clubs of the Regional Federation of Community Unions of older people in the Biobío region of the city of Concepción (Chile), and the objective of the study was explained to them. After management approval, an invitation letter was sent to potential participants for an informational meeting to explain the aim and purpose of the study, the procedure, and their voluntary participation, as well as the confidentiality statement.

After the participants signed the informed consent, the necessary sociodemographic data (age and sex) were self-reported and the participants were randomly assigned to EG and CG. The anthropometric measurements (i.e., height, weight, and BMI following the formula BMI = weight kg/height m^2) and the self-administered questionnaire were collected prior to the start of the intervention. The survey lasted approximately 15 min. Once the initial data was collected, the intervention program was applied to the EG. Once the intervention period was over, data on quality of life were collected using the WHOQOL-

BREF questionnaire for both groups (CG and EG) within one week after completing the intervention program. All research was carried out in accordance with the Declaration of Helsinki. The research protocol was sent and approved by the Ethics Committee of the Universidad Internacional Iberoamericana on 22 June 2022, being approved and registered in file number CR-163.

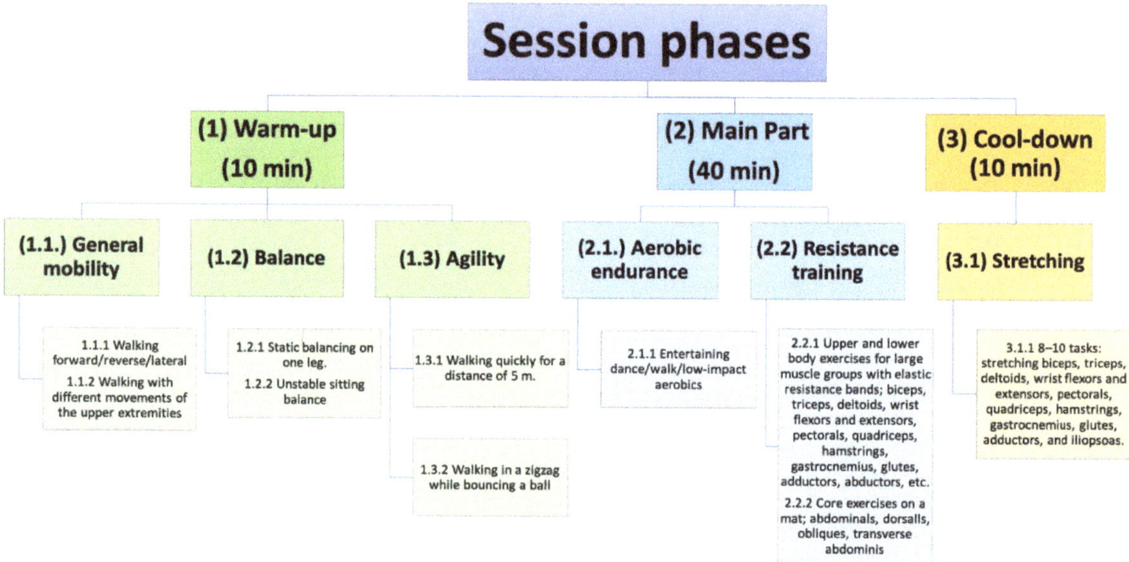

Figure 1. Phases and contents of the sessions and types of exercises of the multicomponent program.

2.5. Statistical Analysis

The IBM SPSS Statistics for Windows program, version 25.0, was used to statistically analyse the data in this study. Measures of central tendency (mean and standard deviation) are used to present the results of the quantitative variables (Overall Quality of Life (OQOL), Overall Health (OH), Physical Health (PH), Psychological Health (PsH), Environment (E), Social Relations (SR), BMI, height, weight, and age); percentages and frequencies are used to present the results of the qualitative variables (sex and degree of overweightness or obesity). The Kolmogorov–Smirnov test was performed to confirm the normality of the data. First, for each dependent variable under investigation, the descriptive statistics (mean and standard deviation) were determined. Second, an independent sample *t*-test was used to determine whether the groups (the experimental group and the control group) were equivalent in terms of age and anthropometry (BMI, height, weight), the Chi square test was used to determine whether the groups were equivalent in terms of the participants' sex and degree of obesity or overweightness, and finally, an independent samples T test was used to check for changes in BMI, height, and weight. Using Time as a repeated measures factor (i.e., Time (pre-test vs. post-test), Group (Control group vs. Experimental group), and Sex (man vs. woman)) to analyse the potential main effect of these factors on the variables of the WHOQOL-BREF questionnaire and their interaction using the statistic Bonferroni, a three-factor ANOVA (time x group x degree of overweight or obesity) was conducted after the six-month intervention. The eta squared ($\eta 2$) was used to calculate the effect size.

3. Results

The sample was divided into two analysis groups, the CG (n = 35), with a mean age of 72.54 years (SD = 5.55), and the EG (n = 35), with a mean age of 73.77 years (SD = 6.32). Regarding the sex variable, 87% of the participants were women (n = 61) and 13% men (n = 9), distributing 33 women and 2 men in the CG and 28 women and 7 men in the EG. The baseline characteristics of the sample (Table 1) indicate that there were no statistically significant differences in any of the variables [i.e., mean age (p = 0.391); gender (p= 0.075); average height (p = 0.685); average weight (p = 0.443); BMI (p = 0.215) and degree of overweight-obesity (p = 528)] between the CG and EG.

Table 1. Sample characterization.

	Control Group	Experimental Group
Variables		
Average age (years)	72.54 ± 5.55	73.77 ± 6.32
Sex		
Man	2 (72.2%)	7 (27.8%)
Woman	33 (27.8%)	28 (72.2%)
Average height (m)	1.538 ± 7.16	1.530 ± 9.16
Average weight (kg)	72.51 ± 11.99	74.80 ± 12.75
Average BMI (kg/m^2)	30.71 ± 4.075	31.88 ± 3.73
Degree of overweight-obesity		
Overweight	17 (24.3%)	11 (15.7%)
Type I Obesity	13 (18.6%)	17 (24.3%)
Type II Obesity	4 (5.7%)	6 (8.6%)
Type III Obesity	1 (1.4%)	1 (1.4%)

Note: Quantitative variables are expressed as mean and standard deviation, and qualitative variables are expressed as frequencies and percentages.

The normality test revealed that the data followed a normal distribution [i.e., OQOL (p = 0.121), OH (p = 0.243), PH (p = 0.516), PsH (p = 0.412), E (p = 0.288), and SR (p = 0.300)].

3.1. *CG and EG Pre-Intervention Comparison*

The results before the intervention indicated that there were no statistically significant differences in any of the variables studied [i.e., OQOL (p = 0.084), OH (p = 0.783), PH (p = 0.175), PsH (p = 0.732), SR (p = 0.715), and E (p = 0.705)] in the comparison between the CG and EG (Table 2).

Table 2. Pre- and post-intervention results of the control and experimental groups.

Variable	CG Pre (n = 35)	EG Pre (n = 35)	CG Post (n = 35)	EG Post (n = 35)
Quality of Life	3.25 ± 1.01	3.80 ± 0.96	3.42 ± 0.91	4.22 ± 0.80
Overall Health	3.00 ± 1.11	3.31 ± 0.96	3.14 ± 0.91	3.62 ± 0.80
Physical Health	3.51 ± 0.67	3.58 ± 0.54	3.46 ± 0.59	3.93 ± 0.51
Psychological Health	3.60 ± 0.74	3.82 ± 0.39	3.58 ± 0.71	4.10 ± 0.52
Social Relations	3.22 ± 0.69	3.49 ± 0.64	3.09 ± 0.72	3.80 ± 0.52
Environment	3.47 ± 0.55	3.68 ± 0.61	3.60 ± 1.26	3.96 ± 0.56

Note: Data are presented as mean ± standard deviation.

Depending on sex (Figure 2), the results indicated that there were no previous statistically significant differences between women in the CG and women in the EG in any of the variables studied [i.e., OQOL (p = 0.067); OH (p = 0.246); PH (p = 0.272); PsH (p = 0.085); SR (p = 0.067); E (p = 0.062)], nor between men from the CG and men from the EG [i.e., OQOL (p = 0.216); OH (p = 0.933); PH (p = 0.077); PsH (p = 0.360); SR (p = 0.330); E (p = 0.318)]. For all these reasons, the groups were equivalent with respect to all the variables studied.

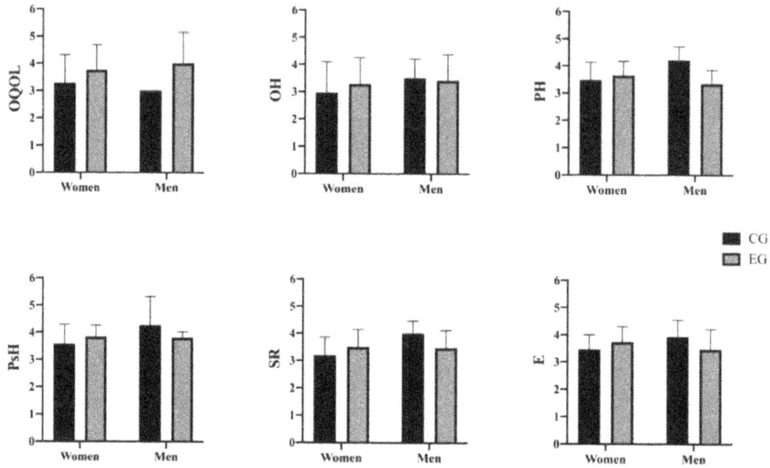

Figure 2. Pre-test differences between CG and EG. CG: control group; EG: experimental group; OQOL: Overall Quality Of Life; OH: Overall Health; PH: Physical Health; PsH: Psychological Health; SR: Social Relations; E: Environment.

3.2. Control Group Results

The pre- and post-intervention results of the CG (Table 1) indicated that there were statistically significant differences in OQOL [$F(1, 66) = 4.423$, $p = 0.039$, $\eta 2 = 0.063$, 95% CI -1.093, -0.028], with the scores being lower before than after 6 months, but not in the rest of the variables [i.e., OH ($p = 0.737$); PH ($p = 0.668$); PsH ($p = 609$); SR ($p = 0.724$); E ($p = 0.827$)].

There were no statistically significant differences in any of the variables studied in the pre–post comparison in the CG, depending on sex (Figure 3), nor in women [i.e., OQOL ($p = 0.345$); OH ($p = 0.164$); PH ($p = 0.071$); PsH ($p = 0.676$); SR ($p = 0.143$); E ($p = 0.363$)], nor in men [i.e., OQOL ($p = 0.058$); OH (1.00); PH ($p = 0.288$); PsH ($p = 0.671$); SR ($p = 1.00$); E ($p = 1.00$)].

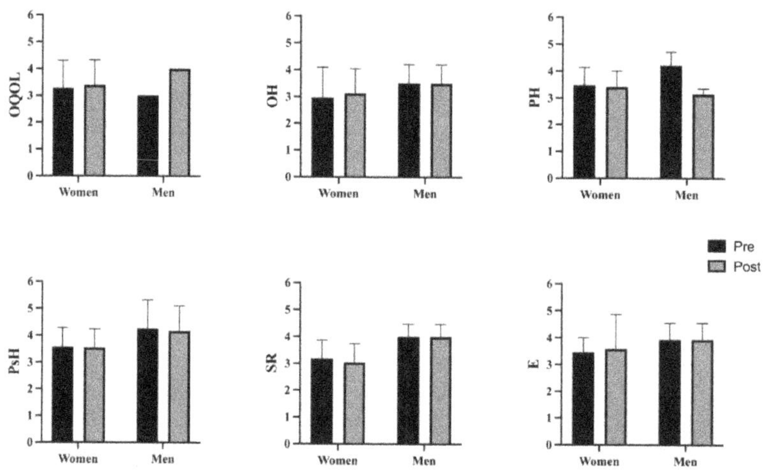

Figure 3. Pre-post-test sex differences in the CG. CG: control group; OQOL: Overall Quality Of Life; OH: Overall Health; PH: Physical Health; PsH: Psychological Health; SR: Social Relations; E: Environment.

3.3. Experimental Group Results

The pre- and post-intervention results of the EG (Table 1) indicated that there were statistically significant differences in all the variables of the questionnaire (i.e., OQOL [F(1, 66) = 11.995, $p < 0.001$, η2 = 0.154, 95% CI −0.845, −0.227]; OH [F(1, 66) = 9.894, $p = 0.002$, η2 = 0.130, 95% CI −0.671, −0.150]; PH [F(1, 66) = 24.187, $p < 0.001$, η2 = 0.268, 95% CI −0.595, −0.252], PsH [F(1, 66) = 48.737, $p < 0.001$, η2 = 0.425, 95% CI −0.524, −0.291]; SR [F(1, 66) = 12.557, $p = 0.001$, η2 = 0.160, 95% CI −0.642, −0.179] and E [F(1, 66) = 6.321, $p = 0.001$, η2 = 0.087, 95% CI −0.793, −0.091]).

In the comparison of pre- and post-intervention in the EG (Figure 4), there were statistically significant differences in all the variables studied between women (OQOL [F(1, 66) = 6.664, $p = 0.012$, η2 = 0.092, 95% CI −0.633, −0.081; OH [F(1, 66) = 4.582, $p = 0.036$, η2 = 0.065, 95% CI −0.483, −0.017]; PH [F(1, 66) = 14.764, $p < 0.001$, η2 = 0.183, 95% CI −0.450, −0.142]; PsH [F(1, 66) = 14.139, $p < 0.001$, η2 = 0.176, 95% CI −0.301, −0.092]; SR [F(1, 66) = 5.1816, $p = 0.019$, η2 = 0.176, 95% CI −0.457, −0.043], except in E ($p = 0.285$); and between men (OQOL [F(1, 66) = 6.664, $p = 0.012$, η2 = 0.092, 95% CI −1.267, −0.162]; OH [F(1, 66) = 5.985, $p = 0.017$, η2 = 0.083, 95% CI −1.038, −0.105]; PH [F(1, 66) = 12.797, $p = 0.001$, η2 = 0.162, 95% CI −0.859, −0.243]; PsH [F(1, 66) = 35.107, $p < 0.001$, η2 = 0.347, 95% CI −0.828, −0.410]; SR [F(1, 66) = 7.596, $p = 0.008$, η2 = 0.347, 95% CI −0.985, −0.157], and E [F(1, 66) = 5.160, $p = 0.026$, η2 = 0.073, 95% CI −1.342, −0.086]).

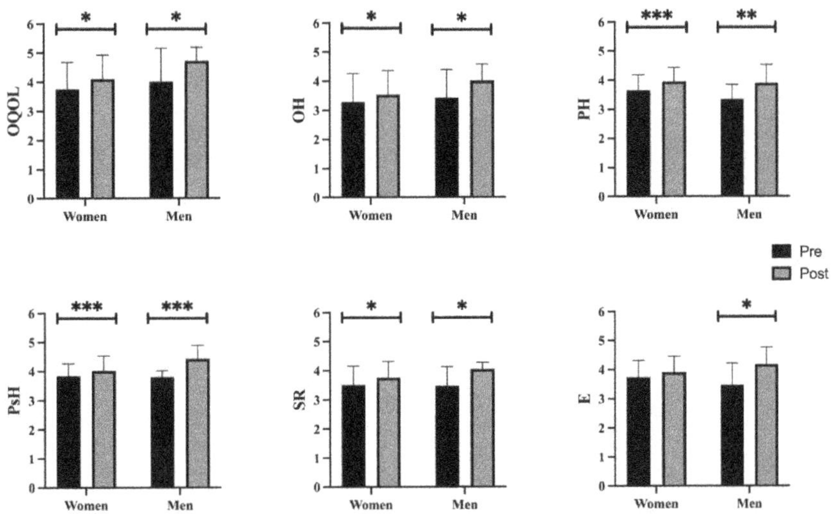

Figure 4. Pre-post-test sex differences in the EG. EG: experimental group; OQOL: Overall Quality Of Life; OH: Overall Health; PH: Physical Health; PsH: Psychological Health; SR: Social Relations; E: Environment. Note: * $p < 0.05$ different between Pre- vs. Post-test; ** $p = 0.001$ different between Pre- vs. Post-test; *** $p < 0.001$ different between Pre- vs. Post-test.

3.4. CG vs. EG Post-Intervention Results

There were statistically significant differences post-intervention results between the CG and EG (Table 1) only in OQOL [F(1, 66) = 3.954, $p = 0.005$, η2 = 0.057, 95% CI −1.430, −0.003]. There were no statistically significant differences in OH ($p = 0.212$), PH ($p = 0.552$), PsH ($p = 0.155$), SR (p =0.149), or E ($p = 0.501$).

In the post-intervention comparison between groups (CG vs. EG) (Figure 5), after carrying out the stratified analysis by gender and analyzing their interaction, there were statistically significant differences in almost all the variables studied between women (OQOL [F(1, 66) = 10.597, $p = 0.002$, η2 = 0.138, 230 95% CI −1.151, −0.276]; PH [F(1, 66) = 13.558, $p < 0.001$, η2 = 0.170, 95% CI −0.808, −0.098]; PsH 231 [F(1, 66) = 9.355, $p = 0.003$, η2 = 0.124,

95% CI −0.800, −0.168]; and SR [$F(1, 66) = 20.080$, $p <$ 232 0.001, $\eta 2 = 0.233$, 95% CI −1.026, −0.393], except in OH ($p = 0.066$) and E ($p = 0.209$).

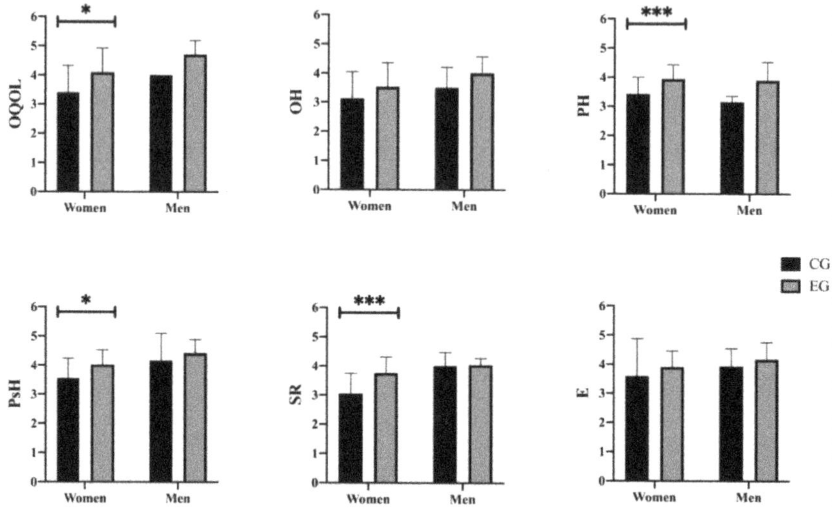

Figure 5. Post-test sex differences between CG and EG. CG: control group; EG: experimental group; OQOL: Overall Quality Of Life; OH: Overall Health; PH: Physical Health; PsH: Psychological Health; SR: Social Relations; E: Environment. Note: * $p < 0.05$ different between Pre- vs. Post-test; *** $p < 0.001$ different between CG vs. EG Post-test.

Regarding men, no statistically significant differences were found in any of the variables studied [i.e., OQOL ($p = 0.300$), OH ($p = 0.472$), PH ($p = 0.583$), PsH ($p = 0.598$), SR ($p = 0.924$), and E ($p = 0.762$)].

4. Discussion

The aim of the present study was to determine the effect of a six-month multicomponent PE program on the perceived quality of life of older Chilean overweight or obese people and whether these effects are similar in women and men. At a general level, the results obtained indicate the beneficial effects of practicing PE in older people [5,27], specifically highlighting that a multicomponent PE program is associated with improvements in the perceived quality of life in older Chilean overweight or obese adults [15,28].

Before the intervention, the CG and the EG presented similar scores in QOL, since there were no statistically significant differences in any of its components (i.e., OQOL; OH; PH; PsH; SR; E), neither globally [28,29] nor based on sex [30]. These results could be due to the fact that the sample was pulled from the same population source and had similar ages and BMIs.

After the intervention using the multicomponent PE program, significant improvements in OQOL were found when comparing CG versus EG. These improvements in the scores given by the EG may be related to the fact that a PE program, such as the one implemented in this research, produces changes and improvements in the functional abilities of the participants [17] and, consequently, in improving the perception of quality of life. These results are consistent with the results obtained by Tricco et al. [31] and Villareal et al. [32], who observed a positive correlation between the increase in performance in general EF with the increase in quality of life in older people with obesity after six months of intervention, as in our case. Depending on sex, the results indicated that there were significant differences between women in the CG and EG after the intervention in OQOL, PH, PsH, and SR. These results may be associated with and related to what was reported in previous studies, which indicates that regular PE can improve results beyond physical health and generate greater social interaction [33]. However, no significant differences were found between men in both groups.

After the intervention using multicomponent PE in the EG, there were significant improvements in all components of the perceived quality of life evaluated with the WHOQOL-BREF questionnaire (i.e., OQOL; OH; PH; PsH; SR; E), globally [34] and in both men [35,36] and women [17], which did not occur in the CG. This improvement in quality of life may be related to participation in PE programs where muscle strength is increased, contributing to the performance of more tasks of daily living with less effort and help. Consequently, participants perceive an improvement in levels of health and physical and psychological well-being, improving social interaction by perceiving that they are more independent [37]. Our results are similar to those reported by Whitehurst et al. [38], who, after applying a multicomponent PE program and evaluating quality of life with the short form health survey (SF-36), observed an improvement in the perceived quality of life, as well as those reported by Maung et al. [34] or Atad and Caspi [39], who showed that performing 2.5 h of PE per week not only produced better physical health but was also associated with a better perceived quality of life.

Regarding the CG, once the intervention period was over, the scores of the different dimensions of quality of life of the components studied were maintained and, in some cases, decreased. These results are consistent with those obtained by Resende-Neto et al. [17] since the improvement in the perception of quality of life occurs alongside participation in systematic PE programs, which was not carried out by this group.

5. Limitations

This research has limitations that we want to note; the first of them is the use of a self-reported questionnaire, which can produce biases in the participants' responses. Another limitation is the size of the sample, due to its limited number and its selection for convenience and the possibility of access. Regarding the sample, it should also be noted that the small number of male participants is very limited due to the characteristics of participation in physical activity programs, and therefore, we cannot extrapolate the results to this group. Thus, more studies would be necessary in which it would be possible to increase the sample size in this regard.

Finally, we must indicate that a long-term follow-up was not carried out to verify whether this multicomponent physical exercise program maintains its long-term effect on the perceived quality of life of overweight or obese older people.

6. Conclusions

As conclusions of this study, we can say that a multicomponent physical exercise program, applied for 6 months, produces significant improvements in self-perceived quality of life and global health, as well as physical and psychological health, social relationships, and the environment, in overweight or obese older people. However, no improvements occurred in older people who did not participate in this multicomponent exercise program.

We can also conclude that a multicomponent physical exercise program produces a greater perception of quality of life in men compared to women in all the variables studied except in physical health, where women give higher scores.

Author Contributions: Conceptualization, Y.P.-R., M.M.-C. and R.N.-P.; methodology, Y.P.-R., M.M.-C. and R.N.-P.; validation, Y.P.-R., V.A.-G., J.R.-N., V.A.-G., M.M.-C. and R.N.-P.; formal analysis, R.N.-P.; investigation, Y.P.-R., M.M.-C. and R.N.-P.; data curation, Y.P.-R.; writing—original draft preparation, Y.P.-R., V.A.-G., J.R.-N., M.M.-C. and R.N.-P.; writing—review and editing, Y.P.-R., V.A.-G., J.R.-N., M.M.-C. and R.N.-P.; visualization, Y.P.-R., V.A.-G., J.R.-N., M.M.-C. and R.N.-P.; supervision, M.M.-C. and R.N.-P.; project administration, Y.P.-R., M.M.-C. and R.N.-P. All authors have read and agreed to the published version of the manuscript.

Funding: This research received no external funding.

Institutional Review Board Statement: The study was conducted according to the guidelines of the Declaration of Helsinki and approved by the Ethics Committee of the Universidad Internacional Iberoamericana (protocol code CR-163 and date of approval 22 June 2022).

Informed Consent Statement: Informed consent was obtained from all subjects involved in the study.

Data Availability Statement: The datasets presented in this article are not available because they are part of a doctoral thesis which has not yet been defended. Requests to access the datasets should be directed to Y.P.-R.

Conflicts of Interest: The authors declare no conflicts of interest.

References

1. Ribera Casado, J.M. Investigación sobre el envejecimiento: Una agenda más allá de la biogerontología—Anales RANM. *An. De. La. Real. Acad. Nac. De. Med. De. España* **2019**, *135*, 281–285. [CrossRef]
2. Sánchez-Rodríguez, M. Envejecimiento En México (ENASEM). Una Herramienta Para El Estudio Del Envejecimiento Saludable. *Casos Y Revis. De. Salud* **2022**, *4*, 39–56. [CrossRef]
3. Marcos-Pardo, P.J.; González-Gálvez, N.; Vaquero-Cristóbal, R.; Sagarra-Romero, L.; López-Vivancos, A.; Velázquez-Díaz, D.; Gea García, G.M.; Ponce-González, J.G.; Esteban-Cornejo, I.; Jiménez-Pavón, D.; et al. Programa de Intervención Multidominio Healthy-Age: Recomendaciones para un envejecimiento saludable: Por la red Healthy-Age. *Cult. Cienc. Deporte* **2021**, *16*, 311–320. [CrossRef]
4. Agudelo-Cuéllar, L.M.; Lancheros-López, F.N. Entorno familiar, social y estado de salud de los adultos mayores: Una revisión sistemática desde el cuidado de enfermería. *Boletín Semillero De. Investig. En. Fam.* **2021**, *3*, e807. [CrossRef]
5. Vázquez, L.Á.; Navarro-Patón, R.; Ramos-Álvarez, O.; Mecías-Calvo, M.; Lago-Fuentes, C. Actividad Física y Calidad de Vida de Adultos Mayores En Argentina: Un Estudio Transversal (Physical Activity and Quality of Life in Argentinian Older Adults: A Cross-Sectional Study). *Retos* **2023**, *48*, 86–93. [CrossRef]
6. Molina Napurí, A.; Cambillo Moyano, E. Validación del Módulo WHOQOL-OLD en personas atendidas en Organizaciones para el Adulto Mayor. *Pesquimat* **2021**, *24*, 9–22. [CrossRef]
7. Queirolo Ore, S.A.; Barboza Palomino, M.; Ventura-León, J. Medición de La Calidad de Vida En Adultos Mayores Institucionalizados de Lima (Perú). *Enfermería Glob.* **2020**, *19*, 259–288. [CrossRef]
8. Rojas, A.; De León, E.; Juárez, A. Actividad Física y Calidad de Vida En El Adulto Mayor. *Eur. Sci. J. ESJ* **2022**, *11*, 365–373. [CrossRef]
9. Bouaziz, W.; Lang, P.O.; Schmitt, E.; Kaltenbach, G.; Geny, B.; Vogel, T. Health Benefits of Multicomponent Training Programmes in Seniors: A Systematic Review. *Int. J. Clin. Pr.* **2016**, *70*, 520–536. [CrossRef]
10. Hammami, N.; Mechraoui, A.; Hattabi, S.; Forte, P.; Sampaio, T.; Sortwell, A.; Teixeira, J.E.; Branquinho, L.; Ferraz, R.; Bouassida, A. Concentric Isokinetic Strengthening Program's Impact on Knee Biomechanical Parameters, Physical Performance and Quality of Life in Overweight/Obese Women with Chronic Meniscal Lesions. *Healthcare* **2023**, *11*, 2079. [CrossRef]
11. Ballin, M.; Lundberg, E.; Sörlén, N.; Nordström, P.; Hult, A.; Nordström, A. Effects of Interval Training on Quality of Life and Cardiometabolic Risk Markers in Older Adults: A Randomized Controlled Trial. *Clin. Interv. Aging* **2019**, *14*, 1589–1599. [CrossRef] [PubMed]
12. Rezaeipour, M. Investigation of Pool Workouts on Weight, Body Composition, Resting Energy Expenditure, and Quality of Life among Sedentary Obese Older Women. *Montenegrin J. Sports Sci. Med.* **2020**, *9*, 67–72. [CrossRef]
13. Fritz, N.B.; Gargallo, P.; Juesas, A.; Flandez, J.; Furtado, G.E.; Teixeira, A.M.; Colado, J.C. High-and Moderate-Intensity Resistance Training Provokes Different Effects on Body Composition, Functionality, and Well-Being in Elderly. *J. Hum. Sport. Exerc.* **2021**, *16*, S335–S352. [CrossRef]
14. Rezaeipour, M.; Apanasenko, G.L.; Banparvari, M. Weight-Loss Parameters and Quality of Life in Obese Aged Women Using WATERinMOTION. *Health Scope* **2021**, *10*, e109478. [CrossRef]
15. Pleticosic-Ramírez, Y.; Mecías Calvo, M.; Navarro-Patón, R. Efectos de Programas de Ejercicio Físico En La Composición Corporal, Condición Física y Calidad de Vida de Personas Mayores Con Sobrepeso u Obesidad: Una Revisión Sistemática (Effects of Physical Exercise Programs on Body Composition, Physical Fitness And. *Retos* **2024**, *56*, 47–62. [CrossRef]
16. Jofré-Saldía, E.; Villalobos-Gorigoitía, Á.; Cofré-Bolados, C.; Ferrari, G.; Gea-García, G.M. Multicomponent Training in Progressive Phases Improves Functional Capacity, Physical Capacity, Quality of Life, and Exercise Motivation in Community-Dwelling Older Adults: A Randomized Clinical Trial. *Int. J. Environ. Res. Public Health* **2023**, *20*, 2755. [CrossRef] [PubMed]
17. De Resende-Neto, A.; do Nascimento, M.A.; Da Silva, D.; Netto, R.; De Santana, J.; Silva, M. Effects of Multicomponent Training on Functional Fitness and Quality of Life in Older Women: A Randomized Controlled Trial. *Int. J. Sport. Exerc. Med.* **2019**, *5*, 2469–5718. [CrossRef]
18. Stolarz, I.; Baszak, E.M.; Zawadka, M.; Majcher, P. Functional Status, Quality of Life, and Physical Activity of Senior Club Members—A Cross-Sectional Study. *Int. J. Environ. Res. Public Health* **2022**, *19*, 1900. [CrossRef] [PubMed]
19. Kim, Y.-J.; Park, H.; Park, J.H.; Park, K.W.; Lee, K.; Kim, S.; Chae, K.; Park, M.H.; Koh, S.-H.; Na, H.R. Effects of Multicomponent Exercise on Cognitive Function in Elderly Korean Individuals. *J. Clin. Neurol.* **2020**, *16*, 612–623. [CrossRef]

20. Cancela, J.M.; Vila, M.H.; Sanchez-Lastra, M.A.; Varela, S. La Socialización Mejora La Adherencia, Pero No La Fuerza, En Programas de Ejercicio Físico Con Componente de Fuerza En Personas Mayores. *Rev. Andal. Med. Deport.* **2021**, *14*, 103–107. [CrossRef]
21. Ato, M.; López-García, J.J.; Benavente, A. A Classification System for Research Designs in Psychology. *Ann. Psychol.* **2013**, *29*, 1038–1059. [CrossRef]
22. Skevington, S.M.; Lotfy, M.; O'Connell, K.A. The World Health Organization's WHOQOL-BREF Quality of Life Assessment: Psychometric Properties and Results of the International Field Trial. A Report from the WHOQOL Group. *Qual. Life Res.* **2004**, *13*, 299–310. [CrossRef] [PubMed]
23. Espinoza, I.; Osorio, P.; Torrejón, M.J.; Lucas-Carrasco, R.; Bunout, D. Validación Del Cuestionario de Calidad de Vida (WHOQOL-BREF) En Adultos Mayores Chilenos. *Rev. Med. Chil.* **2011**, *139*, 579–586. [CrossRef] [PubMed]
24. World Health Organization Obesity and Overweight. Available online: https://www.who.int/news-room/fact-sheets/detail/obesity-and-overweight (accessed on 28 April 2024).
25. Sociedad Internacional para el Avance de la Kinantropometría. *Estándares Internacionales Para La Valoración*; Biblioteca Nacional de Australia: Canberra, ACT, Australia, 2001.
26. Araque-Martínez, M.Á.; Ruiz-Montero, P.J.; Artés-Rodríguez, E.M. Efectos de Un Programa de Ejercicio Físico Multicomponente Sobre La Condición Física, La Autoestima, La Ansiedad y La Depresión de Personas Adultas-Mayores (Effects of a Multicomponent Physical Exercise Program on Fitness, Self-Esteem, Anxiety and Depres. *Retos* **2020**, 1024–1028. [CrossRef]
27. Villarreal Angeles, M.A.; Moncada Jiménez, J.; Ochoa Martínez, P.Y.; Hall López, J.A. Percepción de La Calidad de Vida Del Adulto Mayor En México (Perception of the Quality of Life of Mexican Older Adults). *Retos* **2021**, *41*, 480–484. [CrossRef]
28. Jiménez-Gómez, S.; Sánchez Rojas, I.A.; Castro-Jiménez, L.E.; Rubiano-Espinosa, O.F.; Carrillo-Ramírez, C.E.; Garavito-Peña, F.R.; Barrera-Cobos, N.F. Calidad de Vida En Asistentes a Un Programa de Actividad Física En Bogotá, Colombia. *Rev. Iberoam. De. Cienc. De. La. Act. Física Y El Deporte* **2021**, *10*, 95–111. [CrossRef]
29. Vivaldi, F.; Barra, E. Bienestar Psicológico, Apoyo Social Percibido y Percepción de Salud En Adultos Mayores. *Ter. Psicológica* **2012**, *30*, 23–29. [CrossRef]
30. Rodrigues, M.M.; Quintella Fernandes, R.Á. Calidad de Vida y Morbilidad Referida a Mujeres Productivamente Activas. *Enfermería Glob.* **2017**, *16*, 246–280. [CrossRef]
31. Tricco, A.C.; Thomas, S.M.; Veroniki, A.A.; Hamid, J.S.; Cogo, E.; Strifler, L.; Khan, P.A.; Robson, R.; Sibley, K.M.; MacDonald, H.; et al. Comparisons of Interventions for Preventing Falls in Older Adults: A Systematic Review and Meta-Analysis. *JAMA* **2017**, *318*, 1687–1699. [CrossRef]
32. Villareal, D.T.; Aguirre, L.; Gurney, A.B.; Waters, D.L.; Sinacore, D.R.; Colombo, E.; Armamento-Villareal, R.; Qualls, C. Aerobic or Resistance Exercise, or Both, in Dieting Obese Older Adults. *N. Engl. J. Med.* **2017**, *376*, 1943–1955. [CrossRef]
33. Puciato, D.; Borysiuk, Z.; Rozpara, M. Quality of Life and Physical Activity in an Older Working-Age Population. *Clin. Interv. Aging* **2017**, *12*, 1627–1634. [CrossRef] [PubMed]
34. Maung, T.M.; Jain, T.; Madhanagopal, J.; Naidu, S.R.L.R.; Phyu, H.P.; Oo, W.M. Impact of Aerobic and Strengthening Exercise on Quality of Life (QOL), Mental Health and Physical Performance of Elderly People Residing at Old Age Homes. *Sustainability* **2022**, *14*, 10881. [CrossRef]
35. McAuley, E.; Konopack, J.F.; Motl, R.W.; Morris, K.S.; Doerksen, S.E.; Rosengren, K.R. Physical Activity and Quality of Life in Older Adults: Influence of Health Status and Self-Efficacy. *Ann. Behav. Med.* **2006**, *31*, 99–103. [CrossRef] [PubMed]
36. Pernambuco, C.S.; Rodrigues, B.M.; Bezerra, J.C.P.; Carrielo, A.; Fernandes, A.D.d.O.; Vale, R.G.d.S.; Dantas, E.H.M. Quality of Life, Elderly and Physical Activity. *Health* **2012**, *4*, 88–93. [CrossRef]
37. Roberts, C.E.; Phillips, L.H.; Cooper, C.L.; Gray, S.; Allan, J.L. Effect of Different Types of Physical Activity on Activities of Daily Living in Older Adults: Systematic Review and Meta-Analysis. *J. Aging Phys. Act.* **2017**, *25*, 653–670. [CrossRef] [PubMed]
38. Whitehurst, M.A.; Johnson, B.L.; Parker, C.M.; Brown, L.E.; Ford, A.M. The Benefits of a Functional Exercise Circuit for Older Adults. *J. Strength. Cond. Res.* **2005**, *19*, 647–651. [CrossRef]
39. Atad, O.I.; Caspi, D. Exercise and Perceived Quality of Life among Frail Older Adults. *Qual. Ageing Older Adults* **2020**, *21*, 29–38. [CrossRef]

behavioral sciences

MDPI

Article

Adaptation and Validation of the 3 × 2 Achievement Goals Questionnaire in a Population of Athletes

Cristina García-Romero [1,2], Elkin Eduardo Roldan-Aguilar [3], Carlos Alberto Hurtado-Castaño [3], Josune Rodríguez-Negro [4,5] and Oliver Ramos-Álvarez [5,6,7,8,9,*]

1 Faculty of Education, Camilo José Cela University, 28692 Madrid, Spain; crisgr30@gmail.com
2 Isabel I University, 09003 Burgos, Spain
3 Semillero de Investigación en Fisiología del Fisiología del Ejercicio, Politécnico Colombiano Jaime Isaza Cadavid, Medellín 050022, Colombia; eeroldan@elpoli.edu.co (E.E.R.-A.); carlosahurtado@elpoli.edu.co (C.A.H.-C.)
4 Department of Didactics of Musical, Plastic and Corporal Expression, Faculty of Education, University of the Basque Country (UPV/EHU), 48940 Leioa, Spain; josune.rodriguez@ehu.eus
5 Research Unit of School Sport, Physical Education and Psychomotricity of the University of A Coruña, 15008 A Coruña, Spain
6 Health Economics and Health Services Management Research Group, Marqués de Valdecilla Research Institute (IDIVAL), 39011 Santander, Spain
7 Department of Education, Physical and Sports Education Area, University of Cantabria, Los Castros Avenue, 50, 39005 Santander, Spain
8 Facultad de Ciencias de la Salud, Universidad Europea del Atlántico, 39011 Santander, Spain
9 Facultad de Ciencias Sociales, Universidad Europea del Atlántico, 39011 Santander, Spain
* Correspondence: oliver.ramos@unican.es; Tel.: +34-645951115

Abstract: (1) Background: Sport goals, although widely recognised as crucial for motivation and performance in sport, are multifaceted and can be difficult to measure directly. The present research aims to validate the 3 × 2 achievement goals questionnaire of Mascret in Spanish in a population of athletes. (2) Method: By using a latent factor approach, it is possible to identify the underlying dimensions of these goals and to better understand how they are structured. For this purpose, this questionnaire has been translated and compared with the life satisfaction scale. An exploration of the multifaceted nature of sport goals has been carried out using structural equation modelling. A total of 580 athletes (463 males and 216 females, M = 21.5, SD = 2.36) from different sport disciplines and from 12 autonomous communities in Spain participated in the research. (3) Results: The results show that the questionnaire presents a high scale reliability and that all items contribute significantly to the internal consistency of the scale. (4) Conclusions: The adaptation of this scale to the Spanish population of athletes can be a valid and useful tool to measure and understand motivation and goals in the sport context.

Keywords: motivation; 3 × 2 achievement goals; validation; life satisfaction; sport

1. Introduction

Over the last 30 years, achievement goals have been a reference in motivational research in the context of sport and physical activity. This theory evidences that achievement goals are the reasons that people direct their behaviour towards goals; i.e., individuals' goals lie in striving to demonstrate competence and ability in achievement contexts [1].

The literature on achievement goals has progressed according to an evidenced structure: researchers come up with a conceptual model, theorists develop a measure to assess that model, and finally, the instrument is implemented to analyse its development in different contexts, from which it is extracted whether the model is valid and functional for assessing competence. This procedure has forged a wide network of studies on the understanding of achievement goals [2–6].

The concept of achievement goals emerged in the early 1980s and differentiated between two goals: mastery and performance [1]. In this so-called dichotomous model, mastery goals were oriented towards developing competence through mastery and improvement of tasks, whereas performance goals were interpreted as striving to demonstrate competence in relation to others [7]. Research on the dichotomous model focused on a variety of settings, including school [7,8] and sport [9].

Following research in this field in the 1990s, and after questioning the model both empirically and conceptually, it was proposed to extend the model by incorporating approach–avoidance valences [3]. This model, called the trichotomous model, consisted of the mastery goal (similar to the dichotomous model), the performance-approach goals (focused on doing well in relation to others), and the performance-avoidance goals (focused on not doing badly in relation to others). In this particular model, several measures emerged, for school, work, and sport contexts [10–12].

Years later, Elliot and McGregor (2001) [4] expressed that mastery-based and performance-based goals could be bifurcated, differentiating between the two types of competence definition (mastery and performance) and the two types of competence valence (approach and avoidance). Therefore, the model consisted of four achievement goals, being called the 2 × 2 model: the mastery-approach goals (the traditional mastery goal), the mastery-avoidance goals (focused on not doing badly in relation to the demands of the task), the performance-approach goals (classic performance goal; tries to achieve interpersonal competence), and the performance-avoidance goals (based on avoiding doing worse than others). This measure was tested in different settings, including school [4,13,14] and sports [5,15].

The last model that the achievement goal theory yields, the so-called 3 × 2 model, presents three standards for assessing competence: task, self, and other. Task-based goals use the absolute demand of the task as a reference for assessment; self-based goals use one's own trajectory for competence assessment; and other-based goals are the most complex to adopt, as they assess competence in relation to doing well or poorly in relation to other peers [16]. The model therefore consisted of six achievement goals: the task-approach goals (focused on achieving task-based competence), the task-avoidance goals (focused on avoiding task-based incompetence), the self-approach goals (focused on self-based competence), the self-avoidance goals (focused on avoiding doing worse than how one performed in the past), the other-approach goals (focused on achieving competence based on others), and the other-avoidance goals (focused on avoiding doing worse than one's peers). The instrument of this model was applied in the school context [16,17]; in the French sport context, a validation was conducted by Mascret et al. (2015) [6].

Numerous reasons are evident for carrying out the validation of the 3 × 2 achievement goals questionnaire with a focus on sport in the Spanish language. The first of these is the conceptual aspect, as it is relevant to differentiate between task-based and self-based standards in the sport domain, i.e., to assess whether athletes participating in a sport or physical activity can focus on whether or not they are achieving as a function of the task itself, or how they are doing in relation to how they did in the past or in their future. Empirically, current measures of mastery-approach and mastery-avoidance vary in different terms depending on whether they focus on task-based standards [18], self-based standards [5], or a combination of task-based and self-based standards [19].

The aim of the present study is to adapt, validate, and test the psychometric property of the 3 × 2 achievement goals questionnaire in the sport context in a sample of Spanish athletes.

2. Materials and Methods

2.1. Participants

The sample consisted of 580 athletes (463 males and 216 females, M = 21.5, SD = 2; figure skating, Pilates, powerlifting, rowing, rugby, triathlon, volleyball, and water polo) from 12 autonomous communities in Spain (Asturias, Castilla-La Mancha, Madrid, Cantabria,

Andalusia, Valencia, Basque Country, Castilla y León, Murcia, Catalonia, Aragon, and the Balearic Islands). The athletes completed both questionnaires anonymously in their training sessions.

2.2. Instruments

Achievement Goals in Sport Questionnaire (CML 3 × 2-D): The questionnaire was validated in Spanish based on the one developed by Mascret et al. (2015) [6]. The items were preceded by "In sport my goal is…". This instrument is composed of a total of 18 items grouped into six factors: task-approach (e.g., "…to obtain good results"), task-avoidance (e.g., "…to avoid having bad results"), self-approach (e.g., "…. do better than in the past"), self-avoidance (e.g., "…avoid doing worse than I usually do"), other-approach (e.g., "…do better than others"), and other-avoidance (e.g., "…avoid doing worse than others"). Cronbach's alphas in the Mascret et al. (2015) [6] study ranged from 0.93 (other-avoidance) to 0.80 (task-approach). Participants indicated the degree of agreement with each of these statements using a 7-point Likert scale, ranging from 1 (strongly disagree) to 5 (strongly agree).

2.3. Procedure

The questionnaire was based on the scale of Mascret et al. (2015) [6] and is composed of 18 items grouped into 6 factors. The questionnaire was sent to the sample participating in the research to be completed during their training sessions. Once all the data had been collected, the relevant statistical analyses were carried out for its validation.

2.4. Statistical Analysis

A confirmatory factor analysis was conducted using the R-4.3.3 software package (Lucent Technologies, Alpharetta, GA, USA). A three-factor model was fitted to the questionnaire responses, which consisted of statements related to sport goals, such as "In sport my goal is to perform well" and "In sport my goal is to avoid performing poorly". These items were used to infer three latent factors, interpreted as "personal performance goals", "competitive goals", and "efficacy goals".

Confirmatory factor analysis (CFA) was conducted to assess the structure of the sport goals defined by the variables ML1 to ML18. The theoretical model defined three latent factors: MR1, reflecting goals related to personal performance; MR2, representing competitive goals; and MR3, describing goals related to efficacy.

The proposed model included a total of 129 parameters and was fitted to data from 850 observations using the Diagonally Weighted Least Squares (DWLS) estimator. Convergence was achieved after 41 interactions.

3. Results

Although the aim of this research is confirmatory, it was considered relevant to assess the exploratory results in order to justify the number of latent factors. For this reason, a review of the correlation between the variables was initially carried out, in which the correlations between the different items assessed in the population can be seen (Figure 1).

Of these correlations, while low correlations are expected, the higher-order correlations presented here refer to three groupings that are detailed in the process of constructing latent factors confirmed in the sedimentation plot and the biplot (Figures 2 and 3).

As can be seen from Table 1, the chi-square test of the model was significant ($\chi\hat{}2 = 2056.834$, df = 132, $p < 0.001$), indicating that the proposed model does not exactly reproduce the observed covariance matrix. However, the chi-square test is sensitive to sample size and can be significant even if the discrepancy between the model and the data is trivial. Therefore, other fit indices were also considered.

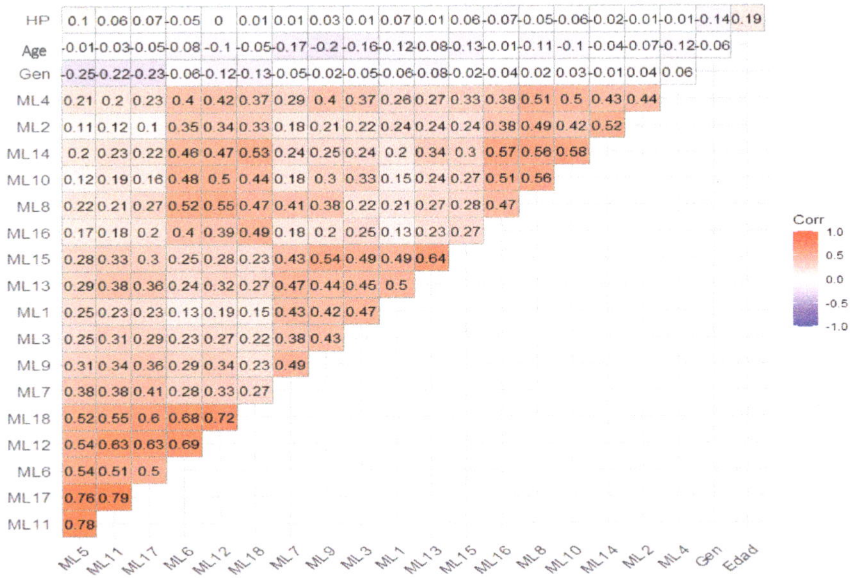

Figure 1. Correlation chart between items.

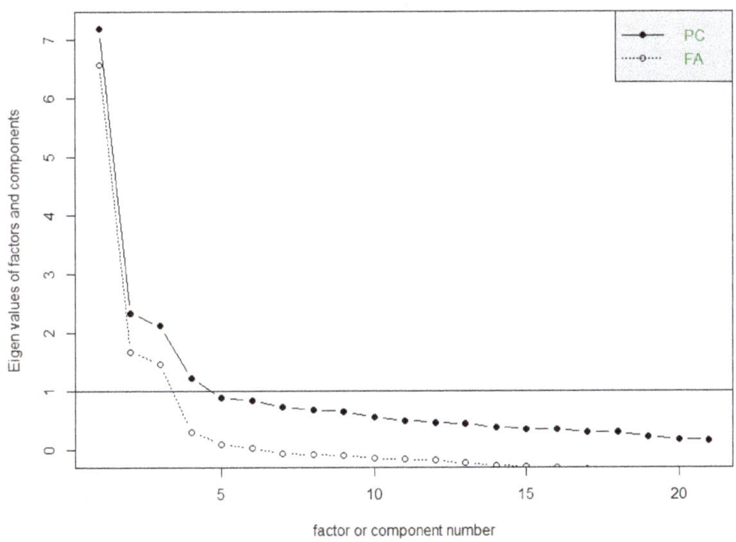

Figure 2. Sedimentation graph.

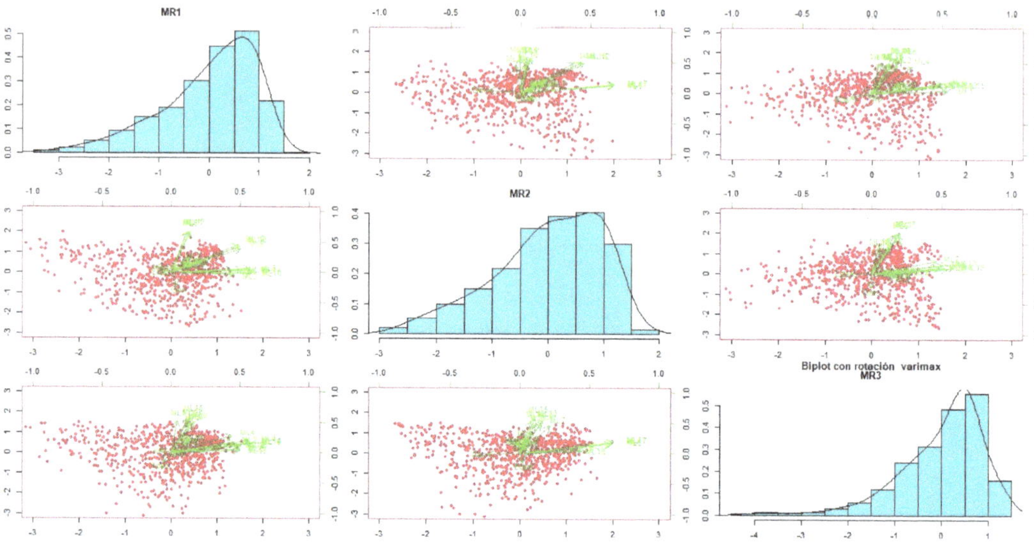

Figure 3. Biplot graph with Varimax rotation.

Table 1. Model fit indices.

Fit Index	Value	Acceptable Fit
Chi-square	2056.834	>0.05
Degrees of freedom	132	-
CFI	0.974	>0.90
TLI	0.970	>0.90
RMSEA	0.131	<0.08
SRMR	0.095	<0.08

Note: CFI: Comparative Fit Index; TLI: Tucker–Lewis Index; RMSEA: Root Mean Square Error of Approximation; SRMR: average difference between the observed correlations and the correlations predicted by the model.

From the same table, it can be seen that the values of the Comparative Fit Index (CFI) and the Tucker–Lewis Index (TLI), which are less sensitive to sample size, were 0.974 and 0.970, respectively. These values are very close to 1, suggesting a good fit of the model to the data. However, the Root Mean Square Error of Approximation (RMSEA) was 0.131, which exceeds the recommended threshold of 0.08 for a good fit. This indicates that the model has an average discrepancy per degree of freedom that is larger than is generally considered acceptable.

The RMSEA is a measure of model fit that takes into account the complexity of the model. Smaller values (usually less than 0.06) indicate a better fit. Here, both the standard and robust RMSEA are above this threshold (0.131 and 0.151), suggesting that the model can be improved.

The SRMR is a measure of the average difference between the observed correlations and the correlations predicted by the model. Values less than 0.08 are generally considered acceptable. In this case, the SRMR is 0.095, which is close to but above the recommended threshold.

Therefore, while some of the model fit metrics seem to suggest that the model fits the data reasonably well, others indicate that there may be room for improvement in the model. In particular, it may be useful to investigate further to identify potential problems with the model, such as variables that do not fit well or complex relationships between variables that are not captured in the current model.

In terms of the variables under study and the latent factors found, these results imply that, although the three latent factors appear to represent distinct aspects of participants' goals in sport, the model may not fully capture the correlation between the different goals.

The discrepancy in the fit indices suggests that, although the model may capture a large proportion of the variance in the data (as indicated by the CFI and TLI), there may also be model specifications that do not fit the data perfectly. These results highlight the importance of using multiple fit indices and considering the results of the CFA in the context of past and future analyses. Table 2 provides the estimation and interpretations of the latent factors in the model.

Table 2. Parameter estimates for latent variables.

	Estimate	Std.Err	z-Value	*P*(>|z|)	Std.lv	Std.all
			MR1			
ML10	1.000	-	-	-	0.727	0.727
ML14	1.049	0.027	39.185	0.000	0.762	0.762
ML8	1.062	0.025	41.870	0.000	0.771	0.771
ML16	0.915	0.028	32.427	0.000	0.665	0.665
ML18	1.164	0.028	41.439	0.000	0.846	0.846
ML6	1.117	0.028	40.177	0.000	0.811	0.811
ML12	1.225	0.027	44.790	0.000	0.890	0.890
ML2	0.856	0.032	26.541	0.000	0.622	0.622
ML4	0.977	0.029	33.415	0.000	0.710	0.710
			MR2			
ML17	1.000	-	-	-	0.924	0.924
ML11	1.002	0.011	90.474	0.000	0.926	0.926
ML5	0.940	0.012	81.133	0.000	0.869	0.869
			MR3			
ML15	1.000	-	-	-	0.829	0.829
ML13	0.955	0.029	33.475	0.000	0.792	0.792
ML1	0.831	0.033	25.421	0.000	0.689	0.689
ML9	0.966	0.029	33.107	0.000	0.801	0.801
ML3	0.870	0.033	26.428	0.000	0.721	0.721
ML7	0.927	0.030	30.867	0.000	0.769	0.769

Note: Std.lv: standardised covariance; Std.Err: standard errors; MR1: personal performance goals; MR2: competitive goals; MR3: efficiency goals.

The characteristics of the three goals analysed can be distinguished, and are as follows:

- Personal performance goals (MR1): This factor includes items that reflect a motivation to improve personal performance as well as to avoid underperformance. Individuals with high scores on this factor may be particularly focused on their personal sport performance, regardless of the performance of others.
- Competitive goals (MR2): This factor reflects the motivation to compete and outperform others in sport performance. Individuals with high scores on this factor may be especially competitive and oriented to outperform their peers.
- Efficacy goals (MR3): This factor is composed of items that refer to being effective and improving effectiveness over time. Individuals with high scores on this factor may be especially motivated to be effective in their sport and improve their effectiveness over time.

Table 3 shows the estimates of the covariances between the latent factors (MR1, MR2, and MR3). The estimated values represent the estimated covariance between each pair of factors, with a higher value indicating a higher relationship. Standard errors (Std.Err) represent the uncertainty in the covariance estimates.

Table 3. Covariances of latent factors in the CFA model.

	Estimate	Std.Err	z-Value	P(>|z|)	Std.lv
MR1 MR2	0.449	0.017	26.309	0.000	0.669
MR1 MR3	0.386	0.019	20.243	0.000	0.640
MR2 MR3	0.439	0.024	18.328	0.000	0.573

Note: Std.lv: standardised covariance; Std.Err: standard errors.

The z-value is a hypothesis test that indicates whether each covariance estimate is significantly different from zero. Large (in absolute terms) z-values and small P(>|z|) values (all 0.000 in this case) provide strong evidence against the null hypothesis that the covariance equals zero. That is, these results indicate that each pair of latent factors has a significant relationship.

The Std.lv value refers to the standardised covariance between the latent factors, indicating the strength of the relationship between them. This shows that the three latent factors (MR1, MR2, and MR3) are significantly related to each other. The strongest covariance is observed between MR1 and MR2, followed by the covariance between MR1 and MR3, and finally the covariance between MR2 and MR3. This suggests that the goals in sport related to these factors are intrinsically linked.

3.1. *Confirmatory Factor Analysis*

The Lavaan plot depicted in Figure 4 shows the factor loadings (the relationships between the latent variables and the observed variables) as well as the correlations between the latent factors, which show how these factors are related to each other.

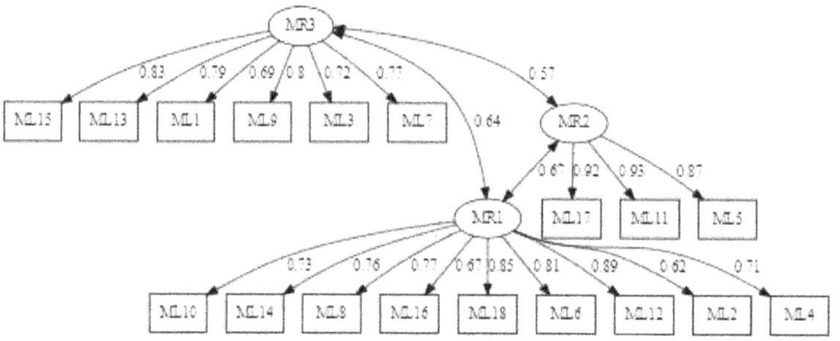

Figure 4. Lavaan chart.

3.2. *Reliability Analysis of the Achievement Goals Test: Dep*

The results are presented in Table 4.

Table 4. Reliability analysis.

Raw_Alpha	Std.Alpha	G6 (smc)	Average_r	S/N	Ase	Mean	Sd	Median_r
0.78	0.89	0.92	0.27	7.9	0.011	9.3	1	0.25

	lower	alpha	upper
Feldt	0.76	0.78	0.8
Duhachek	0.76	0.78	0.8

The reliability of the Sport Goals Test scale was assessed using Cronbach's alpha (α), a measure of internal consistency. The calculation of α is based on the number of items (k) and the ratio of the summed item variances to the total variance of the scale. Formally, α can be represented as

$$\alpha = \frac{k}{k-1}\left(1 - \frac{\sum_{i=1}^{k}\sigma_{Yi}^2}{\sigma_X^2}\right)$$

where σ_{Yi}^2 is the variance of the i-th item, and σ_{Yi}^2 is the total variance of the total observed scores. The raw α obtained for the Dep scale was 0.78.

The standardised α (0.89) was also calculated. This form of α is based on the assumption that all items share the same variance, and is computed as

$$\alpha_{\text{std}} = \frac{k\bar{r}}{1 + (k-1)\bar{r}}$$

where $\bar{r}$ is the average inter-item correlation.

The average inter-item correlation (0.27) and the median inter-item correlation (0.25) were reported. The signal-to-noise ratio, calculated as the ratio of the variance of the true score to the variance of the error, was 7.9.

The standard error of measurement (SEM) of the scale, which reflects the precision of the scale, was also calculated. The SEM is calculated as the standard deviation of the scale scores multiplied by the square root of $(1 - \alpha)$, resulting in a value of 0.011 for the Dep scale.

The reliability of the scale was further assessed using Feldt's confidence interval and Duhachek and Iacobucci's confidence interval, which indicated a range between 0.76 and 0.8 for the α at the 95% confidence level.

Regarding item-to-item reliability, i.e., quantifying how much each item contributes to the overall consistency of the data set, Table 5 can be observed.

Table 5. Reliability if an item is removed.

Item	Raw_Alpha	Std.Alpha	G6 (smc)	Average_r	S/N	Alpha se	Var.r	Med.r
Age-	0.87	0.89	0.92	0.30	8.4	0.0063	0.035	0.27
Gen-	0.78	0.89	0.93	0.30	8.4	0.0115	0.035	0.27
HP	0.81	0.90	0.93	0.30	8.6	0.0100	0.032	0.27
ML1	0.77	0.88	0.92	0.28	7.6	0.0118	0.039	0.27
ML2	0.77	0.88	0.92	0.28	7.6	0.0122	0.038	0.26
ML3	0.77	0.88	0.92	0.27	7.5	0.0119	0.039	0.25
ML4	0.76	0.88	0.92	0.27	7.4	0.0123	0.038	0.24
ML5	0.76	0.88	0.91	0.27	7.4	0.0123	0.036	0.25
ML6	0.76	0.88	0.91	0.27	7.2	0.0128	0.036	0.25
ML7	0.77	0.88	0.92	0.27	7.4	0.0120	0.039	0.25
ML8	0.76	0.88	0.91	0.27	7.3	0.0126	0.037	0.25
ML9	0.77	0.88	0.92	0.27	7.4	0.0121	0.039	0.24
ML10	0.76	0.88	0.91	0.27	7.4	0.0124	0.037	0.25
ML11	0.76	0.88	0.91	0.27	7.3	0.0124	0.036	0.25
ML12	0.75	0.88	0.91	0.26	7.1	0.0130	0.035	0.24
ML13	0.77	0.88	0.91	0.27	7.4	0.0120	0.038	0.25
ML14	0.76	0.88	0.91	0.27	7.4	0.0125	0.037	0.25
ML15	0.77	0.88	0.91	0.27	7.4	0.0120	0.038	0.24
ML16	0.77	0.88	0.92	0.27	7.6	0.0122	0.038	0.25
ML17	0.76	0.88	0.91	0.27	7.3	0.0125	0.036	0.25
ML18	0.76	0.88	0.91	0.26	7.2	0.0128	0.036	0.25

It is notable that, without exception, the alpha calculated for each of the variables inserted into the model exceeded 0.75, which is generally considered acceptable or good, suggesting that the items or scale questions are highly related to each other and therefore likely to measure the same underlying construct [20]. Specifically, a Cronbach's alpha of 0.75 indicates that the construct is reliably measured with relatively high internal consistency. This provides evidence of the reliability of the measure, which is an important aspect of its validity.

In a confirmatory factor analysis (CFA) model, this suggests that the model has identified a coherent underlying latent factor and that the scale items cluster effectively around this factor.

In order to confirm the results presented, the statistics presented in Table 6 were calculated.

Table 6. Other reliability statistics.

Statistic	Value
Cronbach's alpha	0.89
G.6	0.92
Omega hierarchical	0.57
Omega H asymptotic	0.62
Omega total	0.92

From Table 6, it can be noted that G.6 is also a measure of scale reliability and is considered more robust than Cronbach's alpha, especially when item response distributions are not normal. In this case, the value of G.6 is 0.92, which suggests a high level of scale reliability. On the other hand and from the same table, the omega hierarchical indicates the variance that can be explained by a general factor in a set of items. A value of 0.57 indicates that approximately 57% of the variance of the items can be explained by a general factor, suggesting that a general factor underlies most of the items.

Omega H asymptotic is an estimate of the maximum amount of variance that can be attributed to a general factor, based on the upper bound of the variance explained by that factor. A value of 0.62 suggests that up to 62% of the variance of the items could be explained by a general factor.

And finally, omega total represents the total proportion of item variance that can be attributed to all common factors, both general and specific. A value of 0.92 indicates that most of the variance can be explained by the common factors, which is an indication of high reliability.

These results, as well as the calculation of the effects of each variable on each of the estimated underlying factors, can be seen in Figure 5.

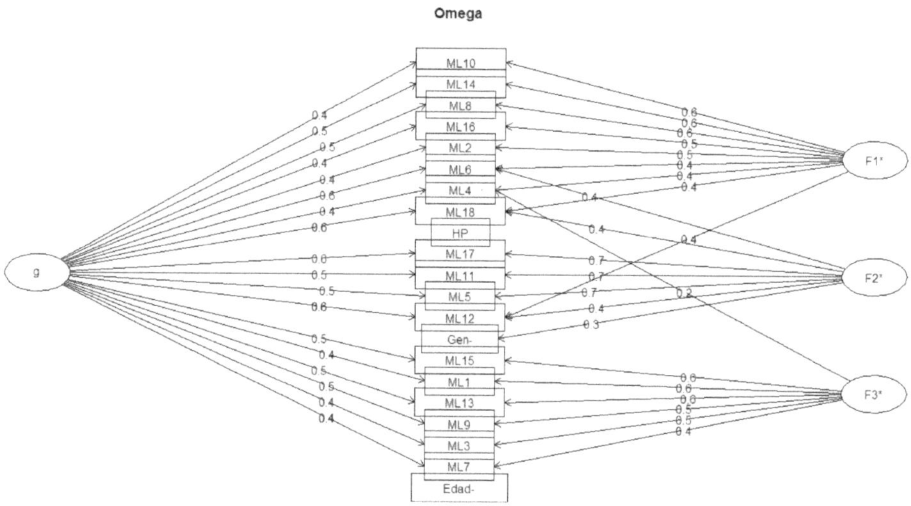

Note: * Common factors.

Figure 5. Graphical representation of the structural CFA model.

4. Discussion

The questionnaire data show that the results of the reliability tests (Cronbach's alpha and McDonald's omega) suggest that the set of items shows high internal consistency, with a Cronbach's alpha of 0.88–0.89 and an omega total of 0.92–0.93. These values above 0.7 indicate that the items consistently measure the same latent construct, providing strong evidence of the scale's reliability; these data are congruent with studies conducted by Mascret et al. (2017) [21] in a sample of teachers, and Ning (2018) [22] and Kadioglu-Akbulut and Uzuntiryaki-Kondakci (2019) [23] in the Hong Kong and Turkish populations, respectively.

With reference to the impact of item deletion, it can also be concluded that the results of the reliability analysis if one item is deleted indicate that all items contribute significantly to the internal consistency of the scale. The removal of any of the items would result in a decrease in Cronbach's alpha or McDonald's omega, so it is suggested to keep all items in the scale.

The data extracted from the study indicate that task- and self-directed goals are distinct goals in the sport context, as Mascret et al. (2015) [6] showed that competence was positively correlated with task-directed goals but was not related to self-goals. The previous authors found problems with some of the stated items, especially with the task-approach and task-avoidance item, regarding their wording, which can sometimes appear ambiguous to the respondent, as one can interpret these items as self- or other-based. Since the domain of sports involves techniques, skills, and strategies, items assessing task goals should involve these three dimensions.

Inter-item correlations show high relationships between items from the other-avoidance goal, whereas inter-construct correlations are highest between task-approach and self-goals and task-avoidance and self-goals, these data being consistent with the studies of Mascret et al. (2015) [6], Cecchini et al. (2021) [24], and García-Romero et al. (2022) [25].

Studies on the achievement goal theory showed that mastery goals were related to positive outcomes, such as high levels of academic achievement and self-efficacy [26–28], personal well-being, relationship building and intrinsic and identified motivation [29], self-determined motivation [30], and autonomy [31]. In contrast, the relationships for the adoption of performance goals were not clearly defined. Some researchers found that these goals were associated with negative and maladaptive outcomes, such as anxiety [32] and burnout [29], because their central focus revolves around outperforming others [33]. However, other studies did not support this hypothesis, as in some achievement contexts, performance goals showed null results, mainly due to their temporally unstable nature [29].

5. Conclusions

Each extension of the dichotomous model adds precision to the achievement goal theory, leading to the current 3 × 2 model. This shows, as indicated in the review by Lochbaum et al. (2023) [34], that the data from the 3 × 2 achievement goals questionnaires are more strongly supported in the sport context than in the education context, with large differences in the significance of the task and other competencies.

Finally, it is important to highlight that, although the scale shows a high degree of reliability, further studies should be conducted to validate it in different contexts and populations. Furthermore, the conclusions obtained so far speak of the scale's reliability, but further research is still needed to examine its content, criterion, and construct validity.

The results obtained so far are promising and suggest that the scale may be a useful tool for measuring and understanding motivation and goals in the sport context.

Author Contributions: Conceptualisation, C.G.-R., E.E.R.-A., C.A.H.-C., J.R.-N. and O.R.-Á.; methodology, C.G.-R., E.E.R.-A., C.A.H.-C., J.R.-N. and O.R.-Á.; validation, C.G.-R., E.E.R.-A., C.A.H.-C., J.R.-N. and O.R.-Á.; formal analysis, C.G.-R., E.E.R.-A., C.A.H.-C., J.R.-N. and O.R.-Á.; investigation, C.G.-R., E.E.R.-A., C.A.H.-C., J.R.-N. and O.R.-Á.; resources, C.G.-R., E.E.R.-A., C.A.H.-C., J.R.-N. and O.R.-Á.; data curation, C.G.-R., E.E.R.-A., C.A.H.-C., J.R.-N. and O.R.-Á.; writing—original draft preparation, C.G.-R., E.E.R.-A., C.A.H.-C., J.R.-N. and O.R.-Á.; writing—review and editing,

C.G.-R., E.E.R.-A., C.A.H.-C., J.R.-N. and O.R.-Á.; visualisation, C.G.-R., E.E.R.-A., C.A.H.-C., J.R.-N. and O.R.-Á.; supervision, C.G.-R., E.E.R.-A., C.A.H.-C., J.R.-N. and O.R.-Á.; project administration, C.G.-R., E.E.R.-A., C.A.H.-C., J.R.-N. and O.R.-Á. All authors have read and agreed to the published version of the manuscript.

Funding: This research received no external funding.

Institutional Review Board Statement: EDUCA Ethics Committee. Authorization Code: 7/2020, approved on 10 January 2020.

Informed Consent Statement: Informed consent was obtained from all subjects involved in this study.

Data Availability Statement: Data are contained within the article.

Conflicts of Interest: The authors declare no conflicts of interest.

References

1. Nicholls, J.G. Achievement motivation: Conceptions of ability, subjective experience, task choice, and performance. *Psychol. Rev.* **1984**, *91*, 328–346. [CrossRef]
2. Ames, C. Achievement Goals, Motivational Climate, and Motivational Processes. In *Motivation in Sport and Exercise*; Roberts, G.C., Ed.; Human Kinetics: Champaign, IL, USA, 1992; pp. 161–176.
3. Elliot, A.J.; Harackiewicz, J.M. Approach and avoidance achievement goals and intrinsic motivation: A mediational analysis. *J. Pers. Soc. Psychol.* **1996**, *70*, 461–475. [CrossRef]
4. Elliot, A.J.; McGregor, H.A. A 2 × 2 achievement goal framework. *J. Pers. Soc. Psychol.* **2001**, *80*, 501–519. [CrossRef] [PubMed]
5. Conroy, D.E.; Elliot, A.J.; Hofer, S.M. A 2 × 2 Achievement Goals Questionnaire for Sport: Evidence for Factorial Invariance, Temporal Stability, and External Validity. *J. Sport. Exerc. Psychol.* **2003**, *25*, 456–476. [CrossRef]
6. Mascret, N.; Elliot, A.J.; Cury, F. Extending the 3 × 2 achievement goal model to the sport domain: The 3 × 2 Achievement Goal Questionnaire for Sport. *Psychol. Sport. Exerc.* **2015**, *17*, 7–14. [CrossRef]
7. Nicholls, J.G.; Patashnick, M.; Cheung, P.C.; Thorkildsen, T.; Lauer, J.M. Can achievement motivation theory succeed with only one conception of success? In *International Perspectives on Achievement and Task Motivation*; Halisch, F., Van den Bercken, J.H.L., Eds.; Swets y Zeitlinger: Lisse, The Netherlands, 1989; pp. 187–208.
8. Meece, J.L.; Anderman, E.M.; Anderman, L.H. Classroom Goal Structure, Student Motivation, and Academic Achievement. *Annu. Rev. Psychol.* **2006**, *57*, 487–503. [CrossRef] [PubMed]
9. Duda, J.L. Motivation in sport: The Relevance of Competence and Achievement Goals. In *Handbook of Competence and Motivation*; Elliot, A.J., Dweck, C.S., Eds.; Guildford Press: New York, NY, USA, 2005; pp. 135–318.
10. Elliot, A.J.; Church, M.A. A hierarchical model of approach and avoidance achievement motivation. *J. Pers. Soc. Psychol.* **1997**, *72*, 218–232. [CrossRef]
11. Middleton, M.J.; Midgley, C. Avoiding the demonstration of lack of ability: An underexplored aspect of goal theory. *J. Educ. Psychol.* **1997**, *89*, 710–718. [CrossRef]
12. Cury, F.; Biddle, S.; Famose, J.P.; Sarrazin, P.; Durand, M.; Goudas, M. Personal and Situational Factors Influencing Intrinsic Interest of Adolescent Girls in School Physical Education: A structural equation modelling analysis. *Educ. Psychol.* **1996**, *16*, 305–315. [CrossRef]
13. Elliot, A.J.; Murayama, K. On the measurement of achievement goals: Critique, illustration, and application. *J. Educ. Psychol.* **2008**, *100*, 613–628. [CrossRef]
14. Méndez-Giménez, A.; Cecchini-Estrada, J.A.; Fernández-Río, J. Perfiles motivacionales y dominancia de metas de logro. *Span. J. Psycologhy* **2014**, *17*, 1–8.
15. Van Yperen, N.W.; Blaga, M.; Postmes, T. A Meta-Analysis of Self-Reported Achievement Goals and Nonself-Report Performance across Three Achievement Domains (Work, Sports, and Education). *PLoS ONE* **2014**, *9*, e93594. [CrossRef] [PubMed]
16. Elliot, A.J.; Murayama, K.; Pekrun, R. A 3 × 2 achievement goal model. *J. Educ. Psychol.* **2011**, *103*, 632–648. [CrossRef]
17. Méndez-Giménez, A.; Cecchini-Estrada, J.A.; Fernández-Río, J. Examinando el modelo de metas de logro 3 × 2 en el contexto de la Educación Física. *Cuad. Psicol. Deporte* **2014**, *14*, 157–168. [CrossRef]
18. Wang, C.K.J.; Biddle, S.J.H.; Elliot, A.J. The 2 × 2 achievement goal framework in a physical education context. *Psychol. Sport. Exerc.* **2007**, *8*, 147–168. [CrossRef]
19. Riou, F.; Boiché, J.; Doron, J.; Romain, A.J.; Corrion, K.; Ninot, G.; D'arripe-Longueville, F.; Gernigon, C. Development and Validation of the French Achievement Goals Questionnaire for Sport and Exercise (FAGQSE). *Eur. J. Psychol. Assess.* **2012**, *28*, 313–320. [CrossRef]
20. Revelle, W.; Zinbarg, R.E. Coefficients Alpha, Beta, Omega, and the glb: Comments on Sijtsma. *Psychometrika* **2009**, *74*, 145–154. [CrossRef]
21. Mascret, N.; Elliot, A.J.; Cury, F. The 3 × 2 Achievement Goal Questionnaire for Teachers. *Educ. Psychol.* **2017**, *37*, 346–361. [CrossRef]

22. Ning, H.K. Psychometric Properties of the 3 × 2 Achievement Goal Questionnaire in a Hong Kong Sample. *J. Psychoeduc. Assess.* **2018**, *36*, 261–272. [CrossRef]
23. Kadioğlu, C.; Uzuntiryaki-Kondakçi, E. Turkish Adaptation of the 3 × 2 Goal Orientation Scale. *Bartın Üniversitesi Eğitim Fakültesi Derg.* **2019**, *8*, 839–866. [CrossRef]
24. Cecchini, J.A.; Méndez-Giménez, A.; García-Romero, C. Intra-individual changes in 3 × 2 achievement goals, friendship goals, motivational regulations and consequences in physical education. *Rev. Latinoam. Psicol.* **2021**, *53*, 180–189. [CrossRef]
25. García-Romero, C.; Méndez-Giménez, A.; Cecchini-Estrada, J.A. Metas de logro 3 × 2 y mediadores psicológicos en estudiantes de Educación Física. *Rev. Int. Med. Cienc. Act. Física Deporte* **2022**, *22*, 455–469. [CrossRef]
26. Gonçalves, T.; Niemivirta, M.; Lemos, M.S. Identificación de los múltiples perfiles de logros y metas sociales de los estudiantes y análisis de su estabilidad y adaptabilidad. *Aprendiz. Difer. Individ.* **2017**, *54*, 149–159.
27. Limpo, T.; Alves, R.A. Relating beliefs in writing skill malleability to writing performance: The mediating role of achievement goals and self-efficacy. *J. Writ. Res.* **2017**, *9*, 97–125. [CrossRef]
28. Zhou, M.; Adesope, O.O.; Winne, P.H.; Nesbit, J.C. Relations of multivariate goal profiles to motivation, epistemic beliefs and achievement. *J. Pac. Rim Psychol.* **2019**, *13*, e1. [CrossRef]
29. Simón-Piqueras, J.A.; Gil-Madrona, P.; Zamorano-García, D.; Torre-Maroto, M.; Fernández-Bustos, J.G. Self-Determined Regulation, Achievement Goals and Sport Commitment in Spanish Masters Swimmers. *Behav. Sci.* **2023**, *13*, 828. [CrossRef] [PubMed]
30. Méndez-Giménez, A.; Cecchini, J.; García-Romero, C. Metas de Logro 3 × 2, Inteligencia Emocional y Relaciones Sociales en el Contexto de la Educación Física. *Rev. Iberoam. Diagn. Eval. Avaliação Psicológ.* **2018**, *49*, 131–141. [CrossRef]
31. García-Romero, C.; Méndez-Giménez, A.; Cecchini-Estrada, J.A. Papel predictivo de las metas de logro 3 ×2 sobre la necesidad de autonomía en Educación Física. *Sport. Sci. J. Sch. Sport Phys. Educ. Psychomot.* **2019**, *6*, 2–17. [CrossRef]
32. Danthony, S.; Mascret, N.; Cury, F. The relationships between the 3 × 2 achievement goal model and test anxiety in Physical Education. *Eur. Phys. Educ. Rev.* **2021**, *27*, 559–573. [CrossRef]
33. Urdan, T. Achievement goal theory: Past results, future directions. In *Advances in Motivation and Achievement*; Maehr, M.L., Pincus, A.L., Eds.; JAI Press: Bingley, UK, 1997; Volume 10, pp. 99–141.
34. Lochbaum, M.; Sisneros, C.; Kazak, Z. The 3 × 2 Achievement Goals in the Education, Sport, and Occupation Literatures: A Systematic Review with Meta-Analysis. *Eur. J. Investig. Health Psychol. Educ.* **2023**, *13*, 1130–1157. [CrossRef]

behavioral sciences

MDPI

Article

Playing for a Healthy Life: Integrating Mobile Exergames in Physical Education

Pablo Sotoca-Orgaz *, Marta Arévalo-Baeza and José A. Navia

Faculty of Medicine and Health Sciences, University of Alcalá, 28805 Alcalá de Henares, Spain; marta.arevalo@uah.es (M.A.-B.); jose.navia@uah.es (J.A.N.)
* Correspondence: pablo.sotoca@uah.es

Abstract: This study aimed to promote a coherent pedagogical framework for integrating mobile exergames into physical education (PE) as a strategy to reduce sedentary behavior. The intervention was grounded in the game-based learning methodology, assessing the impact of exergame practice on the physical and mental well-being of prospective PE teachers. The Borg Rating of Perceived Exertion (RPE) scale and a mental effort scale were used to evaluate perceived exertion across various mini-games, measuring physical intensity, motor engagement, and mental effort with participation from 130 undergraduate students in Physical Activity and Sport Sciences. Additionally, the pedagogical and motivational aspects of the Active Arcade v3.11 video game were analyzed to support its future integration into secondary education PE classes. Participants reported high levels of motor engagement throughout the program, accompanied by moderate physical intensity. They also emphasized the user-friendly nature of these augmented reality exergames and expressed enjoyment during the sessions. The findings suggest that mobile exergames hold considerable potential for enhancing skill acquisition and fundamental motor skills while promoting healthy habits among students in PE classes.

Keywords: exergames; physical education; game-based learning

1. Introduction

The emergence of exergames has introduced a revolutionary concept in video gaming, requiring physical exercise as a mode of interaction (Medeiros et al., 2017; Staiano & Calvert, 2011). In these games, body movement serves as the primary form of engagement (Gómez-Miguel & Calderón-Gómez, 2023). Exergames are defined as video games "that promote (either via using or requiring) players' physical movements (exertion) that is generally more than sedentary and includes strength, balance, and flexibility activities" (Oh & Yang, 2010, p. 9). These active video games represent a new generation of electronic entertainment that challenges the traditional view of passive gaming (Beltrán-Carrillo et al., 2011; Lozano-Sánchez et al., 2019), often criticized for promoting sedentary behaviors by replacing physical activity with prolonged use of computers, video consoles, and mobile devices (Castro-Sánchez et al., 2015), a phenomenon known as "technological sedentarism" (Castro-Sánchez et al., 2015).

This growing concern, highlighted by the World Health Organization (WHO), has prompted physical education professionals to develop innovative strategies to combat sedentary lifestyles. Excessive screen time, particularly among young people, is linked to rising obesity rates and other health issues stemming from insufficient physical activity (Laurson et al., 2008; Shen et al., 2021). In response, the WHO recommended the use of exergames during the COVID-19 quarantine in 2020 to reduce inactivity at home and promote healthy habits (World Health Organization, 2020). Since then, exergames has become increasingly popular as an alternative form of exercise (Luarn et al., 2023; O'Loughlin et al., 2023).

Exergames are designed to encourage movement-based interaction, encompassing a wide range of activities such as sports, active games, and dance (Cerezo-Pizarro et al., 2023). While some require consoles, screens, and platforms, technological advancements have facilitated the development of free-to-play exergames that utilize mobile devices with motion detection (Moller et al., 2023) and augmented reality (Marin-Suelves et al., 2022). This innovation allows users to engage in physical activity in virtually any space, including outdoors (Moller et al., 2023; Marin-Suelves et al., 2022), reflecting a growing preference for portable, multifunctional devices. Mobile phones, once primarily used for passive activities such as chatting or watching movies, now serve as convenient tools for active gaming.

In recent decades, mobile applications offering free-to-play games have emerged as a dominant form of global entertainment. Mobile phones, now widely accessible, are multifunctional tools for communication, expression, leisure, and information (Chóliz et al., 2009). One key motivation for adopting these technologies, particularly among adolescents, is their high entertainment value. Research shows that 94.8% of 15-year-olds in Spain own and use a mobile phone (Spanish Statistical Office, 2023), and 34% of adolescents engage in online gaming daily or almost daily during their leisure time (Hooft-Graafland, 2018). Given adolescents' substantial engagement with mobile applications (Chóliz et al., 2009), mobile exergames present a promising strategy for increasing physical activity levels.

The popularity of active video games has surged over the past decade (Park et al., 2019), with research expanding into fields such as public health, rehabilitation, psychology, neuroscience, and computer science (Benzing & Schmidt, 2018; Gómez-Gonzalvo et al., 2018; Marin-Suelves et al., 2022). Within the educational sector, particularly in physical education, research on exergames has grown considerably (Gómez-Gonzalvo et al., 2018; Marin-Suelves et al., 2022). The pursuit of enhancing learning through active methodologies and the integration of educational technological resources in the classroom has driven novel strategies such as game-based learning (Pellas & Mystakidis, 2020). The proper use of game based learning has been proved to facilitate the assimilation of academic content, as well as the improvement of competencies and skills through a digital game (Pellas & Mystakidis, 2020; Qian & Clark, 2016). Studies suggest that exergames positively impact physical (Ho et al., 2022; Larsen et al., 2013), mental (Andrade et al., 2019; Lee et al., 2017), and social development (Li et al., 2018), while serving as a motivating tool for students (Lyons et al., 2014).

Various exergames have been evaluated for their impact on parameters such as caloric expenditure (Canabrava et al., 2018), motor skill improvement (Comeras-Chueca et al., 2022), cognitive function (Best, 2012), and activity enjoyment (Gu et al., 2023; Moholdt et al., 2017). These games often require full-body involvement, with findings indicating that muscle engagement and cardiovascular demands can meet recommended energy expenditure levels (Haddock et al., 2008; Siegel et al., 2009).

However, in classroom settings, measuring complicated parameters such as heart rate or accessing advanced platforms can be challenging for teachers. Therefore, pre-service physical education teachers would benefit from experience with free-to-play exergames, which require only a mobile phone with a camera and an application to track body movements. For example, the Active Arcade v.3.11 app, used in this study, is freely available. Nonetheless, the presence of digital resources alone does not guarantee skill development. Thus, integrating free-to-play exergames into physical education requires pre-service teachers to be trained (Marin-Suelves et al., 2022) to select, design, facilitate, and adapt these tools to the pedagogical contexts (Monguillot et al., 2018).

Before outlining the study's objectives, it is essential to define key concepts such as motor engagement, practice time, perceived physical and mental effort, and motivational factors in motor activities. These variables are critical for evaluating the effectiveness of exergames in promoting health and well-being. Research consistently shows that sufficient motor engagement time and adequate intensity can significantly enhance physical and mental health (Martínez-Gómez et al., 2007). Motor engagement refers to the time students are actively involved in physical activities during PE classes or other movement-based activities, excluding time spent on organization, instruction, or waiting (Corpas-Ruiz & Villodres, 2023). Practice time denotes the period during which students perform specific motor tasks (Rodríguez-Reyes et al., 2020). Physiological engagement, defined as the time spent working at intensities high enough to induce organic adaptations, maximizes the health benefits of PE classes (Martínez-Gómez et al., 2007). Although various factors influence this relationship, effort can be measured subjectively through physical and mental exertion perception, allowing students to self-assess their engagement (Ouwehand et al., 2021; Rewitz et al., 2024). In addition, motivation and enjoyment are fundamental in achieving long-term benefits through physical activity (Fierro-Suero et al., 2023).

In summary, this study aims to assess the impact of a physical conditioning session using the mobile exergame Active Arcade v3.11 with future PE teachers. The study evaluated participants' motor engagement and perceived effort, along with the app's didactic, motivational, and user-friendly aspects. The following hypotheses were formulated: (i) Active Arcade v3.11 allows each individual to regulate their exerted effort which results in an adjusted perception of physical and mental effort according to their regular fitness; (ii) motor engagement will be significant and suitable for a 60 min session; and (iii) the levels of motivation and enjoyment generated will be high.

2. Materials and Methods

2.1. Participants

A total of 130 students, aged between 18 and 50 years (M = 19.31, MDn = 18, SD = 3.11) were selected. Of these, 68% (n = 89) were male and 32% (n = 41) female. All participants were enrolled in the cross-disciplinary course *Technology and Physical Activity*, a first-year requirement in the Bachelor's Degree in Physical Activity and Sports Sciences at the University of Alcalá, Spain.

Inclusion criteria were as follows: attendance during the preliminary intervention explanations, absence of injuries on the day of the exergame session, and completion of informed consent and data collection questionnaires. The study was approved by the Research and Animal Experimentation Ethics Committee of the University of Alcalá (protocol code CEIP/2024/6/122).

2.2. Procedure

This study forms part of the Teaching Innovation Project titled "Proposals for Game-Based Learning through Exergames and Modern Board Games to Promote Motor Engagement" (Ref. UAH/EV1469) at the University of Alcalá. Before data collection, participants attended a 90 min in-person training session that introduced technologies such as augmented reality (AR) and outlined the research protocol and classroom procedures for the upcoming session.

The practical session, conducted the following day, involved a 90 min Active Arcade v3.11 tournament at the university's sports facilities. Students were divided into groups of 3 to 4, each equipped with personal devices (tablets or smartphones) with the Active Arcade v3.11 app installed. The instructor introduced each mini-game, allocating 12 min per game and a designated space for each group. After each mini-game, participants recorded their highest scores, identified the winning team, and reviewed performance results. The session concluded with certificates awarded to the highest scorers of each mini-game (Figure 1).

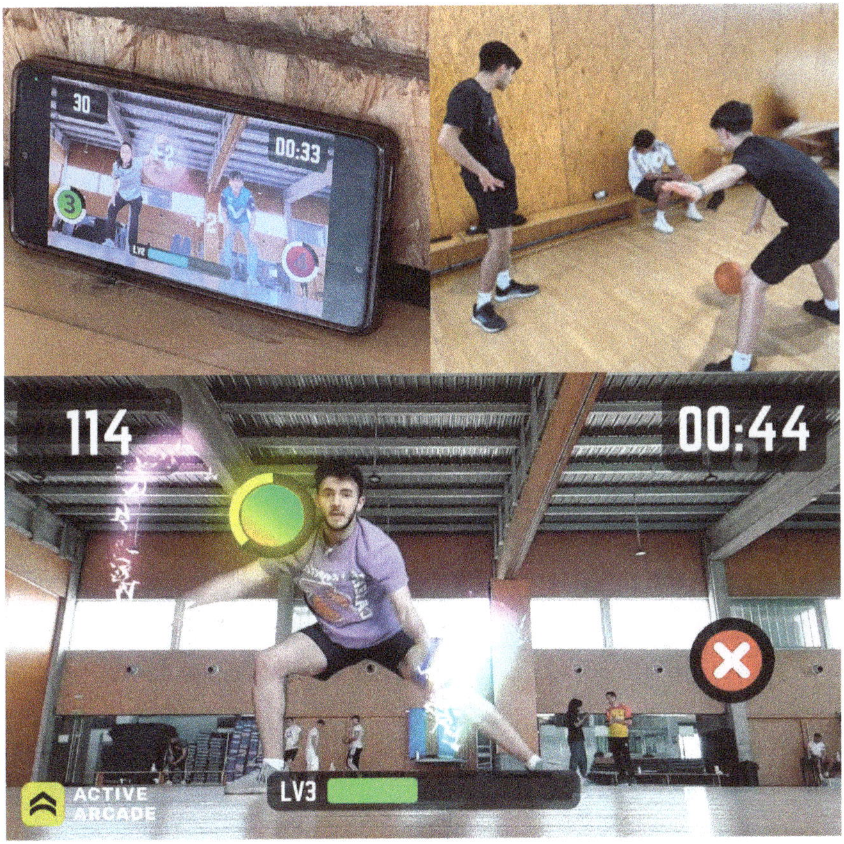

Figure 1. Students playing Active Arcade.

Following the tournament, participants completed an online questionnaire with close and open-ended questions addressing impact and their perceptions of exergames as future physical education teachers in secondary education. The questionnaire data were entered into an Excel database for further analysis.

Game Selection

The exergame app used in this study was Active Arcade v3.11 (NEX Team Inc., San Jose, CA, USA), released in 2021 and available for free on iOS and Android platforms without the need for registration. Active Arcade v3.11 employs motion recognition through the device's camera, enabling users to interact with augmented holographic visuals and sounds via AR technology. This setup requires no peripheral sensors or wearable devices, only an internet connection via Wi-Fi or mobile data.

Active Arcade v3.11 offers 12 mini-games with individual and collaborative modes across multiple difficulty levels. Each mini-game starts with player body recognition through the front camera, initiating the gameplay screen. The primary objective is to perform physical movements to achieve the highest score within a set time limit. Players can review top scores and past gameplay in video format to assess performance accuracy.

Out of the 12 mini-games, six were selected for this study. Each mini-game was repeated up to four times, encouraging participants to improve their scores, compete for the top three class positions, and aim for the tournament record. The selection was made collaboratively by course instructors, who are experts in Physical Activity and Sports Sciences with extensive experience in playful methodologies. The selection was based on four criteria:

- Transferability to school physical education: fostering motor skills development (e.g., movement, jumping, throwing, catching) and enhancing physical attributes such as speed, endurance, and strength.
- Session timing: appropriate intensity level categorized into warm-up, main activity, or cool-down phases.
- Difficulty level: assessed by the application (beginner, intermediate, or advanced) and required space (large or small).
- Game type: gameplay mechanics, competitive or cooperative modes, and individual or team-based play.

Based on these criteria, the following mini-games were selected:

- Cone Knockout (Intermediate Level: Warm-Up Phase)
  Individual agility and speed endurance game. Duration: 60 s.
- Reaction Flow (Beginner Level: Warm-Up Phase)
  Reaction speed game played in pairs. Duration: 60 s.
- DribbleTag (Advanced Level: Main Activity Phase)
  Individual reaction speed and coordination game involving basketball dribbling and passing. Duration: 60 s.
- Box Attack (Advanced Level: Main Activity Phase)
  Individual reaction speed and strength game. Duration: 60 s.
- Galaxy Jumpers (Beginner Level: Cool-Down Phase)
  Team-based jumping game (3–4 players). Duration: until the last player remains active.
- SuperHits (Intermediate Level: Cool-Down Phase)
  Individual rhythm game. Duration: the length of the chosen song.

Certain mini-games were excluded to avoid redundancy:

- High-Kicks and Reaction were omitted due to similarities with Reaction Flow.
- Bunny Hop, Whack a Mole, Fit Pals, and Space Pong were excluded due to their resemblance to Galaxy Jumpers or SuperHits.
- Pose was excluded as it focuses on expressive movement rather than physical exertion.

2.3. Instruments

A questionnaire was developed to assess perceived exertion during the mini-game sessions, utilizing the Borg CR10 Scale, a validated tool for subjective evaluation of physical exertion on a 0–10 scale, where 0 represents minimal exertion and 10 denotes maximum effort (Williams, 2017). This scale was specifically used to measure motor engagement throughout the session. To evaluate mental effort perception, a pictorial scale from similar tools was employed (Ouwehand et al., 2021), corresponding to a 0–10 Likert scale to ensure consistency with the Borg CR-10 Scale results for subsequent analysis.

Building on prior research on digital leisure and exergames in physical education (Chacón-Cuberos et al., 2016), open-ended questions were added to explore participants' familiarity with active video games by asking how frequently they played on digital devices, their experience with video games in the classroom, and their opinion about the potential for integrating these tools into PE curricula. Additionally, consistent with related studies (Hoyos-Quintero et al., 2022), data were collected on participants' frequency of physical exercise during the week, the type of activity performed, and its intensity, using the Borg CR-10 Scale as a reference.

2.4. Data Analysis

This study followed a mixed-methods approach. For the quantitative analysis, descriptive statistics were reported, including the mean (M), standard deviation (SD), and 95% confidence intervals (CIs 95%). Since repeated observations were collected from the same participants, a Repeated Measures Analysis of Variance (RM ANOVA) was conducted. Tukey's post hoc test with adjusted p-values was used for pairwise comparisons. When applicable, an interparticipant factor was added to the model to examine the influence of gender and practice frequency on the measures. Error bars in the ANOVA figures represent the confidence intervals. Effect size was measured using partial eta squared (η_p^2), with values of 0.01, 0.06, and 0.14 indicating small, medium, and large effects, respectively. Additionally, Pearson's r test was used to assess correlations between intensity measures.

For the qualitative analysis, Atlas.ti (v.9.0) was used to examine open-ended responses through thematic and categorical analysis, identifying patterns of meaning in the data (Braun & Clarke, 2006). Based on the coding of responses, the following categories and subcategories were generated, allowing for the identification of broader themes for interpretation: (1) Ease of Use and Potential Applications in the PE Classroom: Opportunities and Limitations, (2) Exergames as Promoters of Motor Skills, (3) Motor Engagement as Effective Practice Time, and (4) Motivation and Enjoyment.

3. Results

To facilitate the analysis of the questionnaire results, responses were organized according to question type. First, data from quantitative questions were presented to provide a structured overview of numerical findings. Subsequently, these results were complemented by an analysis of open-ended questions, examined through a qualitative lens to capture participants' perspectives in greater depth.

3.1. Quantitative Measures

After the session, the measured levels were:

- Physical intensity: $M = 6.55$ [CI 95% 6.27–6.82] $SD = 1.58$.
- Mental intensity: $M = 5.63$ [5.28–5.98] $SD = 2.04$.
- Motor engagement $M = 7.32$ [7.03–7.60] $SD = 1.67$.

ANOVA results revealed significant differences among these measures, $F(2,258) = 64.87$, $p < 0.001$, $\eta_p^2 = 0.33$ (Figure 2). Post hoc pairwise contrasts indicated that motor engagement during the session was significantly higher than physical and mental intensity ($p < 0.01$), and physical intensity exceeded mental intensity ($p < 0.001$).

As depicted in Figure 3, mini-games also differed in intensity, $F(5,645) = 279.40$, $p < 0.001$, $\eta_p^2 = 0.68$. Specifically, Box Attack and Cone Knockout elicited intensities exceeding 7 points, whereas Reaction Flow, Galaxy Jumpers, and SuperHits showed relatively lower intensities (Figure 3). Post hoc pairwise differences among mini-games are detailed in Table 1.

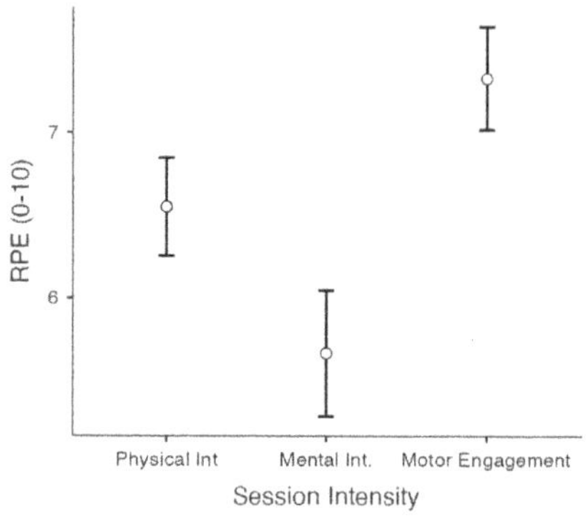

Figure 2. Reported intensity scores of the aspects of the exergames' practice.

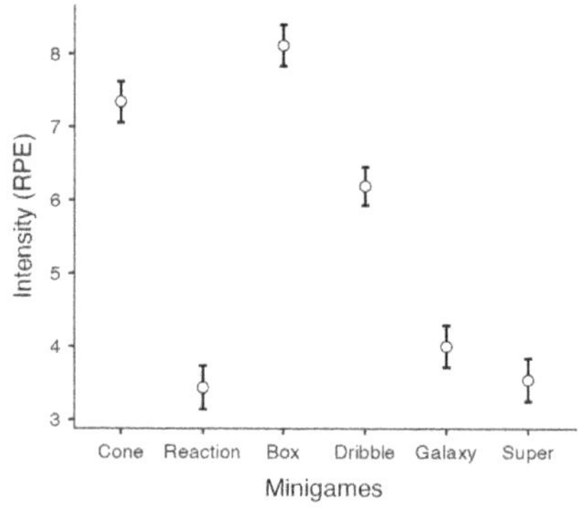

Figure 3. Reported intensity scores of the selected Active Arcade mini-games.

Table 1. Tukey post hoc *p*-values of mini-game intensities.

	Reaction	Box Attack	Dribble	Galaxy	Super
Cone	<0.001	<0.001	<0.001	<0.001	<0.001
Reaction		<0.001	<0.001	0.007	0.986
Box Attack			<0.001	<0.001	<0.001
Dribble				<0.001	<0.001
Galaxy					0.088

The reported intensity of the mini-games was positively correlated with physical and mental intensities, as well as motor engagement during the session (Table 2). For instance, participants who perceived high intensity during the Box Attack game also reported high levels of physical, mental, and motor engagement. Interestingly, motor engagement was found to be more closely related to mini-game intensity than either physical or mental exertion.

Table 2. Pearson correlation matrix between mini-games' intensities and session's intensities.

Active Arcade Mini-Games	Physical Intensity	Mental Intensity	Motor Engagement
Cone Knockout (RPE)	0.38 ***	0.27 **	0.41 ***
Reaction Flow (RPE)	0.17	0.10	0.17
Box Attack (RPE)	0.41 ***	0.33 ***	0.43 ***
Dribble Tag (RPE)	0.47 ***	0.31 ***	0.49 ***
Galaxy Jumpers (RPE)	0.20 *	0.19 *	0.18 *
SuperHits: Catch and Slash (RPE)	0.25 **	0.15	0.23 **

Note. * $p < 0.05$, ** $p < 0.01$, *** $p < 0.001$.

All participants reported engaging in regular weekly sport practice: 22% (n = 29) practiced 1–2 days per week, 49% (n = 63) practiced 3–5 days per week, and 29% (n = 37) practiced 6–7 days per week. The average perceived intensity of their training days was $M = 7.16$ [6.97–7.35] $SD = 1.08$. A repeated measures ANOVA (RM ANOVA) revealed a significant interaction between the number of practice days and the session's overall intensity, F (4,252) = 3.02, $p = 0.018$, $\eta_p^2 = 0.05$. This interaction was primarily driven by mental intensity (Figure 4). Unlike physical intensity or motor engagement, mental intensity was significantly influenced by the frequency of physical practice, F(2,126) = 4.95, $p = 0.009$, $\eta_p^2 = 0.07$ (Figure 4). Participants practicing more than two days per week reported lower mental effort compared to those practicing 1–2 days per week (post hoc $p < 0.05$). Finally, no significant main effects or interactions were found related to gender (all $p > 0.05$), session practice intensities (physical, mental, and motor engagement), mini-game intensities, regular practice frequency, or overall session intensity.

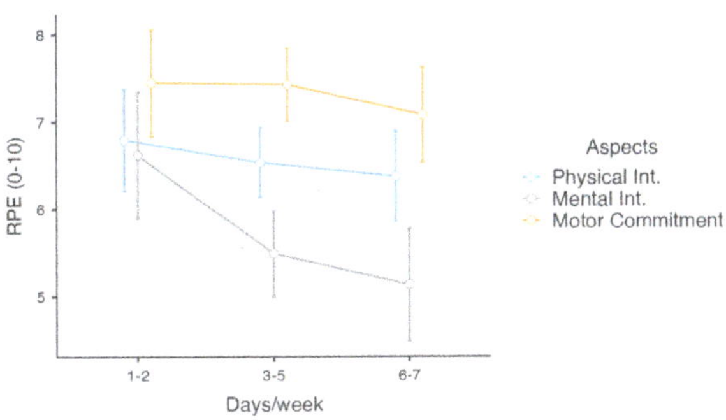

Figure 4. Session's intensities by frequency of practice.

3.2. *Qualitative Measures*

The following section presents the themes identified from the questionnaire responses. The testimonies included are among the most representative, illustrating the most recurrent patterns observed in the analysis of the responses.

3.2.1. Ease of Use and Potential Applications in the PE Classroom: Opportunities and Limitations

Many participants emphasized the importance of integrating exergames like Active Arcade v3.11 into PE classes, noting the potential for coherent technology integration in PE. For instance, E71 stated, "mobile phones should always serve pedagogical purposes in the classroom". Similarly, E14 highlighted that "this type of content is not typically presented in this way in high schools", while E58 pointed out how it can foster "a healthy relationship with technology".

Regarding technical assessment, the application was praised for its intuitive functionality and usability. E107 described it as "intuitive and easy to use", and E22 appreciated the convenience of not needing additional equipment, noting that "it fits in one's pocket". E121 further emphasized its accessibility: "everyone has a mobile phone they usually bring to class, so everyone can download the game and use it". Additionally, E44 noted that the application is widely available as it "can be downloaded on any device, as it is a free resource accessible on both Android and iOS systems".

3.2.2. Exergames as Promoters of Motor Skills

Participants associated the use of Active Arcade with developing motor skills and enhancing physical fitness. E90 noted, "in nearly all the games, you're moving in different ways and have to do so quickly; in others, you jump, and in the basketball game, you control a ball through dribbling while maintaining a continuous bounce". E75 observed, "in the box game, lower-body strength exercises, such as jumps, are combined with upper-body exercises like push-ups". Several participants emphasized the games' speed and reaction requirements. E23 explained, "they are all speed games because you have a limited time to achieve the highest score, and some require reaction time as you don't know where on the screen the elements you need to tap will appear".

Moreover, the games were found to increase enjoyment and participation. E55 remarked, "when exercises like jumps, push-ups, or speed exercises are incorporated into games, they become much more enjoyable and encourage participation without reluctance". This sentiment was echoed by E44, who highlighted the games' versatility beyond PE: "this app can also be used in training sessions. Personally, I'm now considering incorporating it into my basketball practice design at my club".

3.2.3. Motor Engagement as Effective Practice Time

Participants noted high activity levels throughout the session. As E23 explained, "we only rested when it was our teammates' turn". Some admitted finding ways to extend their playtime, such as E33, who said, "we sometimes used two smartphones to play longer". The 60 s duration of most challenges encouraged continuous activity with minimal downtime. E15 remarked, "since the rounds didn't last long and mini-games changed every 15 min or so, we tried to maximize our time by using two or three phones to play and achieve high scores". The structure enabled participants to repeat challenges multiple times. E01 noted, "we completed each challenge about 10 times". E11 highlighted the intensity: "these short, intense series make you want to give your maximum effort, and when you're really focused, class time flies by". Some participants acknowledged taking breaks during game rotations or instructions, while others admitted to stopping due to fatigue. E15 observed that "it seemed to be a low-intensity session, but we were moving for over an hour", while E45 observed, "each person set their own intensity level", with some noting that "there were also more relaxed games at the end of the session" (E18).

3.2.4. Motivation and Enjoyment

Participants frequently highlighted the motivational aspect of integrating video games into physical activity. E74 described it as "intriguing and appealing, making it possible to exercise through video games in the classroom". E65 remarked that this approach "redefines the notion of video games, shifting from sedentary play to active engagement". Participants acknowledged its potential for promoting "healthy leisure" (E92). E103 observed, "you play at an intense level, as reflected by your heart rate; it's exercising without realizing it". E23 added, "if taken seriously, the intensity of many games rivals traditional cardio or strength training sessions".

Competitive and cooperative dynamics also played a role. E67 highlighted the impact of extrinsic motivation on exercise intensity, observing that "Competition drives intensity, as people push to achieve high scores". Meanwhile, E32 emphasized intrinsic motivation: "I didn't focus on others' top scores; I focused on improving my record, competing against myself". Cooperative gameplay was also valued, with E22 noting, "Playing with others adds responsibility—you want to do your best".

4. Discussion

This study evaluated the impact of a mobile exergame (Active Arcade v3.11) on motor skill engagement, perceived physical and mental exertion, and the motivational and usability aspects for training future PE teachers. Results align with previous research (Chow & Mann, 2023; Conde-Cortabitarte et al., 2020; Marin-Suelves et al., 2022; Staiano & Calvert, 2011), demonstrating the benefits of exergames in promoting healthy habits and improving physical, emotional, and cognitive outcomes.

Participants' moderate-to-high weekly physical activity levels reflected their prior training experience, with no significant gender differences in perceived intensity and frequency. These values reflect the participants' experience in physical activity training sessions. Participants reported similar levels of motor engagement accompanied by moderate levels of physical and mental exertion. Lower activity participants reported higher mental exertion, suggesting that cognitive and physical effort are distinct phenomena that require different adaptations (Cárdenas et al., 2015). Ultimately, Active Arcade v3.11 is a video game that can be used by students of any fitness level. The variety of mini-games targeted various skills and abilities—strength development (*Box Attack*), basic motor skills such as jumping and dodging (*Galaxy Jumpers*), reaction speed (*Reaction Flow*), coordination (*SuperHits*), and sport-specific skills (*DribbleTag*)—which highlights the value of this tool in a physical education classroom. This variety sustained high motor engagement without excessive physical demands, favouring practice density over intensity to maximize energy expenditure (Lyons et al., 2011; Sell et al., 2008).

This type of design may result in being more convenient for PE. Instead of higher levels of physical or mental load during PE classes, enough engagement time is necessary. It is not about the amount of intensity but the density of practice (Vaghetti et al., 2018). Additionally, the variety of mini-games promoted sustained engagement, offering a dynamic learning experience (Sheehan et al., 2015). The adequate selection of activities and the use of freely and easily available resources like free-to-play exergames maximize the benefits of physical activity sessions in terms of motor and physiological engagement (Martínez-Gómez et al., 2007). The accessible (Díaz-Barahona, 2020), cost-free nature of exergames (Dixon et al., 2010), combined with their user-friendly and playful approach, encouraged active participation, supporting their integration into PE curricula (Díaz-Barahona, 2020). There is ongoing debate and some controversy regarding the use of technology in educational settings (Wilmer et al., 2017). We, however, consider that its positive or negative impact mostly depends on how well technology is implemented and integrated into pedagogical processes (Fawns, 2022; Selwyn, 2016). In our specific case, mobile devices contributed to the improvement in the practice of physical exercise in a self-regulated and highly motivating manner.

From a motivational perspective, participants reported high enjoyment levels. According to the literature, game-based learning can enhance interest in physical activity (Huang et al., 2019; Marques et al., 2023). Despite concerns about the impact of video games on young people's health and socialization (Gómez-Gonzalvo et al., 2020), an exergame like Active Arcade v3.11 reshapes perceptions of video games. Teachers (or future teachers) can effectively use exergames, with innovations like augmented reality (Omarov et al., 2024), as allies to combat sedentary behaviors among students (Dávila-Morán et al., 2024; Liu et al., 2020; Santos et al., 2021). As has been observed in other studies, motivational aspects, particularly competitive and cooperative elements, enhanced engagement, fostering a positive learning environment (Marker & Staiano, 2015).

Prior experience with digital tools is essential for integrating exergames into PE programs (Conde-Cortabitarte & Rodríguez-Hoyos, 2018). Research indicates that adults often underestimate the potential of technology to improve health outcomes until they encounter its benefits through exergames (Bird et al., 2015). This underscores the importance of training future PE teachers in the pedagogical use of these technologies (Díaz-Barahona, 2020; Meckbach et al., 2013; Naranjo-Harnisth, 2024). Such training fosters critical thinking skills and prepares educators to effectively integrate digital health applications (mHealth) (Fitzpatrick & Russell, 2013; Ubago et al., 2022).

The findings of this study further emphasize the possibility of incorporating technological applications and exergames into PE classrooms (Díaz-Barahona, 2020; Quintero-González et al., 2022; Vaghetti et al., 2018).

The current results indicate the perceived intensity of different exergames. In this regard, a direct practical implication would be that high-intensity mini-games (i.e., Box Attack and Cone Knockout) need to be placed in the middle of the session, whereas lower intensity ones (e.g., Reaction Flow, Galaxy Jumpers, and SuperHits) can be used as warm-up or cool-down exercises. Moreover, future teachers should explore the pedagogical potential of exergames to transform recreational video game use into meaningful educational experiences (Conde-Cortabitarte et al., 2024; Zhao et al., 2024). This intervention serves as a pilot training initiative for prospective PE teachers, enabling them to critically and professionally assess the educational impact of video games in classroom settings.

The results suggest that exergames, when implemented with thoughtful curricular planning, can serve as effective tools for PE instruction. These tools not only support motor skill development and the promotion of healthy habits (Dávila-Morán et al., 2024; Vernadakis et al., 2015), but also enhance enjoyment and motivation towards physical activity through innovative digital resources (Lyons et al., 2014; Marin-Suelves et al., 2022).

5. Conclusions

This study highlights several limitations and potential areas for further research. One major limitation is the current inability to collect real-time physiological fitness data without compromising usability. However, as smartphone technology evolves and heart rate sensors become more integrated, exergames are expected to offer more comprehensive data in the near future.

From a pedagogical standpoint, future research should explore how educators can effectively design and implement exergaming sessions, integrating them into structured lesson plans or extracurricular activities. The intensity levels reported in this study across different mini-games could serve for such planning. Additionally, further research should focus on equipping educators with the skills to incorporate these digital tools into educational environments. Exergames in PE classes can encourage young people to maintain sustained physical throughout their lives, serving as a motivating option that promotes movement in favor of their health.

In conclusion, free-to-play exergames, leveraging mobile devices and interactive games, hold substantial potential to inspire educators to adopt these tools in their teaching practices. Their user-friendliness, engaging nature, and adaptability make them an enjoyable and effective way for students to engage in physical activity, both inside and outside the context of physical education.

Author Contributions: Conceptualization, P.S.-O. and M.A.-B.; methodology, P.S.-O., M.A.-B. and J.A.N.; software, P.S.-O. and J.A.N.; validation, P.S.-O., M.A.-B. and J.A.N.; formal analysis, P.S.-O., M.A.-B. and J.A.N.; investigation, P.S.-O.; resources, P.S.-O.; data curation, P.S.-O., M.A.-B. and J.A.N.; writing—original draft preparation, P.S.-O., M.A.-B. and J.A.N.; writing—review and editing, P.S.-O., M.A.-B. and J.A.N.; visualization, P.S.-O., M.A.-B. and J.A.N.; supervision, P.S.-O., M.A.-B. and J.A.N.; project administration, P.S.-O.; All authors have read and agreed to the published version of the manuscript.

Funding: This research was part of the Innovation Project "Proposals for Game-Based Learning through exergames and modern board games that promote motor engagement" (Ref. UAH/EV1469) funded by the University of Alcalá.

Institutional Review Board Statement: The study was approved by the Research and Animal Experimentation Ethics Committee of the University of Alcalá (protocol code CEIP/2024/6/122, on 13 November 2024).

Informed Consent Statement: Informed consent was obtained from all subjects involved in the study.

Data Availability Statement: The original contributions presented in the study are included in the article; further inquiries can be directed to the corresponding author.

Acknowledgments: We extend our gratitude to all participants for their interest and participation in the subject and their engagement with the proposal involving the use of video games in PE.

Conflicts of Interest: The authors declare no conflicts of interest.

References

Andrade, A., Correia, C. K., & Coimbra, D. R. (2019). The psychological effects of exergames for children and adolescents with obesity: A systematic review and meta-analysis. *Cyberpsychology, Behavior, and Social Networking*, *22*(11), 724–735. [CrossRef]

Beltrán-Carrillo, V. J., Valencia-Peris, A., & Molina-Alventosa, J. P. (2011). Los videojuegos activos y la salud de los jóvenes: Revisión de la investigación. *International Journal of Medicine and Science of Physical Activity and Sport*, *11*(41), 203–219. Available online: https://www.redalyc.org/articulo.oa?id=54222155012 (accessed on 4 June 2024).

Benzing, V., & Schmidt, M. (2018). Exergaming for children and adolescents: Strengths, weaknesses, opportunities and threats. *Journal of Clinical Medicine*, *7*(11), 422. [CrossRef]

Best, J. R. (2012). Exergaming immediately enhances children's executive function. *Developmental Psychology*, *48*(5), 1501–1510. [CrossRef]

Bird, M., Clark, B., Millar, J., Whetton, S., & Smith, S. (2015). Exposure to "exergames" increases older adults' perception of the usefulness of technology for improving health and physical activity: A pilot study. *JMIR Serious Games*, *3*(2), e8. [CrossRef]

Braun, V., & Clarke, V. (2006). Using thematic analysis in psychology. *Qualitative Research in Psychology*, *3*(2), 77–101. [CrossRef]

Canabrava, K., Faria, F., de Lima, J., Guedes, D., & Amorim, P. (2018). Energy expenditure and intensity of active video games in children and adolescents. *Research Quarterly for Exercise and Sport*, *1*(89), 47–56. [CrossRef] [PubMed]

Castro-Sánchez, M., Martínez, A., Zurita, F., Chacón, R., Espejo, T., & Cabrera, Á. (2015). Uso de videojuegos y su relación con las conductas sedentarias en una población escolary universitaria. *Journal for Educators, Teachers and Trainers*, *6*, 40–51.

Cárdenas, D., Conde-González, J., & Perales, J. C. (2015). El papel de la carga mental en la planificación del entrenamiento deportivo. *Revista De Psicología Del Deporte*, *1*(24), 91–100.

Cerezo-Pizarro, M., Revuelta-Domínguez, F., Guerra-Antequera, J., & Melo-Sánchez, J. (2023). The cultural impact of video games: A systematic review of the literature. *Education Sciences*, *13*, 1116. [CrossRef]

Chacón-Cuberos, R., Castro-Sánchez, M., Zurita-Ortega, F., Espejo-Garcés, T., & Martínez-Martínez, A. (2016). Videojuegos activos como recurso TIC en el aula de educación física: Estudio a partir de parámetros de Ocio digital. *Digital Education Review*, *29*, 112–123.

Chóliz, M., Villanueva, V., & Chóliz, M. C. (2009). Ellos, ellas y su móvil: Uso, abuso (¿y dependencia?) del teléfono móvil en la adolescencia. *Revista Española De Drogodependencias*, *1*(34), 74–88. Available online: https://www.researchgate.net/publication/284473053_Ellas_ellos_y_su_movil_Uso_abuso_y_dependencia_del_telefono_movil_en_la_adolescencia (accessed on 4 June 2024).

Chow, D. H. K., & Mann, S. K. F. (2023). Exergaming and education: A relational model for games selection and evaluation. *Frontiers in Psychology*, *14*, 1197403. [CrossRef]

Comeras-Chueca, C., Villalba-Heredia, L., Perez-Lasierra, J. L., Marín-Puyalto, J., Lozano-Berges, G., Matute-Llorente, Á, Vicente-Rodríguez, G., Gonzalez-Aguero, A., & Casajús, J. A. (2022). Active video games improve muscular fitness and motor skills in children with overweight or obesity. *International Journal of Environmental Research and Public Health, 19*(5), 2642. [CrossRef] [PubMed]

Conde-Cortabitarte, I., & Rodríguez-Hoyos, C. (2018). Indagando en las experiencias del profesorado para incorporar los exergames en las aulas de educación física. *EDMETIC, 7*(2), 1–17. [CrossRef]

Conde-Cortabitarte, I., Rodríguez-Hoyos, C., & Calvo-Salvador, A. (2020). Potencialidades y límites educativos de los videojuegos activos: Una investigación basada en entrevistas a docentes de educación física. *Cultura, Ciencia Y Deporte, 15*(43), 43–52. [CrossRef]

Conde-Cortabitarte, I., Rodríguez-Hoyos, C., & Calvo-Salvador, A. (2024). Analizando las posibilidades educativas de los exergames en educación física: Una investigación con estudios de caso. *Revista Española De Educación Física Y Deportes, 438*, 15–29. [CrossRef]

Corpas-Ruiz, J. M., & Villodres, G. C. (2023). Análisis del tiempo de compromiso motor en educación física: Una revisión bibliográfica. *Journal of Sport and Health Research, 15*(3), 455–470. [CrossRef]

Dávila-Morán, R. C., Ruiz Nizama, J. L., Castillo-Sáenz, R. A., Torres Sime, C. L., Saldaña Narro, J. B., & Peña Huertas, J. G. (2024). Impacto de los videojuegos activos en conductas sedentarias en niños en edad escolar. *Retos, 55*, 804–815. [CrossRef]

Díaz-Barahona, J. (2020). Retos y oportunidades de la tecnología móvil en la educación física. *Retos, 37*, 763–773. [CrossRef]

Dixon, R., Maddison, R., Ni Mhurchu, C., Jull, A., Meagher-Lundberg, P., & Widdowson, D. (2010). Parents' and children's perceptions of active video games: A focus group study. *Journal of Child Health Care, 14*(2), 189–199. [CrossRef]

Fawns, T. (2022). An entangled pedagogy: Looking beyond the pedagogy—Technology dichotomy. *Postdigital Science and Education, 4*(3), 711. [CrossRef]

Fierro-Suero, S., Castillo, I., Almagro, B. J., & Saénz-López, P. (2023). The role of motivation and emotions in physical education: Understanding academic achievement and the intention to be physically active. *Frontiers in Psychology, 14*, 1253043. [CrossRef] [PubMed]

Fitzpatrick, K., & Russell, D. (2013). On being critical in health and physical education. *Physical Education and Sport Pedagogy, 20*(2), 159–173. [CrossRef]

Gómez-Gonzalvo, F., Devís-Devís, J., & Molina-Alventosa, P. (2020). Video game usage time in adolescents' academic performance. *Comunicar, 28*(65), 89. [CrossRef]

Gómez-Gonzalvo, F., Molina-Alventosa, J. P., & Devís Devís, J. (2018). Los videojuegos como materiales curriculares: Una aproximación a su uso en Educación Física. *Retos: Nuevas Tendencias en Educación Física, Deporte y Recreación, 34*, 305–310. [CrossRef]

Gómez-Miguel, A., & Calderón-Gómez, D. (Eds.). (2023). *Videojuegos y jóvenes: Lugares, experiencias y tensiones* (1st ed.). Centro Reina Sofía de Fad Juventud. [CrossRef]

Gu, D., Gu, C., Oginni, J., Ryu, S., Liu, W., Li, X., & Gao, Z. (2023). Acute effects of exergaming on young adults' energy expenditure, enjoyment, and self-efficacy. *Frontiers in Psychology, 14*, 1238057. [CrossRef]

Haddock, B. L., Brandt, A. M., Siegel, S. R., Wilkin, L. D., & Kyue, J. (2008). Active video games and energy expenditure in overweight children. *International Journal of Fitness, 4*(2), 17–23. Available online: https://www.ncbi.nlm.nih.gov/pubmed/24683297 (accessed on 10 September 2024). [PubMed]

Ho, R. S., Chan, E. K., Liu, K. K., & Wong, S. H. (2022). Active video game on children and adolescents' physical activity and weight management: A network meta-analysis. *Scandinavian Journal of Medicine & Science in Sports, 32*(8), 1268–1286. [CrossRef]

Hooft-Graafland, J. (2018). New technologies and 21st century children: Recent trends and outcomes. In *OECD education working papers 179* (pp. 1–60). OECD Publishing. [CrossRef]

Hoyos-Quintero, A. M., Yusty Garcia, N., & Flor-Sandon, V. A. (2022). Efecto del uso de videojuegos activos en el nivel de actividad física del adulto joven. *Revisión exploratoria.* Retos, *45*, 888–896. [CrossRef]

Huang, H., Nguyen, H. V., Cheng, T. C. E., Wong, M., Chiu, H., Yang, Y., & Teng, N. I. (2019). A randomized controlled trial on the role of enthusiasm about exergames: Players' perceptions of exercise. *Games for Health Journal, 8*(3), 220–226. [CrossRef]

Larsen, L. H., Schou, L., Lund, H. H., & Langberg, H. (2013). The physical effect of exergames in healthy elderly—A systematic review. *Games for Health Journal, 2*(4), 205–212. [CrossRef] [PubMed]

Laurson, K. R., Eisenmann, J. C., Welk, G. J., Wickel, E. E., Gentile, D. A., & Walsh, D. A. (2008). Combined influence of physical activity and screen time recommendations on childhood overweight. *The Journal of Pediatrics, 153*(2), 209–214. [CrossRef] [PubMed]

Lee, S., Kim, W., Park, T., & Peng, W. (2017). The psychological effects of playing exergames: A systematic review. *Cyberpsychology, Behavior, and Social Networking, 20*(9), 513–532. [CrossRef] [PubMed]

Li, J., Erdt, M., Chen, L., Cao, Y., Lee, S., & Theng, Y. (2018). The social effects of exergames on older adults: Systematic review and metric analysis. *Journal of Medical Internet Research, 20*(6), e10486. [CrossRef] [PubMed]

Liu, W., Zeng, N., McDonough, D. J., & Gao, Z. (2020). Effect of active video games on healthy children's fundamental motor skills and physical fitness: A systematic review. *International Journal of Environmental Research and Public Health, 17*(21), 8264. [CrossRef]

Lozano-Sánchez, A. M., Zurita-Ortega, F., Ubago-Jiménez, J. L., Puertas-Molero, P., & Ramírez-Granizo, I. (2019). Videojuegos, práctica de actividad física, obesidad y hábitos sedentarios en escolares de entre 10 y 12 años de la provincia de Granada. *Retos, 35*, 42–46. [CrossRef]

Luarn, P., Chen, C., & Chiu, Y. (2023). Understanding continuance intention to play exergames during the COVID-19 pandemic: Hedonic and utilitarian aspects. *Managing Sport and Leisure*, 1–14. [CrossRef]

Lyons, E. J., Tate, D. F., Ward, D. S., Bowling, J. M., Ribisl, K. M., & Kalyararaman, S. (2011). Energy expenditure and enjoyment during video game play. *Medicine and Science in Sports and Exercise, 43*(10), 1987–1993. [CrossRef] [PubMed]

Lyons, E. J., Tate, D. F., Ward, D. S., Ribisl, K. M., Bowling, J. M., & Kalyanaraman, S. (2014). Engagement, enjoyment, and energy expenditure during active video game play. *Health Psychology, 33*(2), 174–181. [CrossRef] [PubMed]

Marin-Suelves, D., Guzmán, J. F., & Ramon-Llin, J. (2022). Exergame en Educación Física: Mapeando la investigación Exergame in physical education: Mapping the research. *Retos, 44*, 64–76. [CrossRef]

Marker, A. M., & Staiano, A. E. (2015). Better together: Outcomes of cooperation versus competition in social exergaming. *Games for Health Journal, 4*(1), 25–30. [CrossRef] [PubMed]

Marques, L. M., Uchida, P. M., & Barbosa, S. P. (2023). The impact of Exergames on emotional experience: A systematic review. *Frontiers in Public Health, 11*, 1209520. [CrossRef] [PubMed]

Martínez-Gómez, D., Sampedro, V., & Veiga, Ó. L. (2007). La importancia del compromiso motor y el compromiso fisiológico durante las clases de educación física. *Revista Iberoamericana De Educación, 42*(2), 1–13. [CrossRef]

Meckbach, J., Gibbs, B., Almqvist, J., Öhman, M., & Quennerstedt, M. (2013). Exergames as a teaching tool in physical education? *Sport Science Review, 22*(5–6), 369–385. [CrossRef]

Medeiros, P., Capistrano, R., Zequinão, M. A., Silva, S. A. D., Beltrame, T. S., & Cardoso, F. L. (2017). Exergames como ferramenta de aquisição e desenvolvimento de habilidades e capacidades motoras: Uma revisão sistemática. *Revista Paulista De Pediatria, 35*(4), 464–471. [CrossRef]

Moholdt, T., Weie, S., Chorianopoulos, K., Wang, A. I., & Hagen, K. (2017). Exergaming can be an innovative way of enjoyable high-intensity interval training. *BMJ Open Sport &Amp; Exercise Medicine, 3*(1), e000258. [CrossRef]

Moller, A. C., Sousa, C. V., Lee, K. J., Alon, D., & Lu, A. S. (2023). Active video game interventions targeting physical activity behaviors: Systematic review and meta-analysis. *Journal of Medical Internet Research, 25*, e45243. [CrossRef]

Monguillot, M., Guitert, M., & González-Arévalo, C. (2018). TPACKPEC: Diseño de situaciones de aprendizaje mediadas por TIC en Educación Física. *Movimento (ESEFID/UFRGS), 24*(3), 749–764. [CrossRef]

Naranjo-Harnisth, J. (2024). Uso de aplicaciones tecnológicas en las clases de educación física. *Revista Académica Internacional De Educación Física, 4*(4), 38–65. [CrossRef]

Oh, Y., & Yang, S. (2010). Defining exergames & exergaming. *Proceedings Meaningful Play*, 1–17. Available online: https://meaningfulplay.msu.edu/proceedings2010/mp2010_paper_63.pdf (accessed on 15 September 2024).

O'Loughlin, E. K., Sabiston, C. M., O'rourke, R. H., Bélanger, M., Sylvestre, M., & O'loughlin, J. L. (2023). The change in exergaming from before to during the COVID-19 pandemic among young adults: Longitudinal study. *JMIR Serious Games, 11*, e41553. [CrossRef] [PubMed]

Omarov, N., Omarov, B., Azhibekova, Z., & Omarov, B. (2024). Applying an augmented reality game-based learning environment in physical education classes to enhance sports motivation. *Retos, 60*, 269–278. [CrossRef]

Ouwehand, K., Kroef, A. V. D., Wong, J., & Paas, F. (2021). Measuring cognitive load: Are there more valid alternatives to likert rating scales? *Frontiers in Education, 6*, 702616. [CrossRef]

Park, S., Hwang, J., & Choi, Y. (2019). Effect of mobile health on obese adults: A systematic review and meta-analysis. *Healthcare Informatics Research, 25*(1), 12–26. [CrossRef] [PubMed]

Pellas, N., & Mystakidis, S. (2020). A systematic review of research about game-based learning in virtual worlds. *JUCS—Journal of Universal Computer Science, 26*(8), 1017–1042. [CrossRef]

Qian, M., & Clark, K. R. (2016). Game-based learning and 21st century skills: A review of recent research. *Computers in Human Behavior, 63*, 50–58. [CrossRef]

Quintero-González, L. E., Jiménez-Jiménez, F., & Area Moreira, M. (2022). Claves para la integración y el uso de los dispositivos móviles en las clases de educación física. *Acción Motriz, 1*(20), 17–26. Available online: https://www.accionmotriz.com/index.php/accionmotriz/article/view/111 (accessed on 15 September 2024).

Rewitz, K., Schindler, S., & Wolff, W. (2024). Examining the alignment between subjective effort and objective force production. *PLoS ONE, 19*(8), e0307994. [CrossRef]

Rodríguez-Reyes, A. D., Rivas, J., & Pávez-Adasme, G. (2020). Tiempo de compromiso motor en la clase de educación física motor commitment time in physical education class. *Voces De La Educación, 5*(10), 90–113. Available online: https://www.revista.vocesdelaeducacion.com.mx/index.php/voces/article/view/256/213 (accessed on 15 September 2024).

Santos, I. K. D., Medeiros, R. C. D. S., Cunha De, Medeiros, J. A. D., Almeida-Neto, P. F. D., Sena, D. C. S. D., Cobucci, R. N., Oliveira, R. S., Cabral, B. G. D. A. T., & Dantas, P. M. S. (2021). Active video games for improving mental health and physical fitness—An alternative for children and adolescents during social isolation: An overview. *International Journal of Environmental Research and Public Health, 18*(4), 1641. [CrossRef] [PubMed]

Sell, K., Lillie, T., & Taylor, J. (2008). Energy expenditure during physically interactive video game playing in male college students with different playing experience. *Journal of American College Health, 56*(5), 505–511. [CrossRef]

Selwyn, N. (2016). *Is technology good for education?* Polity Press.

Sheehan, D. P., Katz, L., & Kooiman, B. J. (2015). Exergaming and physical education: A qualitative examination from the teachers' perspectives. *Journal of Case Studies in Education, 4*, 1–14.

Shen, C., Dumontheil, I., Thomas, M., Röösli, M., Elliott, P., & Toledano, M. (2021). Digital technology use and BMI: Evidence from a cross-sectional analysis of an adolescent cohort study. *Journal of Medical Internet Research, 23*(7), e26485. [CrossRef] [PubMed]

Siegel, S. R., Haddock, B., Dubois, A. M., & Wilkin, L. D. (2009). Active Video/arcade games (exergaming) and energy expenditure in college students. *International Journal of Exercise Science, 3*(2), 165–174. Available online: https://www.ncbi.nlm.nih.gov/pubmed/20407622 (accessed on 4 June 2024). [CrossRef]

Spanish Statistical Office. (2023). *Encuesta sobre equipamiento y uso de tecnologías de información y comunicación en los hogares.* Instituto Nacional de Estadística. Available online: https://www.ine.es/dyngs/INEbase/es/operacion.htm?c=estadistica_C&cid=1254736176741&menu=ultiDatos&idp=1254735976608 (accessed on 4 June 2024).

Staiano, A. E., & Calvert, S. L. (2011). Exergames for physical education courses: Physical, social, and cognitive benefits. *Child Development Perspectives, 5*(2), 93–98. [CrossRef] [PubMed]

Ubago, J. L., Puertas, P., González-Valero, G., Melguizo, E., Valverde-Janer, M., & Ortega-Caballero, M. (2022). Uso de los dispositivos móviles (Mhealth) en la práctica deportiva en adolescentes. *International Journal of Developmental and Educational Psychology, 1*(1), 165–170. [CrossRef]

Vaghetti, C. A. O., Monteiro-Junior, R. S., Finco, M. D., Reategui, E., & Silva Da Costa Botelho, S. (2018). Exergames experience in physical education: A review. *Physical Culture and Sport. Studies and Research, 78*(1), 23–32. [CrossRef]

Vernadakis, N., Papastergiou, M., Zetou, E., & Antoniou, P. (2015). The impact of an exergame-based intervention on children's fundamental motor skills. *Computers and Education, 83*, 90–102. [CrossRef]

Williams, N. (2017). The borg rating of perceived exertion (RPE) scale. *Occupational Medicine, 67*(5), 404–405. [CrossRef]

Wilmer, H. H., Sherman, L. E., & Chein, J. M. (2017). Smartphones and cognition: A review of research exploring the links between mobile technology habits and cognitive functioning. *Frontiers in Psychology, 8*, 605. [CrossRef] [PubMed]

World Health Organization. (2020). *Here are some physical activities you can do at home during #COVID19.* World Health Organization (WHO). Available online: https://x.com/WHO/status/1250692858203553793 (accessed on 4 June 2024).

Zhao, M., Lu, X., Zhang, Q., Zhao, R., Wu, B., Huang, S., & Li, S. (2024). Effects of exergames on student physical education learning in the context of the artificial intelligence era: A meta-analysis. *Scientific Reports, 14*(1), 7115. [CrossRef] [PubMed]

behavioral sciences

MDPI

Article

The Effect of Free Weight Resistance Training on Cognitive Function Explored Through Eye Tracking: A Randomized Double-Blind Clinical Trial

Cristián Mateluna-Núñez [1,*], Romualdo Ibáñez-Orellana [2,3], César Campos-Rojas [2,3], Andrea Santana-Covarrubias [2,3], Rodrigo Fuentes Figueroa [1] and Ricardo Martínez-Flores [4]

1 Escuela de Educación Física, Pontificia Universidad Católica de Valparaíso, Valparaíso 2340025, Chile; rodrigoafuentesfigueroa@gmail.com
2 Instituto de Literatura y Ciencias del Lenguaje, Pontificia Universidad Católica de Valparaíso, Valparaíso 2340025, Chile; romualdo.ibanez@pucv.cl (R.I.-O.); cesar.campos@pucv.cl (C.C.-R.); andrea.santana@pucv.cl (A.S.-C.)
3 Instituto de Literatura y Ciencias del Lenguaje, Pontificia Universidad Católica de Valparaíso, Millennium Nucleus for the Science of Learning (MiNSoL), Valparaíso 2340025, Chile
4 IRyS Group, Escuela de Educación Física, Pontificia Universidad Católica de Valparaíso, Valparaíso 2340025, Chile; ricardo.antonio.martinezf@gmail.com
* Correspondence: matelunanc@gmail.com or cristian.mateluna@pucv.cl; Tel.: +56-998721031

Abstract: In this study, we investigated the impact of a 10-week free weight resistance training (RT) program on cognitive function in healthy young adults. In this randomized controlled trial, 18 participants were assigned to either an experimental or control group. We assessed cognitive function by using eye-tracking (ET) technology during text processing tasks. First-pass reading times (FPRTs) and total reading times (TRTs) were measured. Results revealed a significant three-way interaction between group, moment, and syntactic complexity in FPRTs, demonstrating training effects on cognitive processing. The experimental group showed a distinctive shift in processing patterns: from longer times in low complexity pre-intervention to increased times in high complexity post-intervention, particularly in early processing measures (FPRTs). Complementary analyses of strength improvements showed that increased strength was associated with enhanced attention allocation to complex structures and improved processing efficiency for simpler texts, suggesting RT's potential to modulate cognitive function.

Keywords: cognition; resistance training; cognitive function; eye tracking; text processing; exercise; executive function

1. Introduction

Neuromuscular function is one of the most important and determining factors in athletic performance (Cormie et al., 2011; Mateluna-Núñez et al., 2022) and a key objective of resistance training (RT), such as weightlifting; however, RT, defined as a physical exercise program designed to maintain and improve muscular strength, endurance, and lean muscle mass (Ratamess et al., 2009; Liguori & ACSM, 2021), is also vital for maintaining health and enhancing functional capacity in both young and older populations (Hillman et al., 2008; Guizelini et al., 2018). In this regard, RT has been associated with a reduction in all-cause mortality, decreased cardiovascular risk and blood pressure (El-Kotob et al., 2020), improvements in glucose metabolism (Colberg et al., 2016), benefits to bone, tendon health, and cartilage loss prevention (Maestroni et al., 2020), cancer treatment (Hojman et al., 2018), the prevention of muscle loss, and reductions in obesity by promoting fat loss (Westcott,

2012). Alongside physical benefits, there is also evidence suggesting that RT can prevent cognitive and neuronal declines (Chow et al., 2021; Landrigan et al., 2020). The physiological explanation for this cognitive improvement considers the reduction in inflammation (Chupel et al., 2017) and the increase in blood flow to the brain (Barnes, 2015; Wilke et al., 2019). Another reason is that RT enhances the availability of various growth factors on the brain, such as insulin-like growth factor-1 (IGF-1) (El-Kotob et al., 2020) and vascular endothelial growth factor (VEGF) (Chow et al., 2021), which regulate exercise-induced angiogenesis and neurogenesis in the hippocampus. RT also increases the production of brain-derived neurotrophic factor (BDNF), which is involved in neuroplasticity and learning (Cotman et al., 2007).

While the existing literature presents encouraging potential regarding the use of RT as a tool to enhance cognitive function, it also reveals specific aspects within the research domain that warrant further exploration. These aspects include populations, programming parameters, and outcome measures. Most studies have concentrated on populations experiencing age-related or disease-related cognitive decline (Chow et al., 2021), but there are relatively few studies that have specifically targeted healthy young adults and demonstrated a positive impact of RT (Brush et al., 2016; Cassilhas et al., 2007). Regarding programming parameters, existing studies have mainly used exercises with machine weights, or a combination of machine and free weights (FWs), revealing improvements in attention, short- and long-term memory (Cassilhas et al., 2007), inhibitory control (Nagamatsu et al., 2012; Wilke et al., 2020), and general cognitive function (Fiatarone Singh et al., 2014); however, very few have explored the exclusive use of free weights (Chow et al., 2021). With regard to outcome measures, they have frequently been associated with executive functions (EFs) like inhibitory control, working memory, attention, and cognitive flexibility (Coetsee & Terblanche, 2017; Hsieh et al., 2016). These measures have been assessed using various tests, such as the Montreal Cognitive Assessment (MoCA) (Smolarek et al., 2016), the Alzheimer's Disease Assessment Scale–Cognitive Subscale (ADASCog) (Fiatarone Singh et al., 2014), the Wechsler Adult Intelligence Scale (WAIS) (Cassilhas et al., 2007), the Toulouse–Pieron's Concentration Attention Test (Cassilhas et al., 2007), the Rey–Osterrieth Complex Figure (ROCF) (Cassilhas et al., 2007), the Stroop test (Coetsee & Terblanche, 2017), or the Modified Sternberg Task (Hsieh et al., 2016).

In this scenario, it may be worthwhile to explore the potential benefits of chronic RT in healthy young adults, considering the use of a methodology that enables the online evaluation of cognitive performance in higher-order cognitive tasks, such as written-text processing, a multifaceted cognitive process that requires sustained attention, working memory, and the integration of information into a coherent mental representation (Kintsch, 1998; Van den Broek & Kendeou, 2022). One of these methodologies is eye tracking (ET), a device that allows for the measurement of eye movement, gaze behavior, and pupil dilation. ET allows for assessing performance based on various saccadic movements during information processing, assuming that longer fixation and regression times indicate higher processing costs. Eye movement research in the context of reading is grounded in the eye–mind hypothesis (Just & Carpenter, 1980), which posits a strong relation between eye gaze and cognitive processes and assumes that longer fixation times indicate a higher cognitive load imposed by a task. Studies employing this methodology have uncovered important aspects of the interaction between vision and cognition in the reading process, such as the amount of information gathered during a single fixation, the time required for different types of information extraction from words, and the challenges readers encounter in comprehending textual material (Hyönä & Kaakinen, 2019).

Given that at present there is no evidence regarding the impact of RT on the cognitive function of healthy young adults engaged in higher-order processing tasks, the aim of this study is to determine the impact of RT with FWs on written-text processing, utilizing eye-tracking technology. Our methodology relies on the well-established eye–mind hypothesis (Hyönä & Kaakinen, 2019), which directly links eye fixations to cognitive processing. Eye movements during reading provide real-time indicators of cognitive processing effort, as fixation duration reflects the cognitive effort required for information processing. Since readers typically fixate on most words in texts (Hyönä & Kaakinen, 2019), these fixation patterns offer reliable data about the cognitive demands of text processing. Thus, rather than measuring post hoc comprehension, our study focused on the more immediate and objective measures of cognitive processing through eye tracking, following current trends in reading cognition research (Conklin et al., 2018).

2. Materials and Methods

2.1. Experimental Approach to the Problem

To assess the impact of an RT intervention on text processing, we conducted a clinical trial employing an experimental design including both experimental and control groups. Participants were randomly assigned to either group using concealed allocation, facilitated by Excel's randomization function. Moreover, the assessor remained blinded throughout the study, ensuring unbiased evaluation. Cognitive function, assessed through ET metrics (including FPRTs and TRTs), was evaluated at the study's outset and again after 10 weeks of the training intervention in both groups. The experimental group engaged in a 10-week program of free-weight strength training, which encompassed push, pull, and leg exercises. In the second week, the experimental group determined their indirect one-repetition maximum (RM) values as part of a technical learning phase for the exercises and underwent a re-evaluation in the tenth week.

2.2. Participants

Twenty-two students from Pontificia Universidad Católica de Valparaíso (PUCV) participated in this study, consisting of seventeen women and five untrained men aged between 19 and 28. All participants were Chilean, native Spanish speakers, and fourth-year students in the Translation and Interpreting program at PUCV. As fourth-year students, all had achieved a certified B2 English proficiency level and corresponding reading skills. Given that they were all in the same year and program, their academic workload and formal reading hours were similar. As exclusion criteria for the subjects, we considered individuals with health issues that could interfere with training, individuals who had participated in any training programs in the six months prior to the study, and those with abnormal or uncorrected vision that could interfere with eye tracking. This information was collected through a registration form completed by the participants themselves (Table A1).

This study is registered at ClinicalTrials.gov (identifier: NCT06662487). Additionally, the study received ethical approval from the Bioethics and Biosafety Committee at PUCV (BIOEPUCV-HB 546-2022, 8th September 2022), and written consent was obtained from each participant. All participants were randomized after signing the consent form to maintain blinding (Smart et al., 2015). Additionally, the evaluator was also blinded to the group to which the participants belonged. This ensured that the study followed a double-blind design (Smart et al., 2015).

This study represents a first step in exploring the impact of free-weight training on written-text processing, a higher-order cognitive measure. As no prior studies directly comparable to ours are available, and no effect sizes were found in the literature, we followed the recommendations of Beck (2013), who discusses sample size requirements for exercise-based interventions, particularly in studies with strength as a primary outcome, and Faul et al. (2009), who provide guidance on selecting the appropriate method for sample size calculation based on the statistical test. Following these recommendations, we used an effect size (f) of 0.80, an alpha value of 0.05, and a statistical power of 0.80, configured for a repeated-measure ANOVA with two groups and two time points for evaluation, based on the characteristics of our data. Based on this calculation, 12 participants were required. While this approach has limitations, we consider it a useful starting point for this study and an initial guide for future research in this emerging area. Figure 1 shows the distribution of the participants and the blinding of the study design.

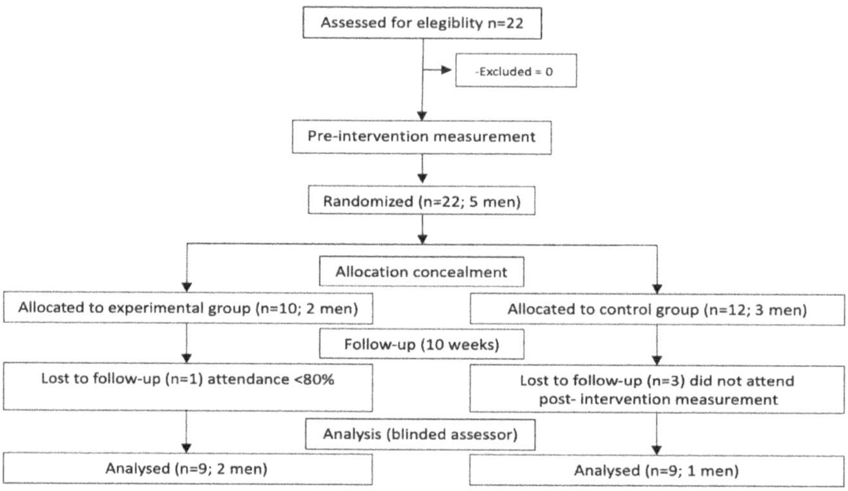

Figure 1. Consort flow chart of the study.

A total of 18 young adult university students completed their participation in this study; overall, significant differences in terms of age were only found between the experimental and control groups. Table 1 shows a description of the baseline values of the participants.

Table 1. Participants' baseline values. *p*-value of *t*-test for independent samples for continuous variables and chi-square for category variables. (cm): centimeters; (kg): kilograms. *p*-value < 0.005 in bold.

Variable	All (n = 18)	Experimental (n = 9)	Control (n = 9)	*p*-Value
Sex				0.555
Women	15 (83.3%)	7 (38.9%)	8 (44.4%)	
Men	3 (16.7%)	2 (11.1%)	1 (5.6%)	
Age (years)	21.0 ± 2.14	20.0 ± 0.86	22.0 ± 2.60	**0.044**
Height (cm)	161 ± 0.07	1.62 ± 0.09	1.59 ± 0.04	0.340
Weight (kg)	58.9 ± 10.3	62.3 ± 12.8	55.4 ± 5.66	0.159
BMI	22.8 ± 3.49	23.6 ± 4.11	22.0 ± 2.75	0.338

2.3. Materials

2.3.1. RT Program

The program lasted 10 weeks, including 2 weeks prior to the intervention, which aimed at learning the exercises and evaluating the maximum strength. The training frequency consisted of 3 sessions per week, with each session comprising 5 exercises (Fiatarone

Singh et al., 2014) organized around push, pull, and leg movement patterns. Free weights targeting large muscle groups were utilized for the exercises (Chow et al., 2021). Specific exercises included bench press, close-grip bench press, military press, dumbbell bench press, dumbbell shoulder press, bar bent-over row, T-grip row, close-grip row, meadow row, dumbbell single-arm row, high-bar squat, deadlift bar, Bulgarian squat, dumbbell lunges, and hip thrust. The program incorporated moderate intensities (Chow et al., 2021), ranging from 60% to 80% of the 1RM (Schoenfeld et al., 2021), with a focus on progressive overload. Additionally, there was an increase in volume from week 5, reaching 2–3 sets per exercise. Table 2 shows a description of the RT program that was implemented with the participants.

Table 2. Resistance training (RT) program.

Exercise	Week 1	Week 2	Week 3	Week 4	Week 5	Week 6	Week 7	Week 8
Day 1								
High-bar squat	Int: 60% RM	Int: 65% RM	Int: 70% RM	Int: 75% RM	Int: 70% RM	Int: 75% RM	Int: 80% RM	
Bar deadlift	Rep: 12	Rep: 10	Rep: 8	Rep: 6	Rep: 8	Rep: 6	Rep: 4	Control
Bulgarian squat	S: 2	S: 2	S: 2	S: 2	S: 3	S: 3	S: 3	1RM
Dumbbell lunge	R: 2′	R: 2′	R: 2′	R: 2′	R: 2′	R: 2′	R: 2′	
Hip thrust								
Day 2								
Bench press	Int: 60% RM	Int: 65% RM	Int: 70% RM	Int: 75% RM	Int: 70% RM	Int: 75% RM	Int: 80% RM	
Close-grip bench press	Rep: 12	Rep: 10	Rep: 8	Rep: 6	Rep: 8	Rep: 6	Rep: 4	Control
Military press	S: 2	S: 2	S: 2	S: 2	S: 3	S: 3	S: 3	1RM
Dumbbell bench press	R: 2′	R: 2′	R: 2′	R: 2′	R: 2′	R: 2′	R: 2′	
Dumbbell shoulder press								
Day 3								
Bent-over bar row	Int: 60% RM	Int: 65% RM	Int: 70% RM	Int: 75% RM	Int: 70% RM	Int: 75% RM	Int: 80% RM	
T-grip row	Rep: 12	Rep: 10	Rep: 8	Rep: 6	Rep: 8	Rep: 6	Rep: 4	Control
Close-grip row	S: 2	S: 2	S: 2	S: 2	S: 3	S: 3	S: 3	1RM
Meadow row	R: 2′	R: 2′	R: 2′	R: 2′	R: 2′	R: 2′	R: 2′	
Dumbbell single-arm row								

Int: intensity; Rep: repetition; S: series; R: rest; and 1RM: one-repetition maximum.

2.3.2. Processing

Six expository texts written in Spanish on general knowledge topics of language, history, and science were utilized (two for each topic). To ensure the suitability of the texts for the readers' characteristics, they were extracted from school textbooks. The length of the texts ranged between 110 and 112 words. Each text had two versions, based on their syntactic complexity (high/low). Syntactic complexity was operationalized based on dependency locality, which refers to the distance between syntactically related elements. In local conditions (low syntactic complexity), syntactically related elements (subject–verb–object) appeared adjacently in the sentence, as in "The student completed the assignment before the end of the semester." In non-local conditions (high syntactic complexity), these elements were separated by an adverbial phrase, increasing processing demands, as in "The student, before the end of the semester, completed the assignment." This manipulation was systematically applied across all experimental texts, maintaining consistent syntactic relationships while varying their locality. The areas of interest where the effects of syntactic complexity were examined correspond to full sentences. This division in terms of syntactic complexity is due to the fact that complex syntactic structures impose greater cognitive demands on the part of the reader, especially in processing and reading comprehension (Kleijn, 2018), which has been supported by different theories (e.g., active filler hypothesis (Clifton & Frazier, 1989); dependency locality theory (Gibson, 1998; Gibson, 2000); and surprisal (Hale, 2001)). Table A2 shows a sample of text in both conditions. Additionally, to ensure that participants were reading attentively, each text was followed by a verification question. Texts were distributed in lists that contained three texts each and were randomly assigned to each participant, ensuring that they did not read the same texts before and after the intervention.

2.4. Procedures

2.4.1. Recording 1RM Procedures

To measure an indirect 1RM, the experimental group performed a general warm-up that included low-intensity aerobic work and joint mobility exercises of the muscle groups involved (Liguori & ACSM, 2021). Subsequently, a specific warm-up was performed with 10 repetitions of the exercises to be performed, with several repetitions in reserve. Finally, the number of repetitions achieved in the last series with the best possible technical execution (less than 10 repetitions) was recorded. The repetitions achieved with each weight were entered into Brzycki's formula to obtain the 1RM for each exercise. These baseline values were then used to schedule the remaining 8 weeks of training, ranging from 60% to 80% intensities. In the tenth week, indirect 1RM measurements were recorded again to assess strength gains.

2.4.2. Training Session Procedures

Each training session was supervised by two certified physical trainers and included both a warm-up and conditioning phase (Liguori & ACSM, 2021). The warm-up consisted of light aerobic activity and joint mobility work aimed at the main muscle groups to be worked on in the session. Three sessions were carried out per week, incorporating different exercises organized by movement patterns. Consequently, each day was composed of five exercises corresponding to specific movement patterns (push–pull and legs).

2.4.3. Eye-Tracking Task

Participants were tested individually and were informed that the task involved reading with eye-tracking equipment. Prior to commencing the experiment, each participant signed an informed consent form. Following this, the eye tracker was set up, and a nine-point calibration screen was carried out for each participant. The participants were instructed to read and comprehend each text, silently, at their own pace, and indicate their readiness to proceed to the (verification) questions by pressing a keyboard button. To prevent the latent learning effect from the first test, before and after the tests the participants read different texts, but care was taken to ensure that they were of the same length in terms of the number of words and syntactic complexity. In addition, in both instances the eye-tracking measurement was performed between 9 and 11 am. Participants were seated 70 cm from the screen, and a chin rest was used to stabilize the head. Eye movements were recorded monocularly by using an EyeLink Portable Duo (SR Research Ltd., Ottawa, ON, Canada) at a sampling frequency of 500 Hz. The stimuli were presented on a 16″ ROG Zephyrus M16 notebook with a refresh rate of 100 Hz and a resolution of 1920 × 1080 pixels.

2.5. Data Preparation

For strength-associated measures, the data preparation procedure encompassed an initial phase of cleaning, involving the identification and removal of outliers. Missing data were managed to ensure the dataset's integrity. Subsequently, variables were transformed, with measurements normalized and adjustments applied to meet the necessary statistical assumptions. The data distribution was checked with the Shapiro–Wilk test and with the visual analysis of residuals and Q-Q plots. Following the recommended procedures for data cleaning in reading experiments with eye tracking (Eskenazi, 2024), fixations shorter than 80 ms were either merged with a nearby fixation (if the distance between the fixations was <1°) or removed from the data. Two eye movement measures associated with particular patterns of text processing were used: FPRTs, which correspond to the sum of the duration of all fixations on the first pass within an area of interest, and TRTs, the sum of the duration of all fixations that fall within an area of interest (Conklin et al., 2018). The reading time measures were skewed and consequently transformed. The best-fitting transformation was selected to normalize the measures; FPRTs were square root transformed and TRTs were logarithmically transformed. A total of 216 eye-tracking observations were analyzed, comprising 108 from before the test, conducted prior to the training, and 108 from after the test, conducted afterward. The dataset included 117 observations from the control group and 99 from the experimental group.

2.6. Data Analysis

To observe the expected differences in reading performance between the experimental and control groups after the intervention period, data were analyzed with linear mixed models (LMMs) by using the lme4 package (Bates et al., 2015) in R statistical software (Version 4.0.1; R Core Team, 2021). Several models were constructed, each focusing on a specific eye movement measure corresponding to individual target sentences within the texts. Variables such as moment (pre vs. post), group (control vs. experimental), and syntactic complexity (low vs. high) were incorporated into these models as fixed effects. Random intercepts for both participants and items were included in the models (Baayen et al., 2008). The models were constructed with a maximal random structure (Barr et al., 2013). In instances where the full random structure led to convergence issues, a top-down trimming process was applied to the random structure, initially considering correlations between factors (Brauer & Curtin, 2018). For two models that failed to converge when using only random intercepts for participants and items, non-significant interaction terms among fixed effects were progressively removed, starting with those associated with the smallest t or z values. Due to difficulties in precisely determining degrees of freedom for statistics estimated by linear mixed models (LMMs), exact p-values or degrees of freedom were not ascertainable. Hence, instead of reporting specific p-values, statistical significance at the 0.05 level was inferred based on $|t \text{ or } z|$ values exceeding 1.96 (Baayen et al., 2008). Given the observed differences between groups and time, subsequent analysis of variance (ANOVA) tests were conducted to confirm that such differences were due to increased strength. This time, strength was categorized into pre–post values in order to compare whether higher levels of post-intervention strength are associated with improvements in eye-tracker measures. The p-value and effect size were computed for each comparison (Hedges' G). The G of edges was used to adjust the effect size to the sample size.

3. Results

To examine the effect of RT on text processing patterns, we conducted a linear mixed model analysis evaluating the effects of group (control vs. experimental), moment (pre vs. post), and syntactic complexity (low vs. high) on FPRTs. The main effect of group was significant, with the experimental group showing higher FPRTs compared to the control group (β = 17.80, SE = 5.38, t = 3.31, CI = [7.19, 28.42]); however, the main effects of moment (β = −1.70, SE = 5.12, t = −0.33, CI = [−11.79, 8.38]) and syntactic complexity (β = 3.12, SE = 5.53, t = 0.56, CI = [−7.79, 14.02]) were not significant. Interaction effects provided further insights into the relationships between factors. The interaction between group and syntactic complexity was significant (β = −27.68, SE = 7.12, t = −3.89, CI = [−41.72, −13.64]), suggesting that the experimental group exhibited reduced FPRTs under high syntactic complexity compared to the control group. Additionally, the three-way interaction among group, moment, and syntactic complexity was significant (β = 25.52, SE = 10.25, t = 2.49, CI = [5.31, 45.73]), highlighting a nuanced relationship among these factors (see Figure 2 and Table A1).

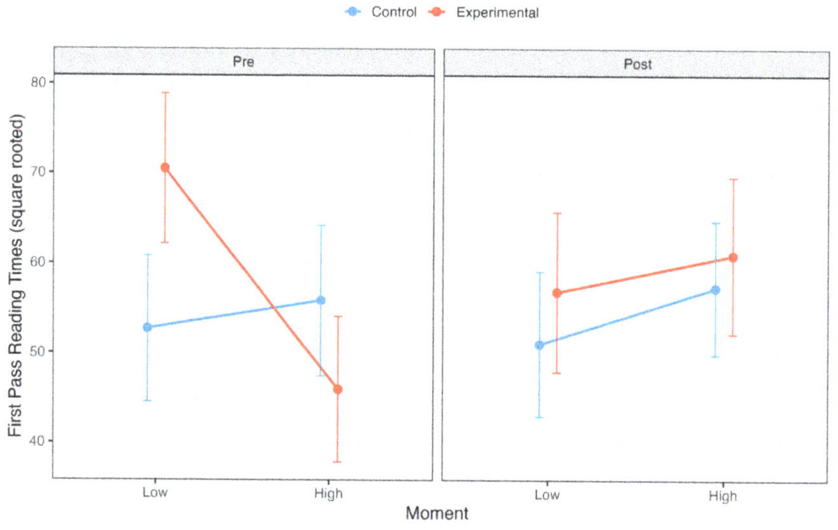

Figure 2. FPRTs (square-rooted) for the control (blue line) and experimental (red line) groups across two moments (pre and post) and two levels of syntactic complexity (low and high). Error bars represent 95% confidence intervals for the mean estimates.

In addition to the linear mixed model analysis, Type III Wald chi-square tests were performed to confirm the significance of main effects and interactions. The main effect of group was significant ($\chi^2(1) = 10.93$, $p < 0.001$), whereas moment ($\chi^2(1) = 0.11$, $p = 0.739$) and syntactic complexity ($\chi^2(1) = 0.32$, $p = 0.573$) were not. A significant interaction was observed between group and syntactic complexity ($\chi^2(1) = 15.10$, $p < 0.001$), and the three-way interaction among group, moment, and syntactic complexity was also significant ($\chi^2(1) = 6.20$, $p = 0.013$).

We conducted a second linear mixed model analysis to assess the effects of group (control vs. experimental), moment (pre vs. post), and syntactic complexity (low vs. high) on TRTs. The main effect of the group was significant, with the experimental group showing longer TRTs compared to the control group (β = 0.41, SE = 0.13, t = 3.14, CI = [0.15, 0.67]). In contrast, the main effects of moment (β = −0.10, SE = 0.12, t = −0.86, CI = [−0.34, 0.13]) and syntactic complexity (β = 0.12, SE = 0.19, t = 0.62, CI = [−0.26, 0.50]) were not significant. Interaction effects provided additional insights into how these factors interacted. A significant group in terms of syntactic complexity interaction (β = −0.36, SE = 0.16, t = −2.26, CI = [−0.68, −0.05]) suggested that participants in the experimental group demonstrated reduced TRTs under conditions of high syntactic complexity compared to the control group; however, the three-way interaction among group, moment, and syntactic complexity was not significant (β = 0.35, SE = 0.23, t = 1.49, CI = [−0.11, 0.81]), indicating no additional complexity in the relationship among these factors (see Figure 3 and Table A3).

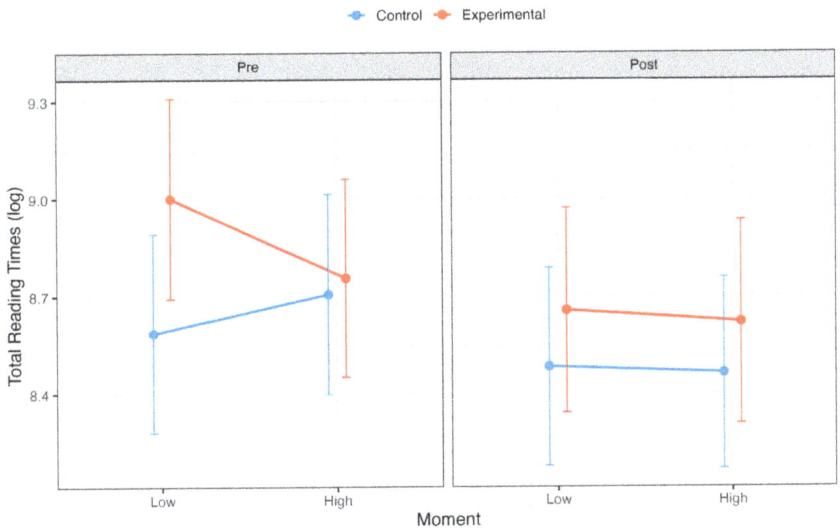

Figure 3. TRTs (log-transformed) for the control (blue line) and experimental (red line) groups across two moments (pre and post) and two levels of syntactic complexity (low and high). Error bars represent 95% confidence intervals for the mean estimates.

To complement the mixed model results, Type III Wald chi-square tests were conducted to evaluate the significance of the main effects and interactions. The main effect of group was confirmed to be significant ($\chi^2(1) = 9.85$, $p = 0.002$), whereas moment ($\chi^2(1) = 0.75$, $p = 0.387$) and syntactic complexity ($\chi^2(1) = 0.38$, $p = 0.538$) were not. The interaction between group and syntactic complexity was significant ($\chi^2(1) = 5.12$, $p = 0.024$), further supporting the reduction in reading times for the experimental group under high syntactic complexity; however, the three-way interaction among group, moment, and syntactic complexity did not reach significance ($\chi^2(1) = 2.22$, $p = 0.137$).

Given our aim to investigate the effect of strength training on participants' cognitive performance, we conducted additional analyses in the experimental group. Specifically, ANOVAs were conducted according to the average strength levels of the pre–post-intervention maximal tests (mean pre = 31.5 ± 9.50; mean post = 42.7 ± 11.1). Figure 4 shows the comparison of the eye-tracker measurements obtained with the pre–post-intervention strength levels globally and separated by syntactic complexity. Overall, in TRTs and FPRTs we found significant differences attributed to the increase in strength after the intervention. In particular, there were significant differences in favor of increased strength in overall reading times and at low syntactic complexity. Similarly, in FPRTs we found significant differences in high and low syntactic complexity.

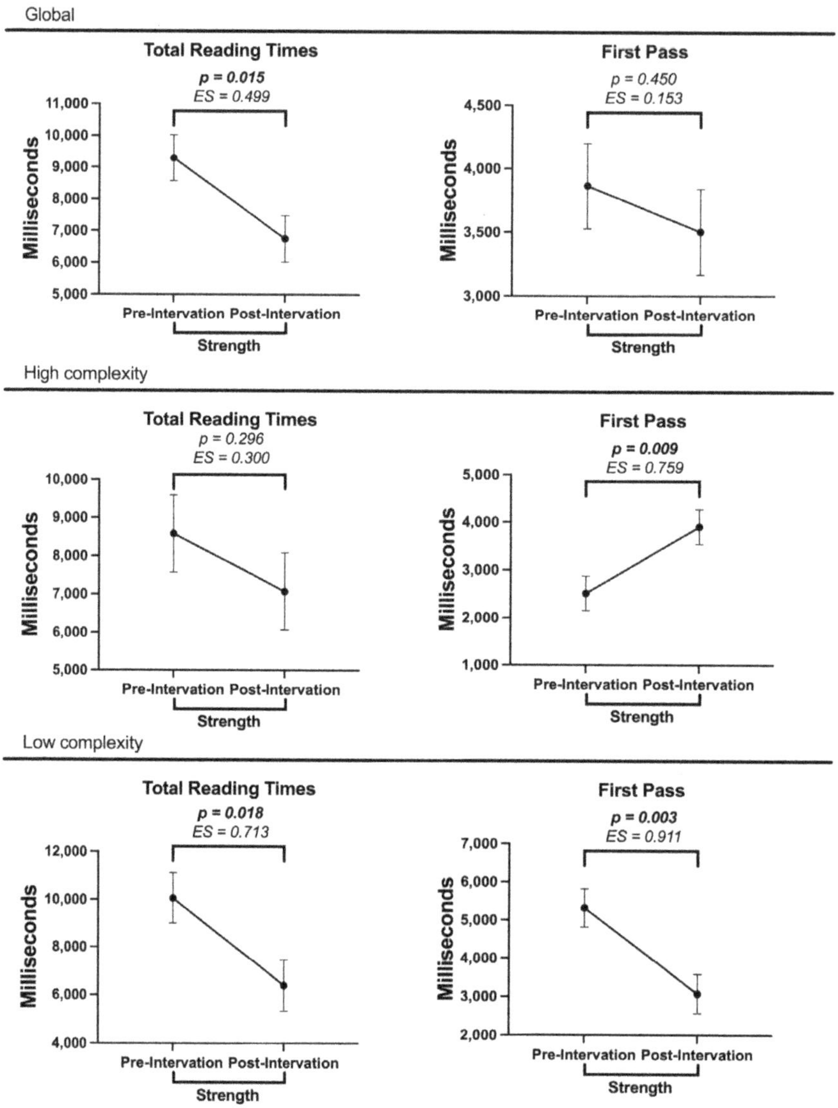

Figure 4. ANOVA results between pre–post-intervention strength values and eye-tracker measurements. In bold, significant *p*-values (<0.05) are presented. ES = effect size (Hedges' g).

4. Discussion

Our analysis of eye movement data revealed distinct patterns of interaction between RT and text processing. For FPRTs, the linear mixed model analysis showed a significant main effect of group, with the experimental group exhibiting higher FPRTs compared to the control group. Neither moment nor syntactic complexity showed significant main effects. The control group maintained consistent processing patterns across pre and post measurements, showing longer processing times in high-complexity conditions compared to low-complexity conditions. Interestingly, the experimental group demonstrated an inverse pattern. Prior to the intervention, they showed longer processing times for low-complexity compared to high-complexity conditions; however, post-intervention, this pattern reversed, with increased processing times in high-complexity conditions. This shift suggests enhanced attention to complex syntactic structures following the training period, particularly as the effect manifests in early processing measures (FPRTs), indicating increased processing focus. Notably, the three-way interaction between group, moment, and syntactic complexity in FPRTs provided compelling evidence of training-induced effects on cognitive processing.

Regarding TRTs, while not showing a significant three-way interaction, the analysis revealed the experimental group's general trend toward decreased reading times between pre and post measurements, particularly in low-complexity conditions, suggesting improved processing efficiency in conditions of no syntactic difficulties, following the resistance training intervention.

Given our aim to investigate the effect of strength training on participants' cognitive performance, we conducted additional analyses in the experimental group. Specifically, ANOVAs were performed according to the average strength levels of the pre–post-intervention maximal tests. The data revealed decreased reading times post-intervention across syntactic complexity levels, suggesting a general improvement in processing efficiency associated with increased strength. Notably, FPRTs increased significantly post-intervention under high-complexity conditions, indicating enhanced attention allocation to complex structures. Additionally, in low-complexity conditions, both TRTs and FPRTs decreased, demonstrating improved processing efficiency for simpler syntactic structures.

One of the findings that encourages further exploration of this relationship is the contrast in FPRTs within the experimental group under the high-syntactic-complexity condition. This condition inherently imposes a higher cognitive load due to the intricate nature of the syntactic structures, which typically require greater cognitive resources and lead to extended reading times compared to low-complexity conditions. While we expected RT to reduce processing times across all complexity conditions, our findings revealed an unexpected pattern: increased early processing times (FPRTs) specifically for high-complexity texts in the experimental group post-intervention. Although seemingly counterintuitive, this pattern likely reflects complex interactions between cognitive mechanisms and training intervention effects.

The increased focus and attentional demands inherent in RT with free weights (FWs) may have selectively enhanced participants' capacity to allocate attentional resources to more-demanding cognitive tasks, such as processing complex syntactic structures. This improvement in high-complexity conditions during early processing suggests that the intervention might have facilitated more effective engagement with intricate structures, potentially mediated by enhancements in EFs like working memory and attentional control. These findings align with prior research indicating that strength training can improve selective attention and inhibitory control, both of which are critical for managing cognitive load during challenging tasks (Nagamatsu et al., 2012; Wilke et al., 2020). The unexpected augmentation of fixation durations following the intervention challenges the expectation of decreased reading times, presumed due to the cognitive advantages gained from strength training. This deviation prompts a critical inquiry into the relationship between strength training and cognitive function, particularly their intricate interplay with discourse processing.

The effects of apparently increased focus on processing texts with high syntactic complexity, reflected in the increased FPRTs found in both the mixed model analysis and ANOVA, along with the decreased reading times of the experimental group in TRTs and FPRTs for texts with low syntactic complexity (ANOVA), could be explained by the positive effects of RT on EFs. Regarding the relationship between RT and EFs, Nagamatsu et al. (2012)'s study, conducted on older adults, showed positive effects on inhibitory control as a result of a chronic RT intervention; however, our results may be more directly associated with findings in young adults, such as those obtained by Wilke et al. (2020), which showed that improvements in inhibitory control are more pronounced in RT with FWs interventions compared to machine-based RT, with the caveat that this study measured acute effects. Another EFs that improves as a result of RT, which could potentially enhance reading and writing performance, is memory, as evidenced by Cassilhas et al. (2007), who reported significant improvements in both short-term and long-term memory in healthy older adults. The same was observed in the study by Nagamatsu et al. (2012), which revealed enhancements in associative memory.

Regarding the relationship between EFs and reading performance, it has been observed (Orozco & Pineda, 2019; Nouwens et al., 2021) that EFs plays a fundamental role in processing and comprehending written texts by orchestrating specific processes, such as information integration, retrieval from the mental lexicon, strategy utilization, and simultaneous engagement in multiple reading tasks. Studies have also demonstrated that updating working memory aids processing by maintaining the activation of relevant information during reading; inhibitory control aids processing by restricting the activation of irrelevant text details and preventing unwanted memory intrusions; and shifting attention supports processing by integrating different types of information and focusing on various text features and situational contexts (Gazzaniga et al., 2014). Therefore, the potential impact of RT on EFs could explain why participants in the experimental group demonstrate greater efficiency as readers, particularly in terms of TRTs and FPRTs under low-syntactic-complexity conditions (ANOVA). Thus, the potential impact of RT on EFs could be related to improvements in reading ability.

Another possible explanation for the positive effects of increased focus on texts with high syntactic complexity and shorter TRTs and FPRTs in low syntactic complexity as a result of RT with FWs refers to the fact that this type of intervention selectively improves aspects of cognition due to differential demands. For example, individuals participating in RT with FWs need to pay constant attention to what they are doing to avoid injuring themselves or those around them. In this sense, these periods of vigilance could act as a form of attentional training and explain why there was an improvement in performance on EFs tests, as many of these tasks assess an individual's ability to attend to specific stimuli (Landrigan et al., 2020). Although significant differences between the effects of RT with FWs and machine-based lifting on athletic performance and muscular architecture have not been found (Hernández-Belmonte et al., 2023), it is evident that attentional demands differ between these two modalities of RT. Exercises using machines isolate muscles and follow predetermined paths; in contrast, FW exercises used in our intervention require individuals to pay attention to a greater number of variables related to coordination and balance to maintain control over the movement of the weights (Liguori & ACSM, 2021). These more complex execution conditions could impact attentional improvement, potentially explaining the effects of the intervention on reading times; however, it would be interesting to evaluate this hypothesis in future studies that directly compare these two forms of RT.

From another perspective, it is plausible that the effects of RT on EFs, and consequently its positive impact on text processing, may be mediated by neurobiological mechanisms unrelated to the specific cognitive demands of the exercise. These mechanisms include increases in molecules such as brain-derived neurotrophic factor (BDNF) and proteins like insulin-like growth factor 1 (IGF-1), which are associated with exercise's effects on learning and depression, as well as the combined action of IGF-1 and vascular endothelial growth factor (VEGF) on hippocampal angiogenesis and neurogenesis (Brush et al., 2016). These molecular changes are thought to induce structural alterations, such as increased gray and white matter volume (Landrigan et al., 2020), which could also lead to cognitive changes, such as an impact on learning and memory, considering the highly plastic nature of the hippocampus (Cassilhas et al., 2016). It is also worth noting that exercise acts as a stimulus for new blood vessel formation, and increased cerebral blood flow correlates with cognitive enhancement (Cassilhas et al., 2007; Bullitt et al., 2009). In fact, Bullitt et al. (2009) demonstrated that physical fitness was positively associated with the number of small blood vessels in older individuals undergoing magnetic resonance angiography, indicating angiogenesis, a phenomenon not observed in sedentary individuals.

It is also possible that neurobiological and cognitive mechanisms work synergistically. For instance, neurobiological mechanisms may enhance neuroplasticity (Cotman et al., 2007; Cassilhas et al., 2016), which in turn might have an impact on EFs that are more consistently engaged during resistance exercises, such as attention (Landrigan et al., 2020), inhibitory control (Orozco & Pineda, 2019), and associative memory (Nagamatsu et al., 2012); however, clear connections between exercise, neurobiological mechanisms, and cognitive changes still need further investigation.

5. Conclusions

RT with FWs showed interesting results, considering the increase in FPRTs for texts with high complexity, which suggests a greater capacity for focus on more intricate texts and a decrease in TRTs and FPRTs for texts with lower complexity. These effects found in the various analyses could be explained by the proven improvements that RT generates in EFs, such as attention, inhibitory control, and memory. These, in turn, relate to improvements in text processing. From a neurobiological perspective, these positive effects could also stem from molecular adaptations and neuroplasticity, elements that should be considered and measured in future research efforts. It can be concluded that RT with free weights has a positive effect on text processing; however, it would be interesting to make a direct comparison between RT with machines to glimpse possible differences. Additionally, there is a small number of studies on the effects of RT on cognitive function in young adults, and even fewer on variables measured through eye tracking. Therefore, this scarcity opens a line of research in which these variables could even intersect with EFs, thus understanding RT as an enhancer of cognitive and academic performance in this age group.

Author Contributions: Conceptualization, C.M.-N. and R.I.-O.; methodology, C.M.-N., R.I.-O., A.S.-C., R.F.F., R.M.-F. and C.C.-R.; formal analysis, C.C.-R. and R.M.-F.; investigation, C.M.-N., R.I.-O., A.S.-C., R.F.F., R.M.-F. and C.C.-R.; data curation, C.C.-R.; writing—original draft, C.M.-N., R.I.-O., C.C.-R., A.S.-C. and R.M.-F.; writing—review and editing, C.M.-N., R.I.-O., A.S.-C., C.C.-R. and R.M.-F. All authors have read and agreed to the published version of the manuscript.

Funding: This work was supported by grants awarded by the National Research and Development Agency (ANID-CHILE). The second, third, and fourth authors were funded by the Fondecyt Regular Project 1240550. Finally, the second and third authors acknowledge the support of the Millennium Science Initiative through an ANID-MILENIO NCS2022_026 grant.

Institutional Review Board Statement: This study received ethical approval from the Bioethics and Biosafety Committee at PUCV (BIOEPUCV-HB 546-2022, on 8 September 2022).

Informed Consent Statement: All participants gave written informed consent.

Data Availability Statement: The data presented in this study are available upon request from the corresponding author.

Acknowledgments: The authors wish to express their gratitude to the administration of the GAF Gymnasium of Physical Conditioning of the School of Physical Education, PUCV, for providing their facilities for the application of the intervention.

Conflicts of Interest: There is no financial support or other benefit from commercial sources for the work reported on in the manuscript. There are no financial interests that any of the authors may have that could create a potential conflict of interest or the appearance of a conflict of interest with regard to the work.

Appendix A

Table A1. Linear mixed model to evaluate the effects of group (control vs. experimental), moment (pre vs. post), and syntactic complexity (low vs. high) on first-pass reading times.

	First-Pass Reading Times				
Predictor	**Estimate**	**Std. Error**	**CI**	**Statistic**	***p***
(Intercept)	52.73	4.12	44.59–60.86	12.78	<0.001
Group [experimental]	17.80	5.38	7.19–28.42	3.31	0.001
Moment [post]	−1.70	5.12	−11.79–8.38	−0.33	0.739
sdl [high]	3.12	5.53	−7.79–14.02	0.56	0.574
Group [experimental] × moment [post]	−12.01	7.77	−27.34–3.31	−1.55	0.124
Group [experimental] × sdl [high]	−27.68	7.12	−41.72–−13.64	−3.89	<0.001
Moment [post] × sdl [high]	3.13	6.94	−10.56–16.82	0.45	0.653
(Group [experimental] × moment [post]) × sdl [high]	25.52	10.25	5.31–45.73	2.49	0.014

Table A2. Fragment of text in two conditions of syntactic complexity.

Low Syntactic Complexity	High Syntactic Complexity
With an immense variety of visual techniques, technology increased the spectacularity of images on the big screen.	Technology, with an immense variety of visual techniques, increased the spectacularity of images on the big screen.

Table A3. Linear mixed model to evaluate the effects of group (control vs. experimental), moment (pre vs. post), and syntactic complexity (low vs. high) on total reading times.

	Total Reading Times				
Predictors	**Estimates**	**Std. Error**	**CI**	**Statistic**	***p***
(Intercept)	8.59	0.15	8.28–8.89	55.45	<0.001
Group [experimental]	0.41	0.13	0.15–0.67	3.14	0.002
Moment [post]	−0.10	0.12	−0.34–0.13	−0.86	0.388
sdl [high]	0.12	0.19	−0.26–0.50	0.62	0.539
Group [experimental] × moment [post]	−0.24	0.19	−0.61–0.13	−1.28	0.202
Group [experimental] × sdl [high]	−0.36	0.16	−0.68–−0.05	−2.26	0.025
Moment [post] × sdl [high]	−0.14	0.16	−0.45–0.17	−0.88	0.381
(Group [experimental] × moment [post]) × sdl [high]	0.35	0.23	−0.11–0.81	1.49	0.138

References

Baayen, R. H., Davidson, D. J., & Bates, D. M. (2008). Mixed-effects modeling with crossed random effects for subjects and items. *Journal of Memory and Language, 59*(4), 390–412. [CrossRef]

Barnes, J. N. (2015). Exercise, cognitive function, and aging. *Advances in Physiology Education, 39*, 55–62. [CrossRef] [PubMed]

Barr, D. J., Levy, R., Scheepers, C., & Tily, H. J. (2013). Random effects structure for confirmatory hypothesis testing: Keep it maximal. *Journal of Memory and Language, 68*(3), 255–278. [CrossRef]

Bates, D., Mächler, M., Bolker, B. M., & Walker, S. C. (2015). Fitting linear mixed-effects models using lme4. *Journal of Statistical Software, 67*(1), 48. [CrossRef]

Beck, T. W. (2013). The importance of a priori sample size estimation in strength and conditioning research. *The Journal of Strength and Conditioning Research, 27*(8), 2323–2337. Available online: www.nsca.com (accessed on 15 September 2024). [CrossRef]

Brauer, M., & Curtin, J. J. (2018). Linear mixed-effects models and the analysis of nonindependent data: A unified framework to analyze categorical and continuous independent variables that vary within-subjects and/or within-items. *Psychological Methods, 23*(3), 389–411. [CrossRef] [PubMed]

Brush, C. J., Olson, R. L., Ehmann, P. J., Osovsky, S., & Alderman, B. L. (2016). Dose-Response and time course effects of acute resistance exercise on executive function. *Journal of Sport and Exercise Psychology, 38*(4), 396–408. [CrossRef]

Bullitt, E., Rahman, F. N., Smith, J. K., Kim, E., Zeng, D., Katz, L. M., & Marks, B. L. (2009). The effect of exercise on the cerebral vasculature of healthy aged subjects as visualized by MR angiography. *American Journal of Neuroradiology, 30*(10), 1857–1863. [CrossRef] [PubMed]

Cassilhas, R. C., Tufik, S., & De Mello, M. T. (2016). Physical exercise, neuroplasticity, spatial learning and memory. *Cellular and Molecular Life Sciences, 73*(5), 975–983. [CrossRef]

Cassilhas, R. C., Viana, V. A. R., Grassmann, V., Santos, R. T., Santos, R. F., Tufik, S., & Mello, M. T. (2007). The impact of resistance exercise on the cognitive function of the elderly. *Medicine and Science in Sports and Exercise, 39*(8), 1401–1407. [CrossRef] [PubMed]

Chow, Z. S., Moreland, A. T., Macpherson, H., & Teo, W. P. (2021). The central mechanisms of resistance training and its effects on cognitive function. *Sports Medicine, 51*(12), 2483–2506. [CrossRef] [PubMed]

Chupel, M. U., Direito, F., Furtado, G. E., Minuzzi, L. G., Pedrosa, F. M., Colado, J. C., Ferreira, J. P., Filaire, E., & Teixeira, A. M. (2017). Strength training decreases inflammation and increases cognition and physical fitness in older women with cognitive impairment. *Frontiers in Physiology, 8*, 377. [CrossRef] [PubMed]

Clifton, C., & Frazier, L. (1989). Comprehending sentences with long-distance dependencies. In G. N. Carlson, & M. K. Tanenhaus (Eds.), *Linguistic structure in language processing. Studies in theoretical psycholinguistics* (Vol. 7, pp. 273–317). Springer.

Coetsee, C., & Terblanche, E. (2017). The effect of three different exercise training modalities on cognitive and physical function in a healthy older population. *European Review of Aging and Physical Activity, 14*(1), 1–10. [CrossRef] [PubMed]

Colberg, S. R., Sigal, R. J., Yardley, J. E., Riddell, M. C., Dunstan, D. W., Dempsey, P. C., Horton, E. S., Castorino, K., & Tate, D. F. (2016). Physical activity/exercise and diabetes: A position statement of the American Diabetes Association. *Diabetes Care, 39*(11), 2065–2079. [CrossRef]

Conklin, K., Pellicer-Sánchez, A., & Carrol, G. (2018). *Eye-tracking. A guide for applied linguistics research*. Cambridge University Press. [CrossRef]

Cormie, P., McGuigan, M., & Newton, R. (2011). Developing maximal neuromuscular power. Part 2—Training considerations for improving maximal power production. *Sports Medicine, 41*(2), 125–146. [CrossRef] [PubMed]

Cotman, C. W., Berchtold, N. C., & Christie, L. A. (2007). Exercise builds brain health: Key roles of growth factor cascades and inflammation. *Trends in Neurosciences, 30*(9), 464–472. [CrossRef] [PubMed]

El-Kotob, R., Ponzano, M., Chaput, J.-P., Janssen, I., Kho, M. E., Poitras, V. J., Ross, R., Ross-White, A., Saunders, T. J., & Giangregorio, L. M. (2020). Resistance training and health in adults: An overview of systematic reviews. *Applied Physiology, Nutrition, and Metabolism, 45*(10)(Suppl. S2), S165–S179. [CrossRef] [PubMed]

Eskenazi, M. A. (2024). Best practices for cleaning eye movement data in reading research. *Behavior Research Methods, 56*(3), 2083–2093. [CrossRef] [PubMed]

Faul, F., Edgar, E., Buchner, A., & Lang, A.-G. (2009). Statistical power analyses using G*Power 3.1: Tests for correlation and regression analyses. *Behavior Research Methods, 41*(4), 1149–1160. [CrossRef] [PubMed]

Fiatarone Singh, M. A., Gates, N., Saigal, N., Wilson, G. C., Meiklejohn, J., Brodaty, H., Wen, W., Singh, N., Baune, B. T., Suo, C., Baker, M. K., Foroughi, N., Wang, Y., Sachdev, P. S., & Valenzuela, M. (2014). The Study of Mental and Resistance Training (SMART) study-resistance training and/or cognitive training in mild cognitive impairment: A randomized, double-blind, double-sham controlled trial. *Journal of the American Medical Directors Association, 15*(12), 873–880. [CrossRef] [PubMed]

Gazzaniga, M. S., Ivry, R. B., & Mangun, G. R. (2014). *Cognitive neuroscience. The biology of the mind* (A. Javsicas, & S. Snavely, Eds.; 4th ed.). W. W. Norton.

Gibson, E. (1998). Linguistic complexity: Locality of syntactic dependencies. *Cognition, 68*(1), 1–76. [CrossRef]

Gibson, E. (2000). The dependency locality theory: A distance-based theory of linguistic complexity. In Y. Miyashita, A. Marantz, & W. O'Neil (Eds.), *Image, language, brain* (pp. 96–126). MIT Press.

Guizelini, P. C., de Aguiar, R. A., Denadai, B. S., Caputo, F., & Greco, C. C. (2018). Effect of resistance training on muscle strength and rate of force development in healthy older adults: A systematic review and meta-analysis. *Experimental Gerontology, 102*, 51–58. [CrossRef] [PubMed]

Hale, J. (2001, June 1–7). *A probabilistic Earley parser as a psycholinguistic model*. Second Meeting of the North American Chapter of the Association for Computational Linguistics (pp. 1–8), Stroudsburg, PA, USA.

Hernández-Belmonte, A., Buendía-Romero, Á., Franco-López, F., Martínez-Cava, A., & Pallarés, J. G. (2023). Adaptations in athletic performance and muscle architecture are not meaningfully conditioned by training free-weight versus machine-based exercises: Challenging a traditional assumption using the velocity-based method. *Scandinavian Journal of Medicine and Science in Sports, 33*(10), 1948–1957. [CrossRef] [PubMed]

Hillman, C., Erickson, K., & Kramer, A. (2008). Be smart, exercise your heart: Exercise effects on brain and cognition. *Nature Reviews | Neuroscience, 9*, 58–65. [CrossRef] [PubMed]

Hojman, P., Gehl, J., Christensen, J. F., & Pedersen, B. K. (2018). Molecular mechanisms linking exercise to cancer prevention and treatment. *Cell Metabolism, 27*(1), 10–21. [CrossRef]

Hsieh, S. S., Chang, Y. K., Hung, T. M., & Fang, C. L. (2016). The effects of acute resistance exercise on young and older males' working memory. *Psychology of Sport and Exercise, 22*, 286–293. [CrossRef]

Hyönä, J., & Kaakinen, J. K. (2019). Eye Movements During Reading. In C. Klein, & U. Ettinger (Eds.), *Eye movement research an introduction to its scientific foundations and applications* (pp. 239–274). Springer International Publishing. [CrossRef]

Just, M. A., & Carpenter, P. A. (1980). A theory of reading: From eye fixations to comprehension. *Psychological Review, 87*(4), 329–354. [CrossRef]

Kintsch, W. (1998). *Comprehension: A paradigm for cognition*. Cambridge University Press.

Kleijn, S. (2018). *Clozing in on readability: How linguistic features affect and predict text comprehension and on-line processing*. Universiteit Utrecht.

Landrigan, J. F., Bell, T., Crowe, M., Clay, O. J., & Mirman, D. (2020). Lifting cognition: A meta-analysis of effects of resistance exercise on cognition. *Psychological Research, 84*(5), 1167–1183. [CrossRef]

Liguori, G., & ACSM. (2021). *ACSM's guidelines for exercise testing and prescription* (11th ed.). ACSM.

Maestroni, L., Read, P., Bishop, C., Papadopoulos, K., Suchomel, T. J., Comfort, P., & Turner, A. (2020). The benefits of strength training on musculoskeletal system health: Practical applications for interdisciplinary care. *Sports Medicine, 50*(8), 1431–1450. [CrossRef]

Mateluna-Núñez, C., Zavala-Crichton, J. P., Monsalves-Álvarez, M., Olivares-Arancibia, J., & Yáñez-Sepúlveda, R. (2022). Effects of weightlifting training on sprint, jump and change of direction performance in athletes: A systematic review. *Retos, 44*, 464–476. [CrossRef]

Nagamatsu, L. S., Handy, T. C., Hsu, C. L., Voss, M., & Liu-Ambrose, T. (2012). Resistance training promotes cognitive and functional brain plasticity in seniors with probable mild cognitive impairment. *Archives of Internal Medicine, 172*(8), 666–668. [CrossRef]

Nouwens, S., Groen, M. A., Kleemans, T., & Verhoeven, L. (2021). How executive functions contribute to reading comprehension. *British Journal of Educational Psychology, 91*(1), 169–192. [CrossRef]

Orozco, P., & Pineda, E. (2019). Evaluación de funciones ejecutivas en estudiantes de primer año universitario que presentan bajo y alto rendimiento en comunicación escrita y producción lectora. *Revista de Lenguas Modernas, 31*, 219–249. [CrossRef]

Ratamess, N. A., Alvar, B. A., Evetoch, T. K., Housh, T. J., Kibler, B. W., Kraemer, W. J., & Triplett, T. N. (2009). Progression models in resistance training for healthy adults. *Medicine and Science in Sports and Exercise, 41*(3), 687–708. [CrossRef]

R Core Team. (2021). *R: A language and environment for statistical computing*. R Foundation for Statistical Computing. Available online: https://www.R-project.org/ (accessed on 1 September 2024).

Schoenfeld, B. J., Grgic, J., Van Every, D. W., & Plotkin, D. L. (2021). Loading recommendations for muscle strength, hypertrophy, and local endurance: A re-examination of the repetition continuum. *Sports, 9*(2), 32. [CrossRef] [PubMed]

Smart, N. A., Waldron, M., Ismail, H., Giallauria, F., Vigorito, C., Cornelissen, V., & Dieberg, G. (2015). Validation of a new tool for the assessment of study quality and reporting in exercise training studies: TESTEX. *International Journal of Evidence-Based Healthcare, 13*(1), 9–18. [CrossRef] [PubMed]

Smolarek, A. de C., Boiko Ferreira, L. H., Gomes Mascarenhas, L. P., McAnulty, S. R., Varela, K. D., Dangui, M. C., de Barros, M. P., Utter, A. C., & Souza-Junior, T. P. (2016). The effects of strength training on cognitive performance in elderly women. *Clinical Interventions in Aging, 11*, 749–754. [CrossRef]

Van den Broek, P., & Kendeou, P. (2022). Reading Comprehension I. In *The science of reading* (pp. 239–260). Wiley. [CrossRef]

Westcott, W. L. (2012). Resistance training is medicine: Effects of strength training on health. *Current Sports Medicine Reports, 11*(4), 209–216. [CrossRef] [PubMed]

Wilke, J., Giesche, F., Klier, K., Vogt, L., Herrmann, E., & Banzer, W. (2019). Acute effects of resistance exercise on cognitive function in healthy adults: A systematic review with multilevel meta-analysis. *Sports Medicine*, *49*(6), 905–916. [CrossRef]

Wilke, J., Stricker, V., & Usedly, S. (2020). Free-weight resistance exercise is more effective in enhancing inhibitory control than machine-based training: A randomized, controlled trial. *Brain Sciences*, *10*(10), 702. [CrossRef] [PubMed]

behavioral sciences

MDPI

Article

Influence of Gender, Parental Control, Academic Performance and Physical Activity Level on the Characteristics of Video Game Use and Associated Psychosocial Problems in Adolescents

Manuel Isorna-Folgar [1], Adrián Mateo-Orcajada [2,*], José María Failde-Garrido [1], María Dolores Dapia-Conde [1] and Raquel Vaquero-Cristóbal [3]

1 Departamento de Análisis e Intervención Psicosocioeducativa, Facultad de Educación y Trabajo Social, Universidad de Vigo, 32004 Ourense, Spain; isorna.catoira@uvigo.es (M.I.-F.); jfailde@uvigo.es (J.M.F.-G.); ddapia@uvigo.es (M.D.D.-C.)

2 Facultad de Deporte, UCAM Universidad Católica de Murcia, 30107 Murcia, Spain

3 Research Group Movement Sciences and Sport (MS&SPORT), Department of Physical Activity and Sport, Faculty of Sport Sciences, University of Murcia, 30100 Murcia, Spain; raquel.vaquero@um.es

* Correspondence: amateo5@ucam.edu

Abstract: Previous research has determined the relevance of video games for adolescents; however, it has not been possible to establish differences in usage patterns and certain psychological variables according to gender, parental control, academic performance, physical activity level or game type, nor the relationship between these variables. For this reason, the aims of this research were as follows: (a) to determine the differences in the gaming variables and the psychological variables related to video games according to gender, the closest environment, the academic performance and the level of physical activity; and (b) to determine which gaming variables and behavioral variables influence psychological variables in adolescents. A descriptive, cross-sectional study was carried out involving 2567 adolescents (mean age: 15.06 ± 2.81 years). Participants completed eight questionnaires on the study variables. The results showed that males play more video games than females; play different types of games and on different platforms; and have more psychological problems than females. Having separated parents and having a greater parental control over video game use is associated with more time spent playing video games. Poorer academic performance is related to playing shooters and open-world games, as well as with a more negative emotional response. However, playing shooters and sport and racing games is related to more physical activity. Playing online games, mainly with strangers, is related to higher addictive and problematic uses. In addition, the times of use during the week and on weekends, especially on weekends, stand out as predictors of most psychological variables related to video games in adolescents. This study provides further scientific evidence on the role of certain behavioral and game-related variables in the relationship between video games and well-being. In addition, it highlights the importance of analyzing in the future those video game players who do not have a problematic or addictive use of video games, but who play frequently without any associated problem. From a practical perspective, the promotion of video games with social and cooperative components, or those that promote physical activity, could be related to social and psychological benefits.

Keywords: academic performance; adolescents; gender; parents; physical activity level; psychology; video games; youth

1. Introduction

Video games have established themselves as one of the main forms of modern leisure, especially for the adolescent population aged between 12 and 17, with between 70 and 75% playing some form of video game on different platforms, reflecting the deep integration of video games into the daily lives of this population [1]. Previous studies have showed that excessive and addictive use can have negative consequences on the mental health and well-being of adolescents [2]. Furthermore, more time spent playing video games could decrease the time spent studying, which could affect the academic performance of adolescents who spend more time playing games [3]. Also, more time spent playing video games could decrease the time available for other activities, such as physical activity, increasing the risk of physical inactivity, sedentary lifestyles and overweight, obesity or other metabolic disorders [4]. However, in both cases, there are studies with contradictory results [5,6], which calls for further research in this area. In addition, it should be noted that patterns of play may depend on different socio-demographic variables [7,8]; but knowledge about the interaction of these variables is still lacking.

1.1. Psychological Theories Explaining the Impact of Video Games on Adolescents

It is important to be aware that the psychological attraction generated by video games is largely due to the ability to satisfy the basic psychological needs for competence, autonomy and social relatedness [9]. This is based on self-determination theory (SDT), which provides a useful theoretical framework for analyzing how satisfying the basic psychological needs increases the intrinsic motivation for a task [10]. As a consequence, there is an increase in the priority the person gives to that activity and the time he/she devotes to it, a phenomenon that has been widely demonstrated to occur during the use of video games [11].

Therefore, in order to understand the reasons why adolescents are attracted to video games, it is necessary to consider the motivations underlying gaming behavior. This approach explains how video games can provide an environment where players experience a sense of achievement, control over their decisions and social relatedness, satisfying these basic needs. This helps to understand why video games not only motivate players to continue playing but can also lead to an improvement in psychological well-being by satisfying these needs [12]. In contrast, a mismatch in this motivation can lead to problematic patterns of use [13,14].

On the other hand, it is worth noting that, according to the uses and gratification theory, players' motivation is key because it influences their behavioral intentions and subsequent choices [15]. Based on this, this theory points out that users structure their behavior in response to their specific needs to obtain gratification [16]. Previous research supported by this theory in the field of video games has shown that personal and social integrative benefits are the best predictors for engagement and purchase [17]. Similarly, enjoyment and achievement are the factors that influence the intention to continue playing, so that hedonic and utilitarian gratifications are the ones that most affect this intention [18,19].

1.2. Impact of Video Games on Academic Performance and Its Relationship with Psychological Variables in Adolescents

In the academic field, it has been observed that addictive video game use decreases academic performance [3], but may also produce benefits in cognition and learning in adolescents [6]. Moreover, previous research has shown that playing video games alone has a minimal influence on academic performance, with other factors such as cyberbullying or exposure to violent content being the most relevant [20]. The timing of play seems to be relevant in this respect, as playing before school seems to produce negative effects on academic performance, but not playing after school [21]. Therefore, there is a lack of studies on the time spent, type and/or form of play that might affect the alterations produced in academic performance [22].

In the psychological field, the importance of academic performance lies in the fact that it is fundamental to adolescent health, as it is related to health-risk behaviors [23], mental health [24] and even sleep quality [25]. However, no previous research has explored the relationship of other psychological variables that could be affected using video games with academic performance, and this is important given the interdependence between these three factors and their influence on future health.

1.3. Impact of Video Games on Physical Activity Level and Its Relationship with Psychological Variables on Adolescents

As for the level of physical activity, previous research has shown a positive association between video game consumption and unhealthy lifestyle habits, such as a decrease in physical activity [26]. It is true that this association occurs mainly with non-active video games, as they keep the player seated for several hours, such as first-person shooter video games [5]. However, it has been observed that ball sport simulators (e.g., FIFA or NBA), even though they are non-active video games, are associated with increased physical activity and participation in sports clubs [5]. Therefore, the results are not consistent across studies, because, although the use of video games is related to higher body mass and lower self-reported general health status, there is not enough evidence to associate gaming time with a worse level of physical activity [27].

In the psychological domain, adolescents with a higher level of physical activity show a better psychological state [28], but the impact of video game use on the psychological health of adolescents by level of physical activity is unclear. In this respect, the use of active video games seems to increase self-esteem and mental health in general, as well as social well-being, but it seems that the type of video game played is very influential [29,30]. On the other hand, sedentary video game use is associated with poorer well-being, isolation and aggressive behavior [31]. Therefore, playing video games and not being physically active seems to be detrimental to psychological health [32], but it is unknown what happens in adolescents who play video games and are also physically active, as well as the psychological variables related to video games that are affected. For this reason, it is important to know which gaming-related variables and which psychological variables in relation to video games, beyond problematic or addictive use, are related to the level of physical activity of the players.

1.4. Socio-Demographic Factors That Determine the Use of Video Games and Their Impact on Psychological Variables in Adolescents

Although motivations and intention to play are important, during adolescence, differences are observed in gaming tendencies (time, type, form of play) and in the psychological impact of video game use as a function of socio-demographic variables such as gender [33] and the influence of the closest environment [34].

1.4.1. Gender as a Determinant of the Use of Video Games and Its Impact on Psychological Variables in Adolescents

According to the gaming variables, it has been observed that the motivations and patterns of play between males and females are different, with males tending to play competitive video games, while females prefer social, non-competitive and simulation video games [7]. In addition, males tend to play for longer periods of time than females, perhaps because they report more fun and motivation [35]. Therefore, differences exist in terms of frequency and type of gaming, although both genders are susceptible to problematic gaming disorders [36].

In the psychological domain, differences are observed between male and female adolescents, with females tending to show greater psychological distress, anxiety and depression compared to males [37]. Furthermore, differences are observed in coping strategies, as well as in the effect of anxiety and stress on well-being and self-esteem in males and females [38]. The higher use of video games leads to males exhibiting more problematic use of video games compared to females (5.8% vs. 3.0%), thus classifying them as more addicted [39]. However, there are no major gender differences in this respect, and in both male and female adolescents, problematic video game use leads to negative psychological consequences such as increased aggression, depression or isolation [40]. Therefore, although gender differences in problematic use are observed, both males and females are affected, but it is not known whether other psychological variables related to video game use differ according to gender.

1.4.2. Closest Environment as a Determinant of the Use of Video Games and Their Impact on Psychological Variables in Adolescents

The closest environment is another aspect of great relevance in the use of video games by adolescents [34]. Regarding the gaming variables, previous studies have shown that adolescents with balanced parental control and a stable family environment develop healthier gaming habits, while those with less supervision or from dysfunctional families are more likely to develop behaviors related to excessive video game use [41]. It is also worth noting that adolescents who play with siblings or friends mitigate the likelihood of excessive play time [8]. However, there are few studies that analyze the relationship between time of use, type of video game or platform used in relation to the closest environment.

According to the psychological domain, it has been observed that high levels of parental involvement, characterized by support and communication, are associated with better well-being, higher self-esteem and lower anxiety [42]; however, dysfunctional families can lead to increased psychological distress [42]. On the video games field, differences are also found in the psychological sphere, highlighting the fact that playing social games, in which one interacts with others, has more positive effects on well-being and is associated with less problematic game use compared to non-social games played individually [43–45]. Similarly, online versus offline play report differences, with online players showing more addictive behaviors, maladaptive cognitions, interpersonal conflicts and social isolation [46,47]. In addition, the people with whom adolescents play video games are also relevant, as playing cooperatively with friends shows more positive and prosocial behavior during play, increasing friendship quality [48], while playing with parents decreases internalizing and aggressive behaviors [49]. The fact that the social environment and the form of play influence psychological variables, such as prosocial behaviors and emotional satisfaction [50], increases the need to look more closely at aspects that may be related to the psychological state of adolescents.

1.5. Research Gap, Research Questions and Aims

Based on the previous scientific literature on the use of video games, it can be observed that the variables of the game itself (time, type of game, type of platform used) differ according to aspects such as gender and closest environment, and these variables may in turn be related to other aspects such as academic performance and level of physical activity [19,24,35,42]. More specifically, previous research has shown that problematic and/or addictive use of video games differs according to gender and closest environment; and this in turn may influence the academic performance and level of physical activity, with the consequences this has for the mental health of adolescents [23,29,38,47]. However, most adolescents do not engage in problematic or addictive video game use, as they play video games in a normal and appropriate way. Furthermore, information on this subject is scarce, with small samples of participants, and it is not possible to draw a reliable conclusion about the relationship between these variables. Therefore, more research is needed to analyze differences in gaming habits as a function of gender, closest environment, physical activity and academic performance with a large sample of adolescents to analyze the interaction between these factors.

On the other hand, psychological variables could also be affected by the use of video games and the variables of the game itself (time, type of game, type of platform used) [31,51]. However, the previous literature has not focused on these variables as influencing the psychological state, focusing on other factors such as gender, immediate environment, academic performance or physical activity [23,28,37,42]. Although there are studies that have analyzed how each of these variables separately affect the psychological state of adolescents, there are no known studies that have analyzed the interaction between these factors and the gaming variables, or the specific weight that these factors could have on mental health of this population. The relevance of this calls for research that focuses on the existing differences in psychological variables related to video games, considering socio-demographic variables such as gender or closest environment, and other behavioral parameters, such as academic performance and level of physical activity.

Based on the previous scientific literature, the research questions posed for this manuscript are (a) 'What factors related to video game use (playing time, game type, platform) show differences according to gender, closest environment, academic performance and physical activity level in adolescents?' (b) 'How are psychological variables related with video game use (playing time, game type, platform), gender, closest environment, academic performance and physical activity level in adolescents?' and (c) What are the factors that determine psychological variables in adolescents: gaming habits, physical activity or academic performance?' The following aims are proposed to provide answers: (a) to determine the differences in the gaming variables and the psychological variables related to video games according to gender, the closest environment, the academic performance and the level of physical activity; and (b) to determine which gaming variables and behavioral variables influence psychological variables in adolescents.

2. Materials and Methods

2.1. Design

The present study was descriptive and cross-sectional and was conducted to measure the level of problematic video game use, addiction, motives for video game use, mood repair, passion scale and emotional and behavioral symptoms of playing video games in the adolescent population. The study design and protocol followed the STROBE statement [52]. All participants and their legal guardians signed the informed consent before the start of the research. They were informed of the procedure to be followed, as well as the questionnaires to be completed, and the aim pursued with the research. They were also informed that the treatment of the data would be completely anonymous and that only the project researchers would use the data. Participation was voluntary, and the participants were informed that they could withdraw from the research at any time, which would result in the elimination of their data collected up to that point. The ethics committee of the University of Vigo approved the research design (code: CE-DCEC-UVIGO-2022-10-04-5109) following the guidelines of the Declaration of Helsinki and the World Medical Association code.

2.2. Participants

The sample size was calculated using the EpiCalc package included in the Rstudio 3.15.0 statistical software (Rstudio Inc., Boston, MA, USA), following the methodology of previous research [53,54]. The standard deviation (SD) of previous research that analyzed the motives for playing video games in the adolescent population was used (SD = 1.07) [55]. Thus, for an estimated error (d) of 0.05, for a 95% confidence interval, the minimum sample needed to carry out the research was 1794 adolescents.

According to data from the Department of Education of the Xunta de Galicia, there are a total of 89,000 students enrolled in Compulsory Secondary Education, Baccalaureate or Vocational Training. From this population, a sample was selected by means of two-stage sampling, by conglomerates, for the selection of the first-level units. In this way, a total of 24 centers were randomly selected, both public and private/subsidized, urban and rural, and belonging to the four Galician provinces, considering the existing quotas at the population level.

All the participants met the following inclusion criteria: (a) age between 12 and 18 years old; (b) attending compulsory secondary education, baccalaureate and vocational studies; (c) volunteering to participate in the research; and (d) not presenting any incapacitating disease that prevented the completion of the questionnaires. The exclusion criteria were (a) not completing all the questionnaires in their entirety.

A total of 2567 adolescents met the inclusion criteria for this research. After applying the exclusion criteria, a total of 2513 adolescents (mean age: 15.06 $\pm$ 2.81 years old) ultimately participated in the research. The socio-demographic characteristics of the sample can be found in Table 1.

Table 1. Socio-demographic characteristics of the study sample.

Variable		n (%)
Gender		
	Males	1286 (51.20)
	Females	1227 (48.80)
Educational level		
	Compulsory secondary education	1825 (72.60)
	Baccalaureate	450 (17.90)
	Vocational studies	238 (9.50)
Physical activity level		
	None	540 (21.50)
	Light	1028 (41.00)
	Moderate	799 (31.70)
	Vigorous	146 (5.80)
Cohabitation of parents		
	Yes	1848 (74.20)
	No	665 (52.80)
Parental control of video game use		
	Never	1483 (60.00)
	Sometimes	340 (12.70)
	Always	690 (27.20)
Academic performance		
	F	183 (6.80)
	D	426 (16.80)
	C	585 (23.40)
	B	906 (36.70)
	A	413 (16.30)
Gaming form		
	Online with friends	1393 (61.50)
	Offline alone	615 (24.40)
	Online with unknown	290 (8.90)
	Offline with friends	215 (5.20)
Type of video game played		
	Sport and racing	1025 (17.08)
	Shooting	979 (16.32)
	Open-world	967 (16.12)
	Strategy	796 (13.27)
	Simulation	584 (9.73)
	Casual	550 (9.17)
	Role Playing	503 (8.38)
	Platforms	346 (5.77)
	Fighting	250 (4.17)

2.3. Instruments

2.3.1. Socio-Demographic, Play Habits and Academic Performance Variables

A socio-demographic ad hoc questionnaire was used, in which participants were asked about their age, gender, academic performance, parental control of time spent playing video games, cohabitation of parents, type of video games played, platform most used to play video games, time spent playing during weekdays and weekends, usual way of playing and money spent per month on video games. This questionnaire was based on the one used in previous research [56].

2.3.2. Physical Activity

A question was used to determine whether adolescents participated in leisure time physical sports activities or not. Those who indicated participation in physical sporting activities answered five additional questions that allowed for the calculation of the index or pattern of the amount of habitual physical sporting activity (Finnish physical sporting activity index) [57,58], which referred to frequency, duration, intensity and participation in organized sports and sports competitions. The Spanish version was used, which was previously validated in previous research, and had an adequate validity and reliability (Cronbach's alpha = 0.81) [35,36]. The responses were recoded into three categories so that all of them had a similar weight for calculating the index or pattern. The resulting value ranged from 5 to 15. Lower scores are characteristic of less active individuals, while higher scores are indicative of more active individuals. In accordance with previous research conducted with adolescents using this same measurement [59,60], and to better represent the patterns of physical activity, the score was used to classify participants into vigorous, moderate, light and insufficient activity.

2.3.3. Experiences Related to Video Games

The questionnaire of experiences related to video games (CERV) was used [37]. This questionnaire was designed in Spanish, and is composed of 17 items that allow the detection of problematic use of video games in adolescents. It is completed with a Likert scale ranging from 1 to 4 points (1: never/almost never; 4: almost always). This questionnaire has two dimensions (dependence/evasion and negative consequences). The dependence/evasion range is between 8 and 32 points, while negative consequences range between 9 and 36 points. Both dimensions showed a Cronbach's alpha above 0.86, making this a valid and reliable instrument for use in adolescents. The total score is obtained by adding the scores of the items belonging to the two subscales. A higher score in the dimensions of the questionnaire, or in the final score, indicates a worse experience of video game use [61].

2.3.4. Video Game Addiction

The video game addiction scale for adolescents (GASA) was used [38,39]. This instrument consists of seven items corresponding to a structure of 7 dimensions (salience, tolerance, emotion, relapse, abstinence, conflict and problems) that are grouped into a higher order factor: addiction. It is completed with a 5-point Likert scale (1: never; 5: very often). The final score ranges between 7 and 35 points. A higher score on this questionnaire indicates greater addiction. The reliability of this instrument is high, with a Cronbach's alpha of 0.86. This instrument was designed and validated by Lemmens et al. [62] and was translated and validated in Spanish by Lloret et al. [63].

2.3.5. Motives for Playing Video Games

The motives for playing video games were analyzed using the video gaming motives questionnaire (VMQ), which was initially designed in Spanish [40]. This questionnaire allows for the analysis of eight motives for playing video games: recreation, competition, cognitive development, coping, social interaction, violent reward, customization and fantasy. It is composed of 24 items, 3 per motive analyzed. It is answered with a 5-point Likert scale (0: do not agree at all; 4: strongly agree). The final score for each motive ranges from 0 to 12 points. A higher score indicates that the motive for gaming is greater. This instrument is considered valid and reliable to determine the motives for playing video games as the Cronbach's alpha for each of the motives ranges between 0.76 and 0.93 [64].

2.3.6. Emotional States

The Trait Meta-Mood Scale (TMMS-24) was used to assess emotional states. The 24-item version was adapted and validated in Spanish [65]. The scale contains three key dimensions: attention to feelings, emotional clarity and repair and regulation of mood, and it is evaluated with a five-point Likert-type scale (1 = strongly disagree, 5 = strongly agree). For this research, the repair dimension that refers to the subject's belief about his/her capacity to interrupt and regulate negative moods and prolong positive ones was measured. This subscale consists of 8 items, with the final score ranging from 8 to 40 points. A higher score indicates a greater ability to interrupt and regulate negative moods. Fernández-Berrocal et al. [65] obtained Cronbach alphas of 0.86 for this dimension of the scale.

2.3.7. Passion Towards the Activity

The passion scale [66] was used to measure passion towards the activity, using the validated Spanish version for this purpose [67]. This scale is divided into two subscales (harmonious and obsessive) composed of six items each. Thus, the scale is composed of a total of twelve items that are rated using a 7-point Likert scale (1: total disagreement; 7: total agreement). Both subscales ranged from 6 to 42 points. A higher score refers to a greater passion demonstrated for the activity. For the Spanish version, the validity and reliability of the scale as a whole, as well as of the subscales, demonstrated an adequate validity and internal consistency (0.81) [67].

2.3.8. Social, Emotional and Behavioral Problems

The strengths and difficulties questionnaire (SDQ) [68] was used in its Spanish version [45]. It is composed of 25 items distributed into five subscales (5 items per subscale): emotional symptoms, conduct problems, hyperactivity, peer problems and prosocial behavior. A 3-point Likert scale (0: not true; 2: certainly true) was used for its completion. The score for each subscale ranges from 0 to 10 points. Higher scores show greater social, emotional and behavioral problems. The Spanish version has been validated, and it has a high reliability (0.88) [69].

2.4. Procedure

The data were collected in the classrooms of the respective education centers, with prior authorization from the management teams in groups of 15 to 25 individuals. For the completion of the questionnaires, the adolescents remained in a room isolated from the noise of the educational center, avoiding any distractions that could alter the answers. A questionnaire was administered, which each participant had to complete individually. The data collection was overseen by researchers, who had experience in conducting this type of task. The researchers present during the completion of the questionnaires did not condition the participants' responses. The researchers simply limited themselves to resolving any doubts that might arise during this process, as well as reminding the participants that there were no good or bad answers to the questionnaires. The order in which the questionnaires were completed was randomized for each participant. The time required to complete the questionnaire ranged from 30 to 45 min.

2.5. Data Analysis

The Kolmogorov–Smirnov test was used to analyze the normality of the data, as well as skewness and kurtosis. Because the variables included followed a normal distribution, parametric tests were used for their analysis. First, the chi-square test ($\chi 2$) was performed to find the differences in the gaming variables as a function of the gender, closest environment, academic performance and physical activity level. Percentages and frequencies were used for the analysis. The corrected standardized residuals were used to determine significance, establishing ± 1.96 as the reference value. Cramer's V was used for the post hoc comparison of the 2×2 tables, and the Contingency Coefficient was used in the $2 \times n$ tables, to obtain the statistical value. The maximum expected value was 0.707; $r < 0.3$ indicated a low association; $r < 0.5$ indicated a moderate association; and $r > 0.5$ indicated a high association [70]. Two Student's *t*-tests were performed to analyze the differences in the psychological variables according to gender (male-female), and the cohabitation of the parents (together-not together). Cohen's d was calculated to determine the effect size in these cases, being small when $d < 0.2$; moderate when $d < 0.8$; and large when $d > 0.8$ [71]. Four ANOVAs were performed to find differences in the psychological variables as a function of parental control of time use, academic performance, level of physical activity and form of play. The Bonferroni post hoc test was used to determine between which groups the differences were significant. Partial eta squared ($\eta p2$) was used to calculate effect size, being small: ES ≥ 0.10; moderate: ES ≥ 0.30; large: ES ≥ 1.2; or very large: ES ≥ 2.0 [72]. Pearson's correlation coefficient was used to determine the relationship between psychological variables, game-related variables and behavior-related variables. For the variables that were statistically significant in the Pearson correlation, a linear regression analysis was performed to predict the variables that could most influence the psychological state of the players. Statistical significance was established for a value of $p < 0.05$. The statistical analyses were performed with the SPSS v.25.0 statistical package (SPSS Inc. IL).

3. Results

3.1. Differences in the Gaming Variables According to Gender, Closest Environment, Academic Performance and Physical Activity Level

Table 2 shows the differences in the type of video games used, the platform of habitual use, the time spent during the week and during the weekend, the way of playing and the money spent per month on video games between males and females. The results show differences in the type of video game played ($p < 0.001$–0.017) and the platform used ($p < 0.001$). Regarding playing habits, males spent more time playing ($p < 0.001$), preferred to play online with friends ($p < 0.001$) and spent more money playing ($p < 0.001$) than females.

Table 2. Differences in the type of video games played, platform used, time spent, form of play and money spent per month according to gender.

Variable	Male (n = 1286)	Female (n = 1227)	Adj. Res	χ2; p	CC
Type of video game					
Platforms	168 (13.06)	176 (14.34)	1.7/−1.7	2.75; 0.098	0.034
Fighting	172 (13.37)	78 (6.36)	−5.3/5.3	28.10; <0.001	0.108
Strategy	487 (37.87)	298 (24.29)	−6.2/6.2	38.60; <0.001	0.126
Role Playing	295 (22.94)	207 (16.87)	−2.9/2.9	8.70; 0.003	0.060
Shooting	785 (61.04)	186 (15.16)	−22.6/22.6	508.82; <0.001	0.419
Casual	161 (12.52)	386 (31.46)	12.6/−12.6	158.51; <0.001	0.249
Simulation	282 (21.93)	297 (24.21)	2.4/−2.4	5.68; 0.017	0.049
Open-world	625 (48.60)	334 (27.22)	−9.8/9.8	95.67; <0.001	0.196
Sport and racing	637 (49.53)	379 (30.89)	−8.2/8.2	68.27; <0.001	0.166
Platform					
Sony	663 (51.56)	215 (17.52)	−17.1/17.1	290.78; <0.001	0.328
PC	489 (38.02)	253 (20.62)	−8.7/8.7	76.40; <0.001	0.175
Nintendo	182 (14.15)	320 (26.08)	8.2/−8.2	68.00; <0.001	0.166
Tablet	79 (6.14)	163 (13.28)	6.6/−6.6	42.90; <0.001	0.132
Mobile Phone	504 (39.19)	714 (58.19)	11.1/−11.1	123.82; <0.001	0.221
Time spent (Weekdays)					
None	418 (32.50)	659 (53.71)	−11.1/11.1	220.32; <0.001	0.288
1 h	189 (14.70)	213 (17.36)	−1.9/1.9		
2 h	127 (9.88)	115 (9.37)	0.4/−0.4		
3 h	119 (9.25)	75 (6.11)	2.9/−2.9		
4 h	88 (6.84)	38 (3.10)	4.3/−4.3		
5 h	81 (6.30)	29 (2.36)	4.8/−4.8		
6 h	79 (6.14)	29 (2.36)	4.6/−4.6		
More than 6 h	148 (11.51)	26 (2.12)	9.2/−9.2		
Time spent (Weekend)					
None	100 (7.78)	492 (40.10)	−19.4/19.4	637.13; <0.001	0.454
1 h	104 (8.09)	204 (16.63)	−6.7/6.7		
2 h	117 (9.10)	153 (12.47)	−2.9/2.9		
3 h	152 (11.82)	98 (7.99)	3.1/−3.1		
4 h	137 (10.65)	80 (6.52)	3.6/−3.6		
5 h	131 (10.19)	56 (4.56)	5.3/−5.3		
6 h	151 (11.74)	41 (3.34)	7.8/−7.8		
More than 6 h	372 (28.93)	63 (5.13)	12.3/−12.3		

Table 2. *Cont.*

Variable	Male (n = 1286)	Female (n = 1227)	Adj. Res	χ2; p	CC
Game form					
Online with friends	849 (66.02)	431 (35.13)	12.1/−12.1	159.86; <0.001	0.267
Online with unknown	91 (7.08)	94 (7.66)	−1.9/1.9		
Offline alone	174 (13.53)	330 (26.89)	−11.1/11.1		
Offline with friends	49 (3.81)	60 (4.89)	−2.4/2.4		
Money spent (month)					
None	857 (66.64)	1046 (85.25)	−14.3/14.3	205.06; <0.001	0.281
<EUR 10	240 (18.66)	61 (4.97)	10.2/−10.2		
EUR 11–20	76 (5.91)	14 (1.14)	6.2/−6.2		
EUR 21–30	37 (2.88)	8 (0.65)	4.0/−4.0		
EUR 31–50	18 (1.40)	4 (0.33)	2.8/−2.8		
EUR 51–100	10 (0.78)	1 (0.08)	2.6/−2.6		
>EUR 100	12 (0.93)	2 (0.16)	2.5/−2.5		

CC: Contingency Coefficient.

Differences according to whether the parents live together or separately are found in Table 3. Differences were found on the platform used (p = 0.020–0.001). The differences were significant in the time spent during the week, with the adolescents whose parents lived together playing less video games (p = 0.002).

As for parental control of time spent, the differences found are shown in Table 4. Differences were found in the type of game (p < 0.001–0.007) and the platform used (p < 0.001–0.019). The adolescents they monitored always played more on weekdays (p < 0.001) and weekends (p < 0.001); played online with friends (p < 0.001); and spent more money per month playing (p < 0.001).

Table 3. Differences in the type of video games played, platform used, time spent, form of play and money spent per month according to the cohabitation of parents.

Variable	Yes (n = 1848)	No (n = 665)	Adj. Res	χ2; p	CC
Type of video game					
Platforms	250 (13.53)	93 (13.98)	0.5/−0.5	0.47; p = 0.793	0.014
Fighting	171 (9.25)	76 (11.43)	1.8/−1.8	3.49; p = 0.175	0.038
Strategy	562 (30.41)	226 (33.98)	2.1/−2.1	5.16; p = 0.076	0.046
Role playing	369 (19.97)	133 (20.00)	0.3/−0.3	0.38; p = 0.826	0.013
Shooting	721 (39.02)	250 (37.59)	−0.1/0.1	1.49; p = 0.475	0.025
Casual	392 (21.21)	154 (23.16)	1.3/−1.3	2.17; p = 0.339	0.030
Simulation	432 (23.38)	148 (22.26)	−0.3/0.3	0.39; p = 0.822	0.013
Open-world	730 (39.50)	229 (34.44)	−1.8/1.8	4.96; p = 0.084	0.046
Sport and racing	764 (41.34)	252 (37.89)	−1.1/1.1	2.87; p = 0.579	0.035
Platform					
Sony	641 (34.69)	238 (35.79)	1.1/−1.1	2.85; p = 0.241	0.034
PC	565 (30.57)	178 (26.77)	−1.4/1.4	2.37; p = 0.306	0.031
Nintendo	368 (19.91)	137 (20.60)	0.7/−0.7	0.81; p = 0.667	0.018
Tablet	199 (10.77)	45 (6.77)	−2.8/2.8	7.87; p = 0.020	0.057
Mobile Phone	863 (46.70)	352 (52.93)	3.5/−3.5	13.55; p = 0.001	0.075
Time spent (Weekdays)					
None	829 (44.86)	245 (36.84)	3.0/−3.0	36.62; p = 0.002	0.123
1 h	294 (15.91)	108 (16.24)	−0.5/0.5		
2 h	167 (9.04)	73 (10.98)	−1.7/1.7		
3 h	152 (8.23)	43 (6.47)	1.2/−1.2		
4 h	91 (4.92)	34 (5.11)	−0.5/0.5		
5 h	73 (3.95)	35 (5.26)	−1.6/1.6		
6 h	69 (3.73)	39 (5.86)	−2.5/2.5		
More than 6 h	128 (6.93)	49 (7.37)	−0.6/0.6		

Table 3. *Cont.*

Variable	Yes (n = 1848)	No (n = 665)	Adj. Res	χ2; p	CC
Time spent (Weekend)					
None	439 (23.76)	147 (22.11)	0.4/−0.4	17.12; p = 0.378	0.084
1 h	217 (11.74)	89 (13.38)	−1.5/1.5		
2 h	202 (10.93)	65 (9.77)	0.5/−0.5		
3 h	188 (10.17)	61 (9.17)	0.3/−0.3		
4 h	173 (9.36)	47 (7.07)	1.5/−1.5		
5 h	145 (7.85)	42 (6.32)	1.0/−1.0		
6 h	142 (7.68)	51 (7.67)	−0.2/0.2		
More than 6 h	312 (16.88)	125 (18.80)	−1.6/1.6		
Game form					
Online with friends	958 (51.84)	319 (47.97)	1.3/−1.3	9.82; p = 0.278	0.069
Online with unknown	122 (6.60)	61 (9.17)	−2.4/2.4		
Offline alone	381 (20.62)	128 (19.25)	0.5/−0.5		
Offline with friends	78 (4.22)	31 (4.66)	−0.6/0.6		
Money spent (month)					
None	1409 (76.24)	482 (72.48)	1.0/−1.0	4.08; p = 0.982	0.041
<EUR 10	218 (11.80)	86 (12.93)	−1.0/1.0		
EUR 11–20	69 (3.73)	20 (3.01)	0.8/−0.8		
EUR 21–30	32 (1.73)	16 (2.41)	−1.2/1.2		
EUR 31–50	17 (0.92)	5 (0.75)	0.3/−0.3		
EUR 51–100	8 (0.43)	3 (0.45)	−0.1/0.1		
>EUR 100	9 (0.49)	5 (0.75)	−0.8/0.8		

CC: Contingency Coefficient.

Table 4. Differences in the type of video games played, platform used, time spent, form of play and money spent per month according to the parental control.

Variable	Never (n = 1483)	Sometimes (n = 340)	Always (n = 690)	Adj. Res	χ2; p	CC
Type of video game						
Platforms	185 (12.47)	36 (10.59)	118 (17.10)	−3.1/3.1	9.92; p = 0.007	0.065
Fighting	133 (8.97)	33 (9.71)	78 (11.30)	1.6/−1.6	2.68; p = 0.262	0.034
Strategy	446 (30.07)	99 (29.12)	241 (34.93)	−2.1/2.1	4.56; p = 0.102	0.044
Role Playing	281 (18.95)	60 (17.65)	156 (22.61)	−2.0/2.0	3.85; p = 0.146	0.041
Shooting	502 (33.85)	140 (41.18)	330 (47.83)	6.2/−6.2	40.65; p < 0.001	0.132
Casual	355 (23.94)	59 (17.35)	127 (18.41)	−3.5/3.5	12.27; p = 0.002	0.072
Simulation	339 (22.86)	68 (20.00)	164 (23.77)	0.9/−0.9	0.87; p = 0.647	0.019
Open-world	530 (35.74)	124 (36.47)	308 (44.64)	−3.7/3.7	14.53; p < 0.001	0.079
Sport and racing	558 (37.63)	156 (45.88)	295 (42.75)	3.2/−3.2	14.58; p = 0.006	0.079
Platform						
Sony	454 (30.61)	135 (39.71)	287 (41.59)	−5.7/5.7	32.58; p < 0.001	0.118
PC	441 (29.74)	76 (22.35)	224 (32.46)	−2.6/2.6	7.92; p = 0.019	0.058
Nintendo	288 (19.42)	68 (20.00)	145 (21.01)	0.9/−0.9	0.90; p = 0.639	0.019
Tablet	120 (8.09)	55 (16.18)	65 (9.42)	4.9/−4.9	25.05; p < 0.001	0.103
Mobile Phone	726 (48.95)	151 (44.41)	310 (44.93)	−1.9/1.9	3.88; p = 0.144	0.041
Time spent (Weekdays)						
None	669 (45.11)	153 (45.00)	198 (28.70)	−7.3/7.3	95.60; p < 0.001	0.200
1 h	230 (15.51)	60 (17.65)	113 (16.38)	−1.4/1.4		
2 h	134 (9.04)	35 (10.29)	74 (10.72)	−1.7/1.7		
3 h	102 (6.88)	19 (5.59)	72 (10.43)	3.3/−3.3		
4 h	63 (4.25)	6 (1.76)	55 (7.97)	−2.7/2.7		
5 h	68 (4.59)	9 (2.65)	33 (4.78)	−1.5/1.5		
6 h	50 (3.37)	10 (2.94)	49 (7.10)	4.3/−4.3		
More than 6 h	113 (7.62)	12 (3.53)	49 (7.10)	−2.4/2.4		

Table 4. *Cont.*

Variable	Never (n = 1483)	Sometimes (n = 340)	Always (n = 690)	Adj. Res	χ2; p	CC
Time spent (Weekend)						
None	455 (30.68)	39 (11.47)	38 (5.51)	13.6/−13.6		
1 h	211 (14.23)	45 (13.24)	50 (7.25)	−4.5/4.5		
2 h	156 (10.52)	49 (14.41)	65 (9.42)	2.8/−2.8		
3 h	109 (7.35)	46 (13.53)	95 (13.77)	−5.6/5.6	289.07; p < 0.001	0.347
4 h	100 (6.74)	35 (10.29)	83 (12.03)	−4.5/4.5		
5 h	78 (5.26)	31 (9.12)	77 (11.16)	−5.3/5.3		
6 h	101 (6.81)	15 (4.41)	77 (11.16)	4.2/−4.2		
More than 6 h	230 (15.51)	45 (13.24)	165 (23.91)	4.1/−4.1		
Game form						
Online with friends	673 (45.38)	189 (55.59)	415 (60.14)	−5.0/5.0		
Online with unknown	115 (7.75)	21 (6.18)	49 (7.10)	1.5/−1.5	28.97; p < 0.001	0.118
Offline alone	326 (21.98)	62 (18.24)	121 (17.54)	3.7/−3.7		
Offline with friends	70 (4.72)	17 (5.00)	20 (2.90)	−2.4/2.4		
Money spent (month)						
None	1163 (78.42)	244 (71.76)	467 (67.68)	−5.5/5.5		
<EUR 10	149 (10.05)	38 (11.18)	113 (16.38)	4.2/−4.2		
EUR 11–20	39 (2.63)	10 (2.94)	40 (5.80)	3.8/−3.8		
EUR 21–30	26 (1.75)	5 (1.47)	18 (2.61)	1.5/−1.5	40.83; p < 0.001	0.132
EUR 31–50	14 (0.94)	3 (0.88)	5 (0.72)	−0.5/0.5		
EUR 51–100	8 (0.54)	0 (0.00)	3 (0.43)	−1.3/1.3		
>EUR 100	9 (0.61)	2 (0.59)	3 (0.43)	−0.5/0.5		

CC: Contingency Coefficient.

Table 5 shows the differences according to academic performance. There were differences in the type of video game (p < 0.001–0.003) and the platforms used (p < 0.001). Adolescents with lower academic performance spent more hours gaming on weekdays (p < 0.001) and weekends (p < 0.001) and spent more money playing (p < 0.001). Adolescents with a higher academic performance played more offline (p < 0.001).

Table 5. Differences in the type of video games played, platform used, time spent, form of play and money spent per month according to academic performance.

Variable	F (n = 183)	D (n = 426)	C (n = 585)	B (n = 906)	A (n = 413)	Adj. Res	χ2; p	CC
Type of video game								
Platforms	29 (15.85)	62 (14.55)	86 (14.70)	101 (11.15)	61 (14.77)	2.9/−2.9	8.86; p = 0.065	0.062
Fighting	22 (12.02)	44 (10.33)	61 (10.43)	87 (9.60)	27 (6.54)	2.1/−2.1	6.43; p = 0.169	0.053
Strategy	46 (25.14)	122 (28.64)	184 (31.45)	298 (32.89)	114 (27.60)	1.6/−1.6	4.30; p = 0.367	0.043
Role Playing	35 (19.13)	93 (21.83)	114 (19.49)	160 (17.66)	79 (19.13)	−1.8/1.8	4.59; p = 0.332	0.044
Shooting	74 (40.44)	174 (40.85)	238 (40.68)	351 (38.74)	105 (25.42)	−5.2/5.2	29.95; p < 0.001	0.114
Casual	25 (13.66)	76 (17.84)	114 (19.49)	222 (24.50)	100 (24.21)	2.5/−2.5	16.71; p = 0.002	0.085
Simulation	49 (26.78)	94 (22.07)	128 (21.88)	198 (21.85)	88 (21.31)	2.0/−2.0	4.05; p = 0.399	0.042
Open-world	71 (38.80)	176 (41.31)	207 (35.38)	355 (39.18)	120 (29.06)	3.3/−3.3	16.40; p = 0.003	0.084
Sport and racing	72 (39.34)	166 (38.97)	237 (40.51)	353 (38.96)	156 (37.77)	−0.8;0.8	4.25; p = 0.834	0.043
Platform								
Sony	73 (38.89)	160 (37.56)	207 (35.38)	299 (33.00)	100 (24.21)	3.9/−3.9	24.30; p < 0.001	0.102
PC	65 (35.52)	118 (27.70)	182 (31.11)	258 (28.48)	83 (20.10)	−3.6/3.6	21.34; p < 0.001	0.095
Nintendo	21 (11.48)	67 (15.73)	94 (16.07)	206 (22.74)	89 (21.55)	3.2/−3.2	21.22; p < 0.001	0.095
Tablet	12 (6.56)	23 (5.40)	45 (7.69)	99 (10.93)	54 (13.08)	3.2/−3.2	21.33; p < 0.001	0.096
Mobile Phone	90 (49.18)	198 (46.48)	277 (47.35)	418 (46.14)	188 (45.52)	1.6/−1.6	3.24; p = 0.519	0.037

Table 5. *Cont.*

Variable	F (*n* = 183)	D (*n* = 426)	C (*n* = 585)	B (*n* = 906)	A (*n* = 413)	Adj. Res	χ2; *p*	CC
Time of use (Weekdays)								
None	52 (28.42)	170 (39.91)	219 (37.44)	401 (44.26)	206 (49.88)	4.3/−4.3	75.55; *p* < 0.001	0.179
1 h	24 (13.11)	52 (12.21)	103 (17.61)	156 (17.22)	53 (12.83)	−2.0/2.0		
2 h	18 (9.84)	38 (8.92)	55 (9.40)	80 (8.83)	41 (9.93)	−0.8/0.8		
3 h	13 (7.10)	31 (7.28)	53 (9.06)	67 (7.40)	22 (5.33)	1.7/−1.7		
4 h	9 (4.92)	27 (6.34)	23 (3.93)	51 (5.63)	10 (2.42)	−2.4/2.4		
5 h	8 (4.37)	25 (5.87)	30 (5.13)	29 (3.20)	17 (4.12)	−2.2/2.2		
6 h	13 (7.10)	22 (5.16)	25 (4.27)	34 (3.75)	12 (2.91)	2.3/−2.3		
More than 6 h	22 (12.02)	34 (7.98)	46 (7.86)	48 (5.30)	18 (4.36)	3.4/−3.4		
Time of use (Weekend)								
None	34 (18.58)	80 (18.78)	128 (21.88)	194 (21.41)	136 (32.93)	5.8/−5.8	91.28; *p* < 0.001	0.196
1 h	10 (5.46)	33 (7.75)	77 (13.16)	136 (15.01)	43 (10.41)	3.4/−3.4		
2 h	22 (12.02)	45 (10.56)	57 (9.74)	94 (10.38)	46 (11.14)	1.0/−1.0		
3 h	17 (9.29)	35 (8.22)	60 (10.26)	92 (10.15)	30 (7.26)	−1.4/1.4		
4 h	12 (6.56)	33 (7.75)	53 (9.06)	82 (9.05)	32 (7.75)	0.7/−0.7		
5 h	11 (6.01)	37 (8.69)	38 (6.50)	72 (7.95)	21 (5.08)	−1.6/1.6		
6 h	14 (7.65)	35 (8.22)	52 (8.89)	68 (7.51)	23 (5.57)	−1.6/1.6		
More than 6 h	42 (22.95)	101 (23.71)	98 (16.75)	134 (14.79)	49 (11.86)	2.2/−2.2		
Game form								
Online with friends	91 (49.73)	216 (50.70)	303 (51.70)	459 (50.66)	168 (40.68)	−2.7/2.7	41.18; *p* < 0.001	0.143
Online with unknown	13 (7.10)	45 (10.56)	44 (7.52)	54 (5.96)	28 (6.78)	2.7/−2.7		
Offline alone	33 (18.03)	72 (16.90)	113 (19.32)	189 (20.86)	94 (22.76)	2.5/−2.5		
Offline with friends	1 (0.55)	15 (3.52)	14 (2.39)	54 (5.96)	21 (5.08)	3.1/−3.1		
Money spent (month)								
None	112 (61.20)	300 (70.42)	434 (74.19)	684 (75.50)	315 (76.27)	−2.6/2.6	54.01; *p* < 0.001	0.153
<EUR 10	23 (12.57)	54 (12.68)	66 (11.28)	98 (10.82)	48 (11.62)	−1.0/1.0		
EUR 11–20	6 (3.28)	16 (3.76)	24 (4.10)	36 (3.97)	5 (1.21)	−2.7/2.7		
EUR 21–30	8 (4.37)	5 (1.17)	14 (2.39)	17 (1.88)	3 (0.73)	2.8/−2.8		
EUR 31–50	2 (1.09)	8 (1.88)	5 (0.85)	5 (0.55)	1 (0.24)	2.6/−2.6		
EUR 51–100	2 (1.09)	6 (1.41)	0 (0.00)	3 (0.33)	0 (0.00)	3.3/−3.3		
>EUR 100	3 (1.64)	2 (0.47)	3 (0.51)	4 (0.44)	1 (0.24)	2.4/−2.4		

CC: Contingency Coefficient.

The differences according to the level of physical activity practiced are shown in Table 6. Differences were found in the type of video game played ($p < 0.001$–0.007) and the platform used ($p < 0.001$–0.035). The adolescents who practiced more physical activity played more video games during the weekend ($p < 0.001$); played more online with friends ($p < 0.001$); and spent between EUR 10 and 20 more than the rest ($p = 0.036$).

Table 6. Differences in the type of video games played, platform used, time spent, form of play and money spent per month according to the physical activity level.

Variable	Insufficient (*n* = 540)	Light (*n* = 1028)	Moderate (*n* = 799)	Vigorous (*n* = 146)	Adj. Res	χ2; *p*	CC
Type of video game							
Platforms	76 (14.07)	156 (15.18)	91 (11.39)	21 (14.38)	−2.3/2.3	5.65; *p* = 0.130	0.048
Fighting	44 (8.15)	109 (10.60)	78 (9.76)	18 (12.33)	−1.5/1.5	3.00; *p* = 0.392	0.035
Strategy	174 (32.22)	317 (30.84)	258 (32.29)	46 (31.51)	−0.8/0.8	0.784; *p* = 0.853	0.018
Role Playing	116 (21.48)	230 (22.37)	129 (16.15)	28 (19.18)	−3.3/3.3	12.18; *p* = 0.007	0.071
Shooting	147 (27.22)	391 (38.04)	354 (44.31)	83 (56.85)	4.4/−4.4	57.99; *p* < 0.001	0.155
Casual	153 (28.33)	226 (21.98)	152 (19.02)	18 (12.33)	4.4/−4.4	27.29; *p* < 0.001	0.106

Table 6. *Cont.*

Variable	Insufficient (n = 540)	Light (n = 1028)	Moderate (n = 799)	Vigorous (n = 146)	Adj. Res	χ2; p	CC
Simulation	139 (25.74)	259 (25.19)	158 (19.77)	26 (17.81)	−2.8/2.8	13.03; p = 0.005	0.074
Open-world	205 (37.96)	430 (41.83)	293 (36.67)	37 (25.34)	−3.6/3.6	18.02; p < 0.001	0.086
Sport and racing	141 (26.11)	372 (36.19)	421 (52.69)	89 (60.96)	8.4/−8.4	144.00; p < 0.001	0.244
Platform							
Sony	121 (22.41)	340 (33.07)	346 (43.30)	77 (52.74)	−6.9/6.9	82.80; p < 0.001	0.185
PC	150 (27.78)	324 (31.52)	234 (29.29)	39 (26.71)	1.5/−1.5	2.97; p = 0.397	0.035
Nintendo	117 (21.67)	228 (22.18)	141 (17.65)	19 (13.01)	−2.3/2.3	11.50; p = 0.009	0.069
Tablet	41 (7.59)	108 (10.51)	85 (10.64)	9 (6.16)	−1.8/1.8	6.29; p = 0.098	0.051
Mobile Phone	276 (51.11)	520 (50.58)	356 (44.56)	70 (47.95)	−2.8/2.8	8.62; p = 0.035	0.060
Time of use (Weekdays)							
None	249 (46.11)	419 (40.76)	348 (43.55)	68 (46.58)	−2.0/2.0	24.73; p = 0.420	0.101
1 h	87 (16.11)	179 (17.41)	111 (13.89)	27 (18.49)	−2.0/2.0		
2 h	52 (9.63)	94 (9.14)	78 (9.76)	18 (12.33)	1.1/−1.1		
3 h	34 (6.30)	82 (7.98)	69 (8.64)	10 (6.85)	−1.5/1.5		
4 h	25 (4.63)	46 (4.47)	48 (6.01)	7 (4.79)	1.6/−1.6		
5 h	19 (3.52)	51 (4.96)	37 (4.63)	3 (2.05)	−1.4/1.4		
6 h	27 (5.00)	50 (4.86)	28 (3.50)	4 (2.74)	−1.4/1.4		
More than 6 h	35 (6.48)	79 (7.68)	55 (6.88)	6 (4.11)	−1.4/1.4		
Time of use (Weekend)							
None	188 (34.81)	218 (21.21)	158 (19.77)	30 (20.55)	6.9/−6.9	80.63; p < 0.001	0.181
1 h	62 (11.48)	133 (12.94)	91 (11.39)	19 (13.01)	1.1/−1.1		
2 h	51 (9.44)	130 (12.65)	73 (9.14)	17 (11.64)	2.6/−2.6		
3 h	56 (10.37)	91 (8.85)	91 (11.39)	13 (8.90)	1.6/−1.6		
4 h	40 (7.41)	84 (8.17)	80 (10.01)	15 (10.27)	1.5/−1.5		
5 h	23 (4.26)	78 (7.59)	74 (9.26)	13 (8.90)	−3.2/3.2		
6 h	41 (7.59)	75 (7.30)	69 (8.64)	10 (6.85)	1.1/−1.1		
More than 6 h	24 (4.44)	85 (8.27)	70 (8.76)	18 (12.33)	−3.3/3.3		
Game form							
Online with friends	214 (39.63)	501 (48.74)	467 (58.45)	105 (71.92)	5.6/−5.6	90.11; p < 0.001	0.207
Online with unknown	38 (7.04)	101 (9.82)	42 (5.26)	5 (3.42)	3.7/−3.7		
Offline alone	151 (27.96)	220 (21.40)	118 (14.77)	20 (13.70)	6.0/−6.0		
Offline with friends	23 (4.26)	48 (4.67)	38 (4.76)	1 (0.68)	−2.4/2.4		
Money spent (month)							
None	439 (81.30)	768 (74.71)	591 (73.97)	111 (76.03)	3.3/−3.3	30.19; p = 0.036	0.112
<EUR 10	51 (9.44)	134 (13.04)	101 (12.64)	17 (11.64)	−2.2/2.2		
EUR 11–20	13 (2.41)	31 (3.02)	36 (4.51)	10 (6.85)	2.2/−2.2		
EUR 21–30	4 (0.74)	24 (2.33)	20 (2.50)	1 (0.68)	−2.3/2.3		
EUR 31–50	3 (0.56)	13 (1.26)	6 (0.75)	0 (0.00)	1.8/−1.8		
EUR 51–100	3 (0.56)	4 (0.39)	3 (0.38)	1 (0.68)	0.5/−0.5		
>EUR 100	5 (0.93)	3 (0.29)	5 (0.63)	1 (0.68)	−1.5/1.5		

CC: Contingency Coefficient.

3.2. *Differences in the Psychological Variables According to Gender*

Table 7 shows the differences in the psychological variables according to the gender of the adolescents. Males showed a higher problematic use of video games ($p < 0.001$), higher gaming addiction ($p < 0.001$); higher scores in all categories in terms of gaming motives ($p < 0.001$), except for customization ($p = 0.132$); higher mood repair with the use of video games ($p < 0.001$) and higher scores in the passion scale ($p < 0.001$). Females showed higher scores in emotional symptoms ($p < 0.001$) and prosocial behavior ($p < 0.001$).

Table 7. Differences in the psychological variables according to gender.

Variable	Male (n = 1286)	Female (n = 1227)	t	95% CI	d	p
CERV						
Evasion	14.68 ± 4.16	10.92 ± 3.54	24.21	3.45; 4.06	0.39	<0.001
Negative consequences	13.74 ± 3.58	11.03 ± 2.77	21.05	2.46; 2.96	0.32	<0.001
Total	28.42 ± 7.26	21.95 ± 6.02	24.14	5.94; 6.99	0.67	<0.001
Gaming addiction	6.49 ± 4.79	2.87 ± 4.16	20.09	3.27;3.98	0.45	<0.001
VMQ						
Recreation	10.13 ± 2.52	8.73 ± 2.98	10.72	1.15; 1.67	0.27	<0.001
Competition	8.26 ± 3.08	6.03 ± 3.23	14.54	1.92; 2.52	0.31	<0.001
Cognitive development	5.52 ± 3.24	3.58 ± 2.91	12.79	1.65; 2.25	0.31	<0.001
Coping	6.01 ± 3.65	3.61 ± 2.68	18.62	2.15; 2.65	0.32	<0.001
Social interaction	5.81 ± 3.25	3.60 ± 3.07	14.28	1.91; 2.52	0.32	<0.001
Violent reward	4.87 ± 3.70	2.47 ± 3.24	13.94	2.07; 2.74	0.35	<0.001
Customization	7.20 ± 3.73	6.92 ± 3.77	1.53	−0.08; 0.64	0.04	0.132
Fantasy	6.45 ± 3.66	5.48 ± 3.86	5.30	0.61; 1.32	0.37	<0.001
Mood repair	25.77 ± 7.00	23.48 ± 7.11	8.10	1.74; 2.85	0.71	<0.001
Passion scale						
Harmonious	9.71 ± 2.91	7.50 ± 2.18	21.43	2.01; 2.41	0.26	<0.001
Obsessive	10.49 ± 3.02	7.96 ± 2.49	22.71	2.30; 2.74	0.28	<0.001
SDQ						
Emotional symptoms	12.43 ± 4.23	16.15 ± 4.63	−20.99	−4.07; −3.37	0.44	<0.001
Conduct problems	12.33 ± 3.01	12.27 ± 2.98	0.55	−0.17; 0.30	0.03	0.581
Peer relationship problem	15.57 ± 2.57	15.65 ± 2.56	−0.77	−0.28; 0.12	0.02	0.440
Hyperactivity/inattention	16.30 ± 3.13	16.16 ± 2.81	1.20	−0.09; 0.38	0.03	0.234
Prosocial behavior	20.63 ± 3.33	21.66 ± 3.05	−8.03	−1.28; −0.78	0.32	<0.001

3.3. Differences in the Psychological Variables According to the Closest Environment

Table 8 shows the differences in the psychological variables according to whether the parents live together. It is observed that in those adolescents whose parents live together, mood repair was higher (p = 0.005). In the adolescents whose parents live apart, the score was higher in emotional symptoms (p < 0.001), conduct problems (p < 0.001) and peer relationship problems (p < 0.001).

It was also observed that adolescents whose parents always monitored them showed greater problematic use of video games (p < 0.001), greater gaming addiction (p < 0.001) as well as higher scores in all gaming motives (recreation: p = 0.003–0.048) and passion (p < 0.001). On the other hand, adolescents who were never monitored showed higher scores in competition (p = 0.022), violent reward (p < 0.001), emotional symptoms (p = 0.008) and prosocial behavior (p = 0.015); and lower scores in mood repair (p < 0.001) (Figure 1).

3.4. Differences in the Psychological Variables According to the Academic Performance of the Adolescents

The differences as a function of academic performance are found in Table 9. Adolescents who failed or passed with a low grade showed higher scores in problematic use of the video games (p < 0.001–0.035); gaming addiction (p < 0.001); passion (p < 0.001–0.034); emotional symptoms (p < 0.001); conduct problems (p < 0.001–0.002); and their main gaming motives were coping (p = 0.022–0.035), social interaction (p < 0.001–0.002) and violent reward (p < 0.001). They only showed lower scores than adolescents with good grades (A or B) in prosocial behavior (p < 0.001–0.003) (Figure 2).

3.5. Differences in the Psychological Variables According to the Level of Physical Activity

The differences in the psychological variables according to the level of physical activity of the adolescents are shown in Table 10. Adolescents with insufficient and light physical activity showed lower competitiveness ($p < 0.001$–0.022), cognitive development ($p < 0.001$–0.017), social interaction ($p < 0.001$–0.021) and violent reward ($p < 0.001$–0.005). In addition, these adolescents showed lower mood repair ($p < 0.001$–0.044), greater emotional symptoms ($p < 0.001$) and peer relationship problems ($p < 0.001$–0.026) as well as less hyperactivity/inattention ($p < 0.001$–0.026) (Figure 3).

3.6. Differences in the Psychological Variables According to the Game Form

Table 11 shows the differences according to game form. Problematic video game use, gaming addiction and passion for video games were higher in adolescents who played online as compared to those who played offline ($p < 0.001$–0.009). Regarding the motives for gaming, recreation ($p < 0.001$–0.002), competition ($p < 0.001$–0.009), cognitive development ($p < 0.001$), coping ($p < 0.001$–0.046), social interaction ($p < 0.001$) and violent reward ($p < 0.001$–0.007) were the main motives for gaming for those who played online. Mood repair was higher only when comparing adolescents who played online with friends compared to those who played alone offline ($p = 0.045$). And in emotional and behavioral symptoms, players who played online with strangers showed higher emotional symptoms ($p < 0.001$–0.014), higher conduct problems ($p = 0.012$) and peer relationship problems ($p < 0.001$) (Figure 4).

Table 8. Differences in the psychological variables according to cohabitation of parents and parental control of time spent on video games.

Variable	Cohabitation of Parents						Parental Control of Time Use						
	Yes (n = 1848)	No (n = 665)	t	95% CI	d	p	Never (n = 1483)	Sometimes (n = 340)	Always (n = 690)	F	95% CI	ES	p
CERV													
Evasion	12.85 ± 4.30	12.86 ± 4.30	−0.05	−0.40; 0.38	0.04	0.960	14.12 ± 4.35	13.37 ± 3.82	14.87 ± 3.77	13.22	13.90; 14.34	0.02	<0.001
Negative consequences	12.35 ± 3.37	12.66 ± 3.79	−1.94	−0.62; 0.00	0.03	0.053	13.16 ± 3.65	13.05 ± 3.15	13.97 ± 3.34	11.48	13.21; 13.58	0.01	<0.001
Total	25.20 ± 7.31	25.52 ± 7.72	−0.94	−0.99; 0.35	0.07	0.351	27.28 ± 7.54	26.42 ± 6.57	28.84 ± 6.57	13.44	27.14; 27.89	0.02	<0.001
Gaming addiction	4.68 ± 4.78	4.95 ± 5.05	−1.20	−0.70; 0.17	0.05	0.234	5.72 ± 4.90	5.77 ± 4.82	7.07 ± 4.57	15.45	5.93; 6.44	0.02	<0.001
VMQ													
Recreation	9.66 ± 2.75	9.53 ± 2.88	0.87	−0.16; 0.42	0.03	0.390	9.54 ± 2.85	9.27 ± 2.91	9.95 ± 2.57	6.68	9.44; 9.73	0.01	0.001
Competition	7.41 ± 3.32	7.60 ± 3.30	−1.05	−0.53; 0.16	0.03	0.307	7.56 ± 3.36	6.94 ± 3.41	7.56 ± 3.16	3.91	7.18; 7.53	0.00	0.020
Cognitive development	4.82 ± 3.27	4.86 ± 3.26	−0.25	−0.39; 0.30	0.03	0.801	4.86 ± 3.35	4.37 ± 3.16	4.95 ± 3.12	3.08	4.56; 4.90	0.00	0.050
Coping	4.84 ± 3.43	4.91 ± 3.46	−0.42	−0.37; 0.24	0.03	0.685	5.42 ± 3.86	5.00 ± 3.87	5.88 ± 3.63	5.39	5.23; 5.63	0.01	0.005
Social interaction	5.01 ± 3.32	5.10 ± 3.49	−0.49	−0.44; 0.27	0.04	0.632	4.86 ± 3.44	4.77 ± 3.46	5.41 ± 3.13	5.77	4.84; 5.19	0.01	0.003
Violent reward	3.95 ± 3.66	4.23 ± 3.87	−1.40	−0.67; 0.11	0.04	0.166	4.29 ± 3.97	3.30 ± 3.49	3.88 ± 3.32	7.79	3.63; 4.02	0.01	<0.001
Customization	7.19 ± 3.73	6.85 ± 3.80	−1.71	−0.05; 0.74	0.04	0.093	6.94 ± 3.88	7.45 ± 3.75	7.17 ± 3.53	2.14	6.99; 7.39	0.00	0.[illegible]24
Fantasy	6.07 ± 3.75	6.24 ± 3.80	−0.85	−0.57; 0.22	0.04	0.397	6.02 ± 3.82	5.88 ± 3.70	6.27 ± 3.71	1.19	5.86; 6.26	0.00	0.312
Mood repair	24.88 ± 7.13	23.96 ± 7.20	2.79	0.27; 1.56	0.71	0.005	24.08 ± 7.23	26.25 ± 7.33	25.38 ± 6.54	12.52	24.86; 25.61	0.01	<0.001
Passion scale													
Harmonious	8.58 ± 2.75	8.81 ± 2.93	−1.78	−0.48; 0.02	0.02	0.087	9.30 ± 2.95	8.93 ± 2.63	9.86 ± 2.67	12.10	9.21; 9.51	0.01	<0.001
Obsessive	9.23 ± 3.01	9.35 ± 3.15	−0.83	−0.39; 0.16	0.03	0.416	10.05 ± 3.05	9.62 ± 2.80	10.66 ± 2.85	13.38	9.95; 10.27	0.02	<0.001
SDQ													
Emotional symptoms	14.00 ± 4.77	14.95 ± 4.84	−4.33	−1.38; −0.52	0.48	<0.001	14.07 ± 4.86	13.07 ± 5.02	13.61 ± 4.57	5.01	13.33; 13.84	0.01	0.007
Conduct problems	12.19 ± 2.95	12.64 ± 3.09	−3.27	−0.72; −0.18	0.30	<0.001	12.50 ± 3.02	12.28 ± 3.21	12.41 ± 2.98	0.59	12.24; 12.56	0.00	0.565
Peer relationship problem	15.53 ± 2.51	15.87 ± 2.67	−2.88	−0.57; −0.11	0.26	<0.001	15.79 ± 2.61	15.41 ± 2.81	15.59 ± 2.44	2.70	15.46; 15.74	0.00	0.073
Hyperactivity/ inattention	16.20 ± 2.97	16.29 ± 3.03	−0.68	−0.36; 0.17	0.03	0.496	16.21 ± 3.07	16.46 ± 3.46	16.37 ± 2.84	0.96	16.18; 16.51	0.00	0.334
Prosocial behavior	21.19 ± 3.15	20.96 ± 3.47	1.54	−0.06; 0.52	0.03	0.138	20.72 ± 3.45	21.38 ± 3.64	20.99 ± 3.10	4.23	20.85; 21.21	0.01	0.026

Table 9. Differences in psychological variables according to academic performance.

Variable	Academic Performance								
	F (n = 183)	D (n = 426)	C (n = 585)	B (n = 906)	A (n = 413)	F	95% CI	ES	p
CERV									
Evasion	15.08 ± 4.59	15.04 ± 4.16	14.37 ± 4.31	13.79 ± 3.88	13.75 ± 3.92	7.09	14.18; 14.63	0.02	<0.001
Negative consequences	14.62 ± 4.37	14.35 ± 3.89	13.55 ± 3.59	12.98 ± 3.14	12.40 ± 2.66	17.51	13.39; 13.77	0.04	<0.001
Total	29.70 ± 8.35	29.39 ± 7.58	27.92 ± 7.42	26.77 ± 6.56	26.15 ± 6.20	12.64	27.60; 28.37	0.03	<0.001
Gaming addiction	7.46 ± 5.56	7.30 ± 5.16	6.28 ± 4.86	5.59 ± 4.61	5.20 ± 3.99	11.46	6.11; 6.63	0.03	<0.001
VMQ									
Recreation	9.62 ± 2.76	9.72 ± 2.72	9.44 ± 2.90	9.69 ± 2.76	9.76 ± 2.67	0.79	9.49; 9.80	0.00	0.532
Competition	8.07 ± 3.37	7.56 ± 3.36	7.56 ± 3.36	7.28 ± 3.27	7.25 ± 3.26	1.98	7.36; 7.73	0.01	0.095
Cognitive development	4.86 ± 3.16	4.98 ± 3.33	4.79 ± 3.39	4.71 ± 3.14	4.89 ± 3.23	0.43	4.67; 5.02	0.00	0.786
Coping	5.94 ± 4.03	6.05 ± 3.82	5.53 ± 3.77	5.29 ± 3.70	5.05 ± 3.78	3.42	5.37; 5.78	0.01	0.009
Social interaction	5.84 ± 3.62	5.64 ± 3.35	5.21 ± 3.39	4.64 ± 3.27	4.49 ± 3.15	8.51	4.98; 5.35	0.02	<0.001
Violent reward	5.44 ± 3.98	4.65 ± 3.86	4.01 ± 3.70	3.67 ± 3.53	3.17 ± 3.60	11.47	3.99; 4.39	0.03	<0.001
Customization	6.74 ± 3.71	7.15 ± 3.81	6.78 ± 3.80	7.22 ± 3.77	7.41 ± 3.48	1.63	6.85; 7.26	0.00	0.163
Fantasy	6.23 ± 3.73	6.12 ± 3.76	5.87 ± 3.78	6.08 ± 3.78	6.22 ± 3.74	0.48	5.90; 6.31	0.00	0.754
Mood repair	23.41 ± 8.13	24.04 ± 7.25	24.93 ± 6.86	25.25 ± 7.01	25.47 ± 6.44	3.34	24.23; 25.00	0.01	0.100
Passion scale									
Harmonious	10.51 ± 3.53	10.15 ± 2.93	9.60 ± 2.89	8.96 ± 2.57	8.75 ± 2.43	18.36	9.44; 9.75	0.04	<0.001
Obsessive	10.77 ± 3.26	10.81 ± 3.24	10.24 ± 3.07	9.92 ± 2.78	9.65 ± 2.63	7.87	10.12; 10.44	0.02	<0.001
SDQ									
Emotional symptoms	14.77 ± 4.87	14.41 ± 4.71	14.01 ± 4.84	13.64 ± 4.79	12.44 ± 4.85	7.59	13.59; 14.12	0.02	<0.001
Conduct problems	13.44 ± 3.68	12.90 ± 3.16	12.58 ± 3.05	12.12 ± 2.81	11.76 ± 2.80	10.40	12.40; 12.72	0.02	<0.001
Peer relationship problem	16.06 ± 3.27	15.80 ± 2.75	15.87 ± 2.63	15.53 ± 2.40	15.46 ± 2.43	2.32	15.60; 15.88	0.01	0.055
Hyperactivity/inattention	16.72 ± 3.27	16.42 ± 3.23	16.49 ± 3.00	16.13 ± 3.03	15.94 ± 2.92	2.43	16.17; 16.51	0.01	0.056
Prosocial behavior	20.04 ± 3.66	20.24 ± 3.75	20.93 ± 3.27	21.22 ± 3.12	21.39 ± 3.27	7.88	20.58; 20.95	0.02	<0.001

Table 10. Differences in psychological variables according to the level of physical activity of the adolescents.

Variable	Level of Physical Activity							
	Insufficient (n = 540)	Light (n = 1028)	Moderate (n = 799)	Vigorous (n = 146)	F	95% CI	ES	p
CERV								
Evasion	14.07 ± 4.51	14.33 ± 4.05	14.33 ± 4.01	13.88 ± 4.10	0.67	13.91; 14.40	0.00	0.568
Negative consequences	13.27 ± 3.70	13.58 ± 3.52	13.32 ± 3.37	13.12 ± 3.51	1.15	13.11; 13.53	0.00	0.327
Total	27.34 ± 7.73	27.91 ± 7.06	27.65 ± 6.91	27.00 ± 7.28	0.84	27.05; 27.90	0.00	0.474
Gaming addiction	6.09 ± 5.13	6.25 ± 4.69	6.19 ± 4.85	5.82 ± 4.76	0.30	5.80; 6.38	0.00	0.823
VMQ								
Recreation	9.30 ± 3.00	9.53 ± 2.72	9.92 ± 2.70	9.81 ± 2.71	4.26	9.48; 9.81	0.01	0.052
Competition	6.52 ± 3.40	7.15 ± 3.27	8.19 ± 3.18	8.60 ± 2.94	26.17	7.42; 7.81	0.04	<0.001
Cognitive development	4.34 ± 3.38	4.70 ± 3.13	5.23 ± 3.31	4.99 ± 3.56	6.03	4.62; 5.01	0.01	<0.001
Coping	5.07 ± 3.77	5.59 ± 3.77	5.71 ± 3.78	5.16 ± 4.00	2.48	5.16; 5.61	0.00	0.059
Social interaction	4.23 ± 3.39	5.00 ± 3.34	5.47 ± 3.35	5.29 ± 3.08	10.09	4.80; 5.20	0.02	<0.001
Violent reward	3.40 ± 3.69	3.75 ± 3.61	4.54 ± 3.80	5.01 ± 3.74	11.00	3.96; 4.40	0.02	<0.001
Customization	7.25 ± 3.82	7.20 ± 3.64	7.07 ± 3.75	6.03 ± 4.11	3.49	6.66; 7.11	0.01	0.055
Fantasy	6.09 ± 3.79	6.17 ± 3.78	6.11 ± 3.73	5.45 ± 3.84	1.19	5.73; 6.18	0.00	0.311
Mood repair	22.76 ± 7.11	24.74 ± 6.93	25.76 ± 6.96	26.62 ± 7.09	15.69	24.55; 25.39	0.03	<0.001
Passion scale								
Harmonious	9.29 ± 2.90	9.54 ± 2.89	9.42 ± 2.74	9.01 ± 2.75	1.47	9.15; 9.49	0.00	0.220
Obsessive	9.96 ± 3.25	10.24 ± 2.89	10.25 ± 2.90	10.10 ± 3.11	0.84	9.96; 10.32	0.00	0.471
SDQ								
Emotional symptoms	15.11 ± 4.87	14.34 ± 4.67	12.73 ± 4.63	11.74 ± 4.76	29.57	13.20; 13.76	0.05	<0.001
Conduct problems	12.43 ± 3.05	12.48 ± 3.09	12.39 ± 2.93	12.46 ± 3.27	0.09	12.26; 12.63	0.00	0.964
Peer relationship problem	15.86 ± 2.63	15.89 ± 2.61	15.36 ± 2.48	15.38 ± 2.77	5.93	15.47; 15.78	0.01	<0.001
Hyperactivity/inattention	15.84 ± 2.95	16.35 ± 2.97	16.30 ± 3.14	17.23 ± 3.27	6.04	16.25; 16.61	0.01	<0.001
Prosocial behavior	20.48 ± 3.55	20.93 ± 3.33	21.09 ± 3.25	21.05 ± 3.65	2.43	20.69; 21.09	0.00	0.064

Table 11. Differences in psychological variables according to the game form.

Variable	Game Form				F	95% CI	ES	*p*
	Online with Friends (*n* = 1393)	Online with Unknown (*n* = 290)	Offline Alone (*n* = 615)	Offline with Friends (*n* = 215)				
CERV								
Evasion	14.70 ± 4.15	15.13 ± 4.09	12.93 ± 3.66	12.31 ± 3.47	26.67	13.47; 14.06	0.05	<0.001
Negative consequences	13.70 ± 3.55	14.29 ± 3.75	12.28 ± 2.82	12.46 ± 3.22	21.48	12.93; 13.43	0.04	<0.001
Total	28.40 ± 7.20	29.42 ± 7.25	25.21 ± 6.06	24.77 ± 6.33	27.42	26.44; 27.46	0.05	<0.001
Gaming addiction	6.50 ± 4.88	7.42 ± 4.88	4.82 ± 4.11	4.73 ± 4.70	17.96	5.52; 6.21	0.03	<0.001
VMQ								
Recreation	9.92 ± 2.58	9.79 ± 2.83	8.87 ± 3.05	9.38 ± 2.90	14.13	9.29; 9.69	0.02	<0.001
Competition	8.02 ± 3.18	7.96 ± 3.08	5.70 ± 3.10	6.59 ± 3.42	52.47	6.84; 7.30	0.09	<0.001
Cognitive development	5.05 ± 3.22	5.35 ± 3.15	4.02 ± 3.05	4.42 ± 3.63	11.31	4.48; 4.94	0.02	<0.001
Coping	5.82 ± 3.77	5.96 ± 3.70	4.59 ± 3.71	4.59 ± 3.85	12.15	4.97; 5.52	0.02	<0.001
Social interaction	5.98 ± 3.06	4.80 ± 3.39	2.50 ± 2.84	3.94 ± 2.61	125.26	4.08; 4.53	0.18	<0.001
Violent reward	4.40 ± 3.70	4.63 ± 3.76	2.67 ± 3.36	3.02 ± 3.39	24.67	3.42; 3.95	0.04	<0.001
Customization	6.95 ± 3.70	7.66 ± 3.59	7.27 ± 3.93	6.84 ± 4.05	2.16	6.90; 7.45	0.00	0.091
Fantasy	6.01 ± 3.75	6.67 ± 3.57	6.18 ± 3.91	5.60 ± 3.60	1.97	5.84; 6.39	0.00	0.117
Mood repair	25.23 ± 6.95	23.96 ± 7.31	24.09 ± 7.02	24.68 ± 7.35	3.35	23.98; 25.00	0.01	0.018
Passion scale								
Harmonious	9.70 ± 2.90	10.04 ± 2.80	8.55 ± 2.38	8.21 ± 2.46	23.66	8.92; 9.33	0.04	<0.001
Obsessive	10.50 ± 3.01	10.84 ± 3.07	9.16 ± 2.48	8.93 ± 2.43	27.68	9.64; 10.07	0.05	<0.001
SDQ								
Emotional symptoms	13.24 ± 4.71	15.39 ± 5.08	14.84 ± 4.86	13.41 ± 4.36	17.08	13.87; 14.57	0.03	<0.001
Conduct problems	12.45 ± 3.01	13.04 ± 3.33	12.15 ± 2.96	12.16 ± 3.05	3.43	12.23; 12.67	0.01	0.017
Peer relationship problem	15.43 ± 2.52	16.48 ± 2.82	16.00 ± 2.60	15.64 ± 2.12	10.81	15.70; 16.08	0.02	<0.001
Hyperactivity/inattention	16.31 ± 3.13	16.25 ± 2.87	16.28 ± 2.88	16.10 ± 3.12	0.13	16.01; 16.46	0.00	0.943
Prosocial behavior	20.98 ± 3.30	20.39 ± 3.85	21.04 ± 3.48	20.68 ± 2.85	1.73	20.52; 21.02	0.00	0.159

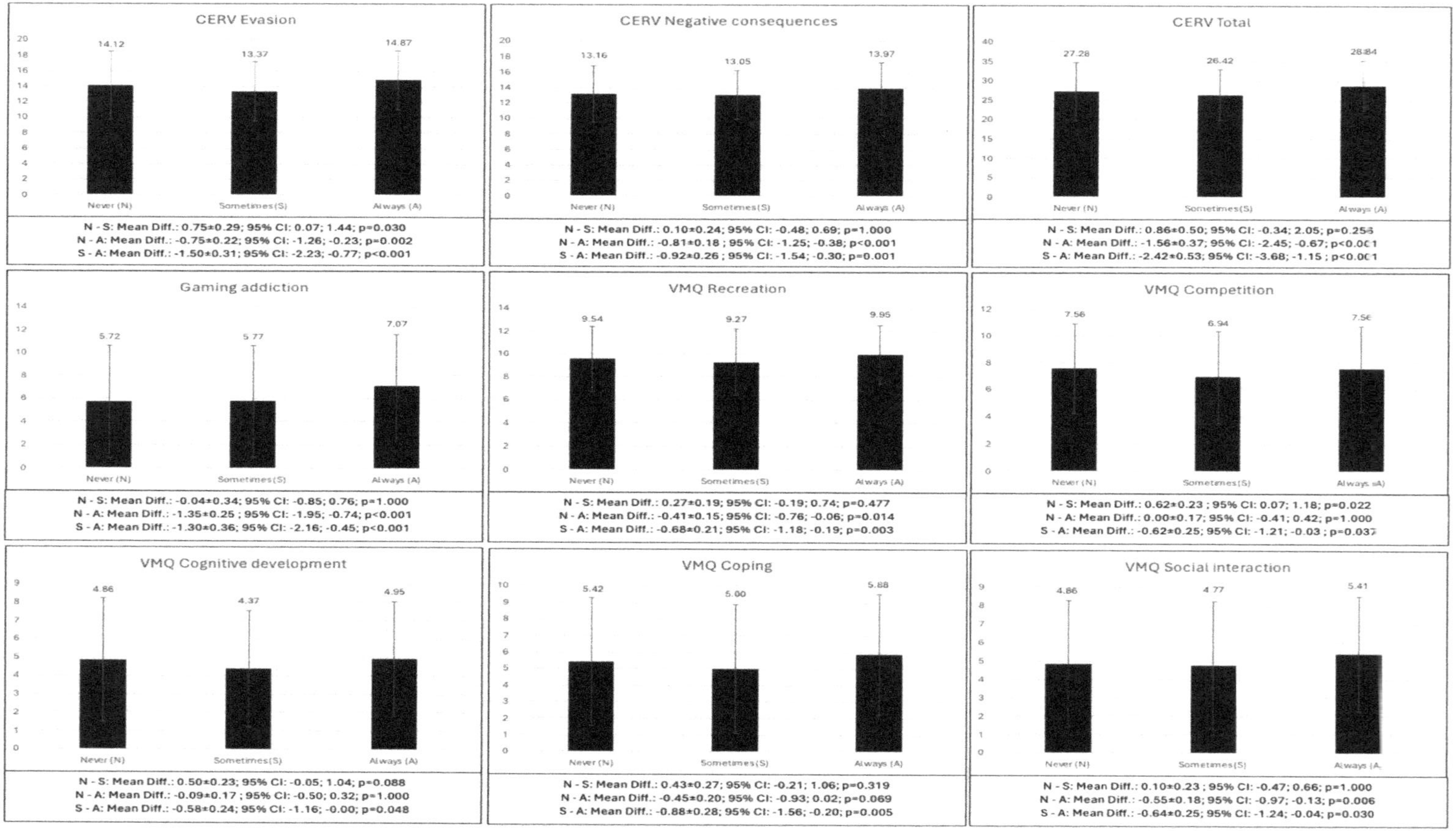

Figure 1. *Cont.*

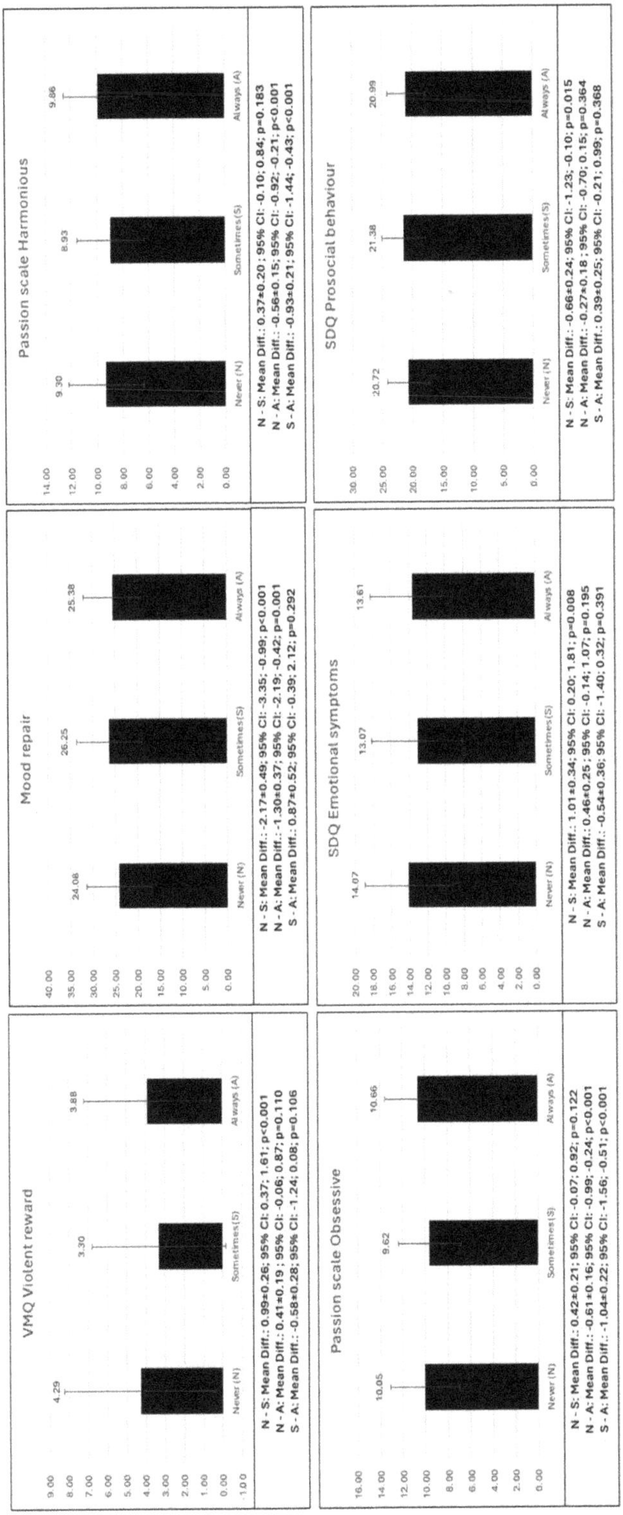

Figure 1. Bonferroni post hoc of the differences in the psychological variables according to the parental control of time spent.

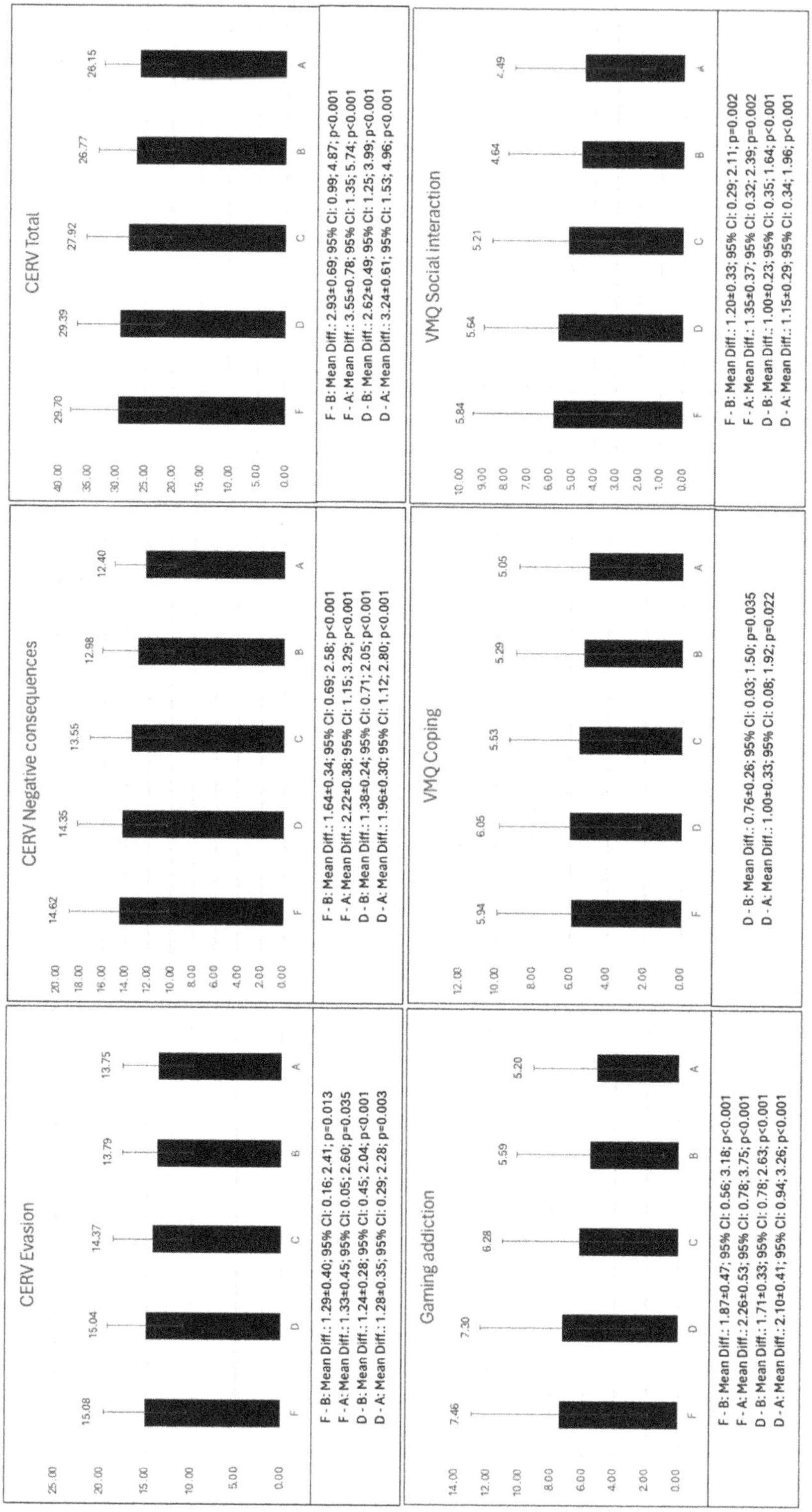

Figure 2. *Cont.*

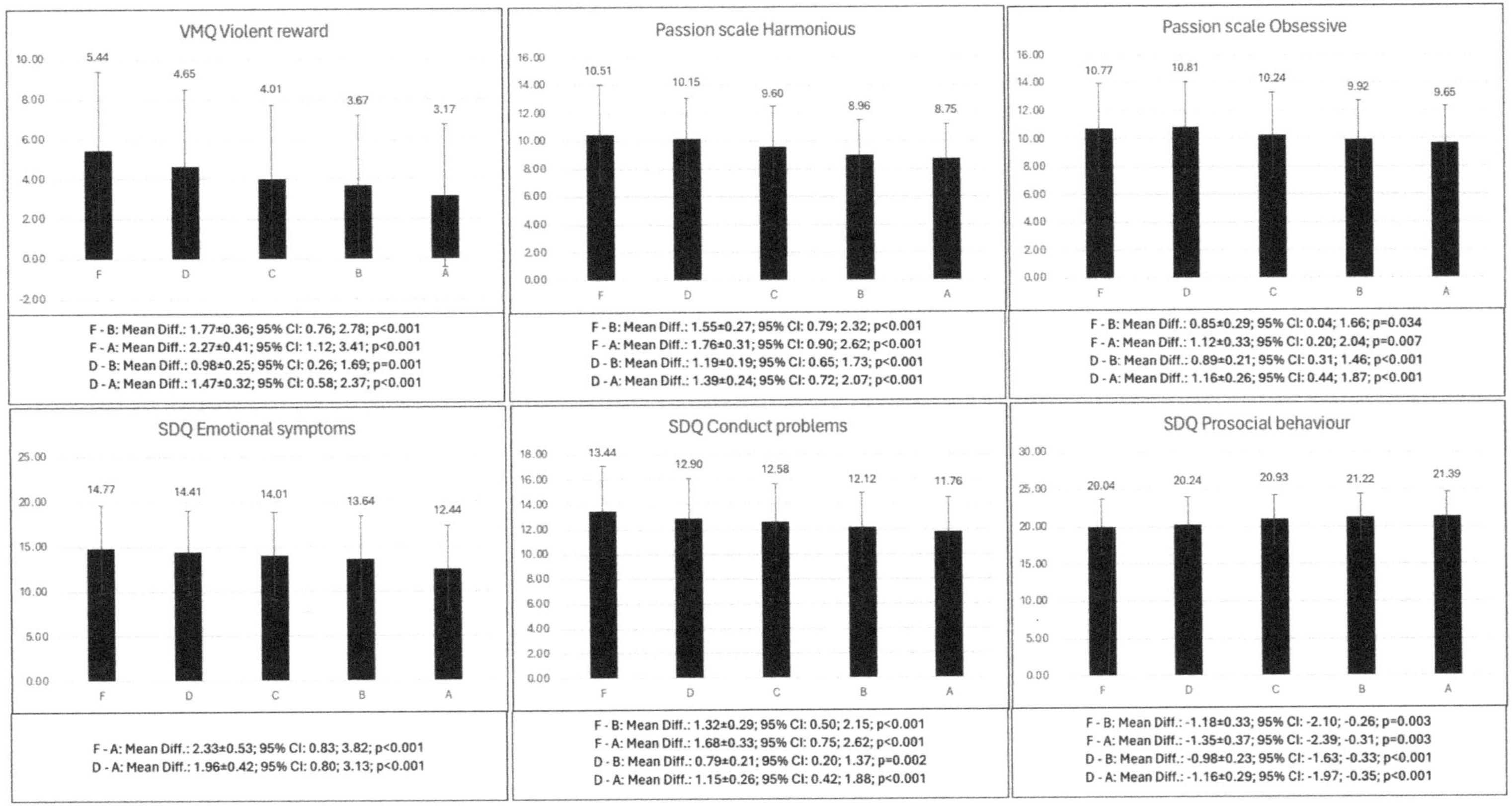

Figure 2. Bonferroni post hoc of the differences in the psychological variables according to academic performance (continued).

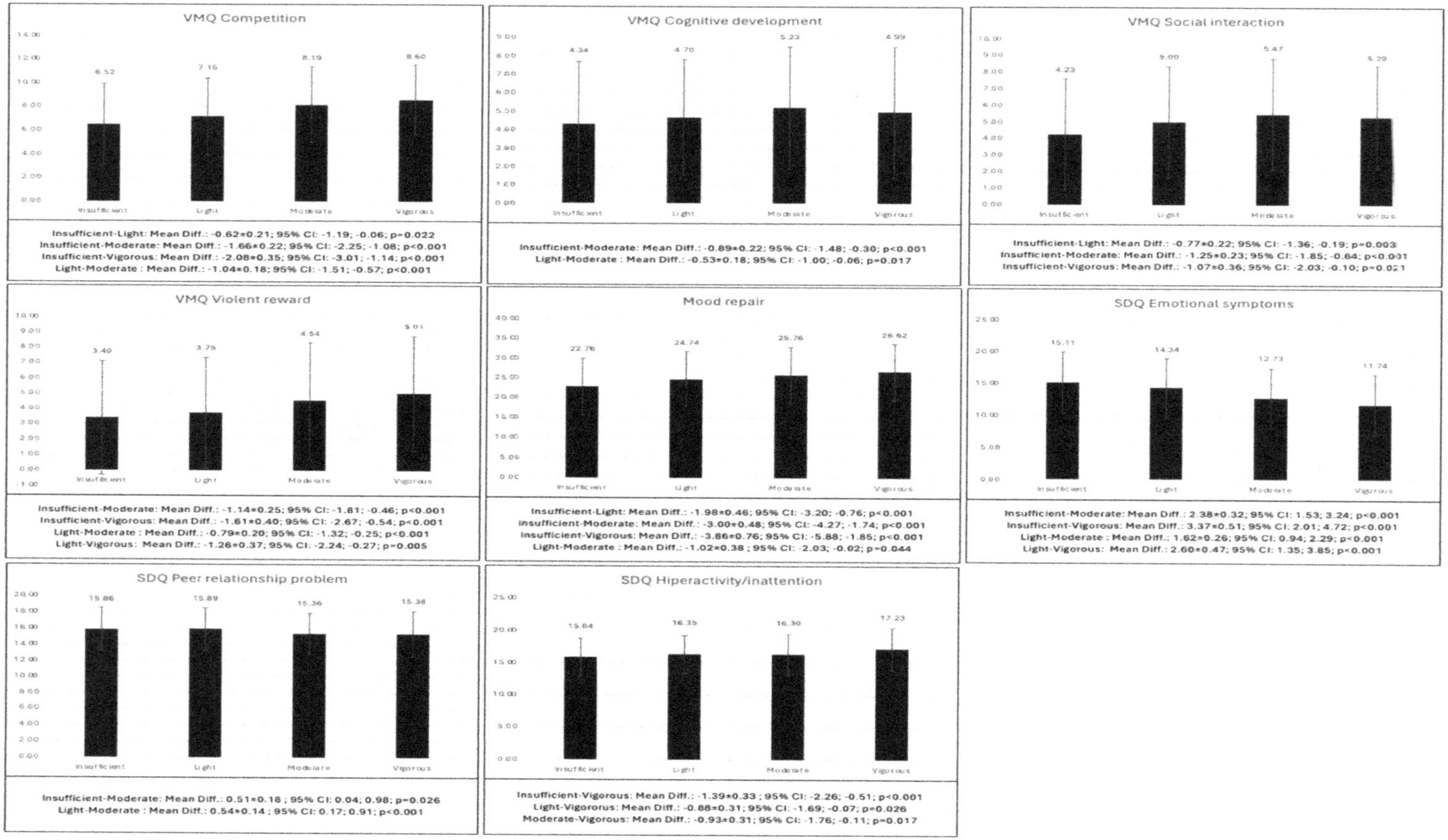

Figure 3. Bonferroni post hoc of the differences in the psychological variables according to the level of physical activity.

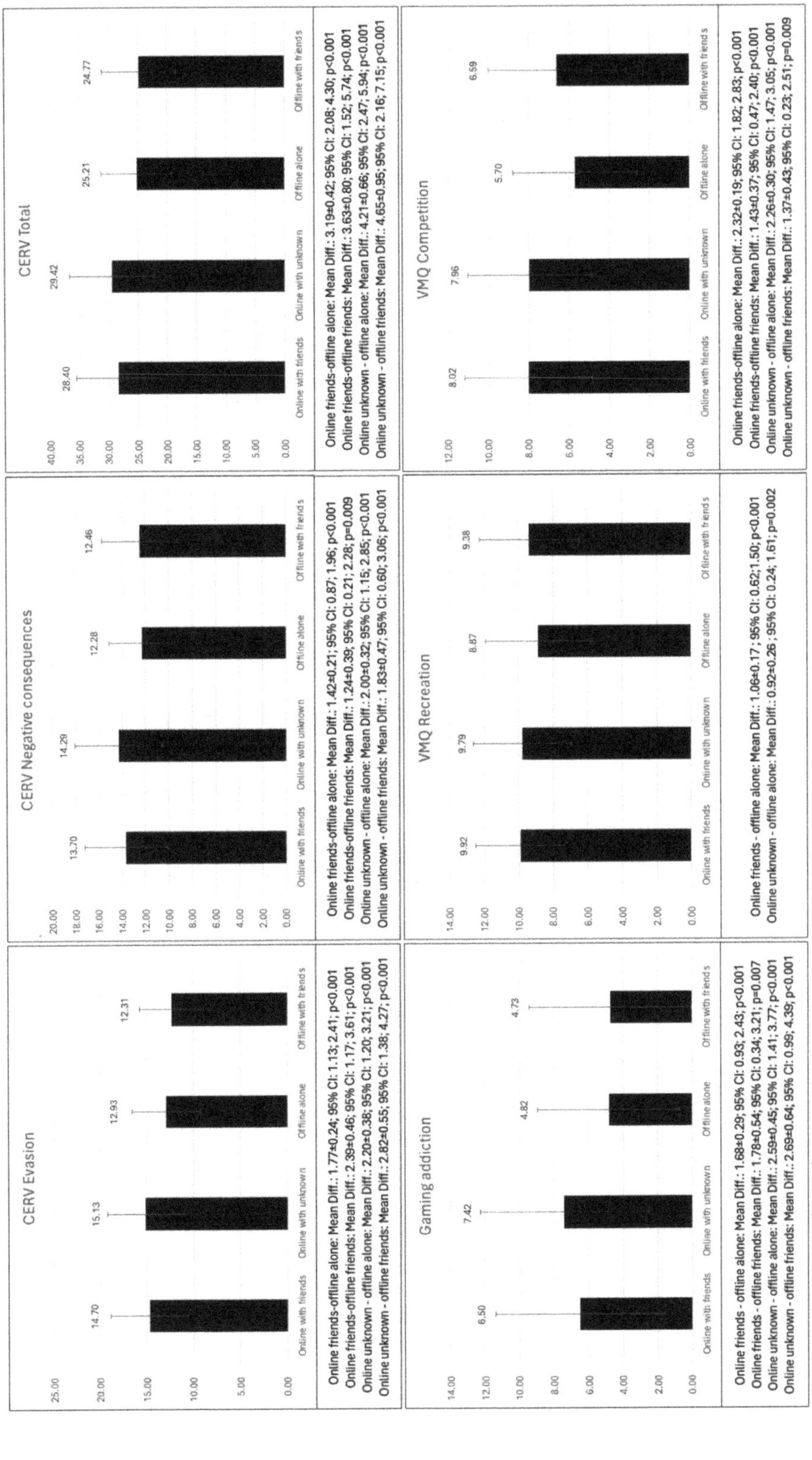

Figure 4. *Cont.*

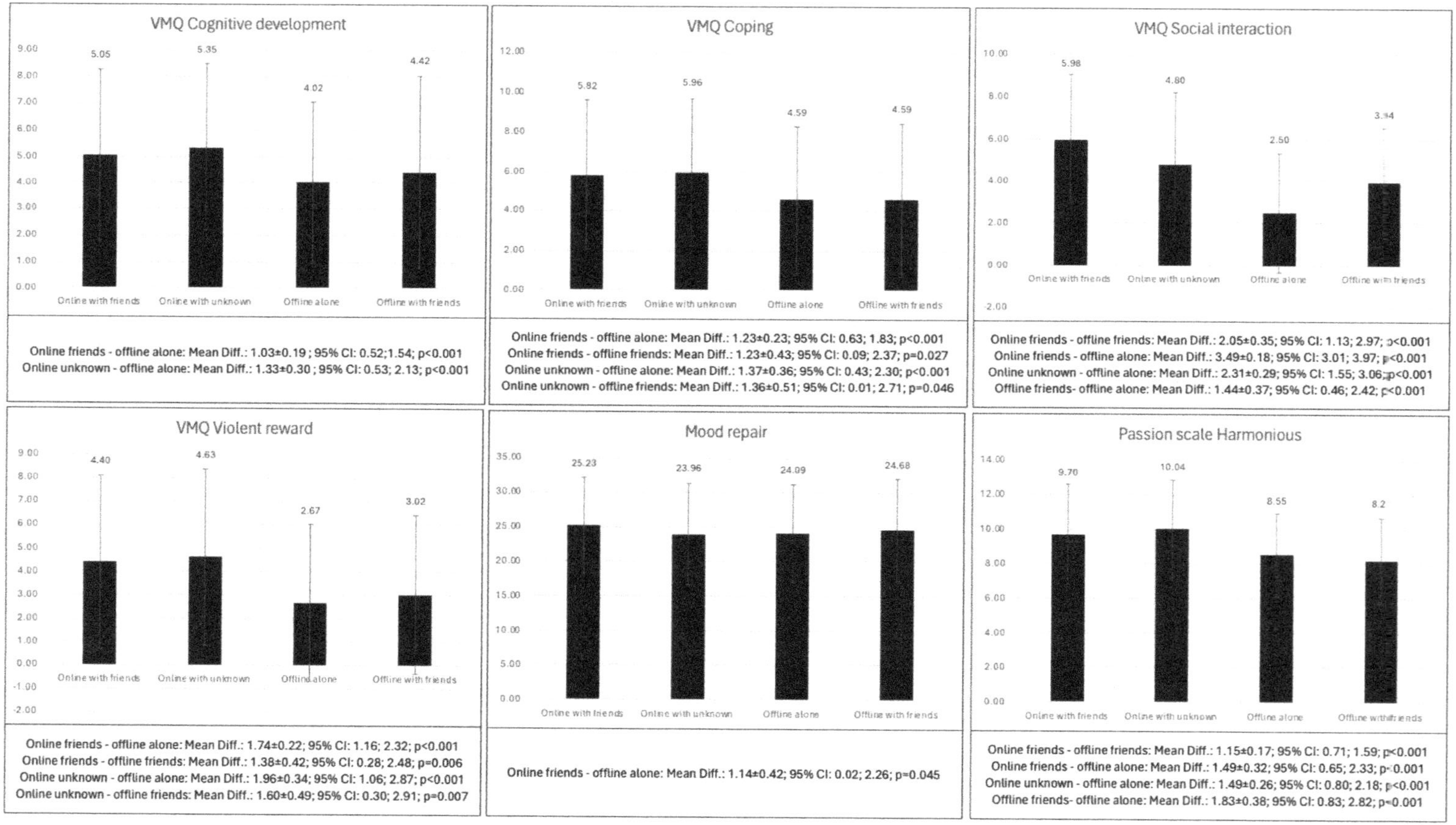

Figure 4. *Cont.*

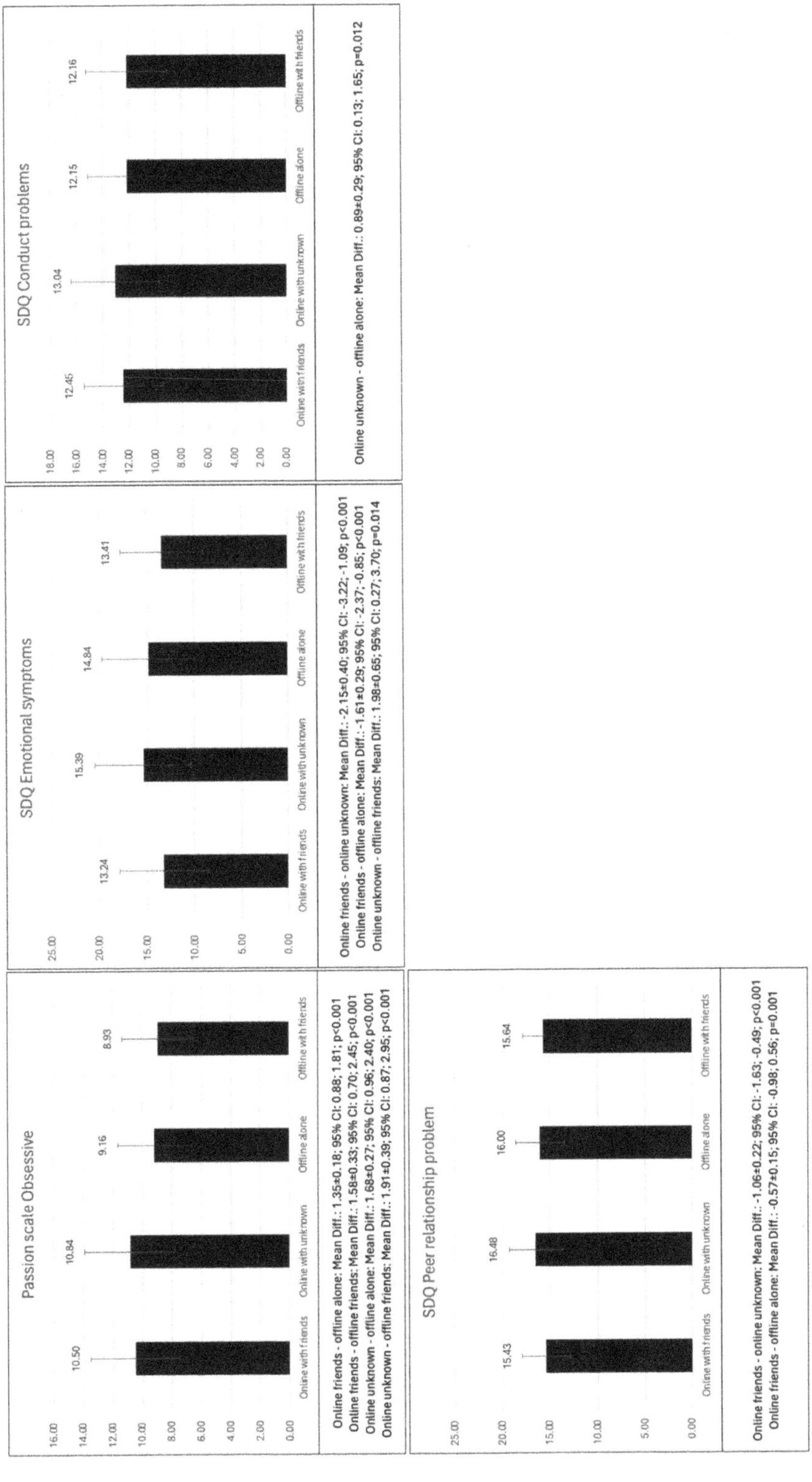

Figure 4. Bonferroni post hoc of the differences in the psychological variables according to the game form.

3.7. Relationship Between Psychological, Game-Related and Behavioral Variables

Correlational analysis between psychological variables and gaming variables, physical activity level and academic performance is shown in Table 12. It was found that physical activity level was positively related to gaming-related experiences ($p < 0.001$–0.004); gaming addiction ($p = 0.004$); gaming motives ($p < 0.001$–0.004); mood repair ($p < 0.001$); passion scale ($p < 0.001$–0.018); and most of the social, emotional and behavioral problems ($p < 0.001$–0.010). Academic performance was inversely related to gaming-related experiences ($p < 0.001$); gaming addiction ($p < 0.001$); all gaming motives ($p < 0.001$–0.016); the passion scale ($p < 0.001$); and social, emotional and behavioral problems ($p < 0.001$). Weekday and weekend play time correlated positively with all variables in both cases ($p < 0.001$–0.003) except for emotional symptoms ($p < 0.001$) and prosocial behavior ($p < 0.001$). Monthly money spent on video games correlated positively with all psychological variables ($p < 0.001$), with the exception of emotional symptoms ($p = 0.002$) and prosocial behavior ($p < 0.001$), with which it was inversely related.

Table 13 shows the linear regression analysis that identifies the game-related variables and the behavioral variables that could predict the psychological state. Although a predictor model was identified for all the variables, the explanatory capacity in some cases was very low. Therefore, it should be noted that gaming-related experiences, as well as gaming addiction, were predicted by time spent playing, money spent and academic performance. Regarding gaming motives, recreation, competition and coping were predicted by time spent, academic performance and physical activity level. Mood repair was predicted by physical activity level, academic performance and time spent on video games on the weekend. With respect to the passion scale, time spent, money spent and academic performance were found to be predictors. And attending to social, emotional and behavioral problems, academic performance, physical activity level, time and money spent on video games were predictors.

Table 12. Correlational analysis between psychological variables and gaming variables, physical activity level and academic performance.

	Physical Activity Level	Academic Performance	Time Spent (Weekdays)	Time Spent (Weekend)	Money Spent (Month)
CERV—Evasion	0.067; $p < 0.001$	−0.152; $p < 0.001$	0.546; $p < 0.001$	0.709; $p < 0.001$	0.354; $p < 0.001$
CERV—Negative consequences	0.057; $p = 0.004$	−0.194; $p < 0.001$	0.489; $p < 0.001$	0.640; $p < 0.001$	0.361; $p < 0.001$
CERV—Total	0.066; $p = 0.001$	−0.179; $p < 0.001$	0.546; $p < 0.001$	0.711; $p < 0.001$	0.376; $p < 0.001$
Gaming addiction	0.057; $p = 0.004$	−0.170; $p < 0.001$	0.531; $p < 0.001$	0.666; $p < 0.001$	0.352; $p < 0.001$
VMQ—Recreation	0.078; $p < 0.001$	0.013; $p = 0.591$	0.238; $p < 0.001$	0.464; $p < 0.001$	0.177; $p < 0.001$
VMQ—Competition	0.207; $p < 0.001$	−0.058; $p = 0.016$	0.267; $p < 0.001$	0.395; $p < 0.001$	0.217; $p < 0.001$
VMQ—Cognitive development	0.103; $p < 0.001$	−0.012; $p = 0.616$	0.275; $p < 0.001$	0.401; $p < 0.001$	0.214; $p < 0.001$
VMQ—Coping	0.058; $p = 0.004$	−0.102; $p < 0.001$	0.380; $p < 0.001$	0.535; $p < 0.001$	0.286; $p < 0.001$
VMQ—Social interaction	0.114; $p < 0.001$	−0.133; $p < 0.001$	0.295; $p < 0.001$	0.496; $p < 0.001$	0.294; $p < 0.001$
VMQ—Violent reward	0.146; $p < 0.001$	−0.158; $p < 0.001$	0.244; $p < 0.001$	0.347; $p < 0.001$	0.237; $p < 0.001$
VMQ—Customization	−0.055; $p = 0.019$	0.040; $p = 0.093$	0.188; $p < 0.001$	0.226; $p < 0.001$	0.092; $p < 0.001$
VMQ—Fantasy	−0.023; $p = 0.316$	0.001; $p = 0.952$	0.218; $p < 0.001$	0.314; $p < 0.001$	0.143; $p < 0.001$
Mood repair	0.157; $p < 0.001$	0.101; $p < 0.001$	0.029; $p = 0.145$	0.083; $p < 0.001$	0.034; $p = 0.100$
Passion scale—Harmonious	0.047; $p = 0.018$	−0.205; $p < 0.001$	0.510; $p < 0.001$	0.649; $p < 0.001$	0.336; $p < 0.001$
Passion scale—Obsessive	0.075; $p < 0.001$	−0.154; $p < 0.001$	0.520; $p < 0.001$	0.673; $p < 0.001$	0.348; $p < 0.001$
SDQ—Emotional symptoms	−0.206; $p < 0.001$	−0.093; $p < 0.001$	−0.088; $p < 0.001$	−0.187; $p < 0.001$	−0.064; $p = 0.002$
SDQ—Conduct problems	0.006; $p = 0.751$	−0.148; $p < 0.001$	0.078; $p < 0.001$	0.079; $p < 0.001$	0.071; $p < 0.001$
SDQ—Peer relationship problems	−0.049; $p = 0.014$	−0.072; $p < 0.001$	0.060; $p = 0.003$	0.008; $p = 0.709$	−0.016; $p = 0.430$
SDQ—Hyperactivity/inattention	0.104; $p < 0.001$	−0.069; $p < 0.001$	−0.008; $p = 0.707$	−0.007; $p = 0.713$	−0.010; $p = 0.617$
SDQ—Prosocial behavior	0.052; $p = 0.010$	0.133; $p < 0.001$	−0.150; $p < 0.001$	−0.151; $p < 0.001$	−0.145; $p < 0.001$

Table 13. Linear regression analysis of the psychological variables depends on gaming variables, physical activity level and academic performance.

Analysis	R^2	p	Independent Variables Included	Standardized Coefficients (B)	p
CERV—Evasion					
Model 1	0.519	<0.001	Time spent (weekend)	0.565	<0.001
			Time spent (weekdays)	0.157	<0.001
			Money spent (month)	0.089	<0.001
			Academic performance	−0.038	0.010
CERV—Negative consequences					
Model 1	0.441	<0.001	Time spent (weekend)	0.496	<0.001
			Money spent (month)	0.124	<0.001
			Time spent (weekdays)	0.127	<0.001
			Academic performance	−0.094	<0.001
CERV—Total					
Model 1	0.532	<0.001	Time spent (weekend)	0.562	<0.001
			Time spent (weekdays)	0.151	<0.001
			Money spent (month)	0.110	<0.001
			Academic performance	−0.067	<0.001
Gaming addiction					
Model 1	0.471	<0.001	Time spent (weekend)	0.502	<0.001
			Time spent (weekdays)	0.176	<0.001
			Money spent (month)	0.099	<0.001
			Academic performance	−0.069	<0.001
VMQ—Recreation					
Model 1	0.228	<0.001	Time spent (weekend)	0.474	<0.001
			Academic performance	0.070	0.001
			Physical activity level	0.049	0.023
VMQ—Competition					
Model 1	0.207	<0.001	Time spent (weekend)	0.294	<0.001
			Physical activity level	0.203	<0.001
			Time spent (weekdays)	0.113	<0.001
			Money spent (month)	0.087	<0.001
VMQ—Cognitive development					
Model 1	0.185	<0.001	Time spent (weekend)	0.321	<0.001
			Time spent (weekdays)	0.107	<0.001
			Physical activity level	0.089	<0.001
			Money spent (month)	0.083	<0.001
VMQ—Coping					
Model 1	0.299	<0.001	Time spent (weekend)	0.457	<0.001
			Money spent (month)	0.100	<0.001
			Time spent (weekdays)	0.061	0.007
VMQ—Social interaction					
Model 1	0.277	<0.001	Time spent (weekend)	0.402	<0.001
			Money spent (month)	0.137	<0.001
			Physical activity level	0.107	<0.001
			Time spent (weekdays)	0.058	0.017
			Academic performance	−0.082	<0.001
VMQ—Violent reward					
Model 1	0.174	<0.001	Time spent (weekend)	0.239	<0.001
			Physical activity level	0.144	<0.001
			Money spent (month)	0.128	<0.001
			Time spent (weekdays)	0.089	<0.001
			Academic performance	−0.124	<0.001

Table 13. *Cont.*

Analysis	R^2	*p*	Independent Variables Included	Standardized Coefficients (B)	*p*
VMQ—Customization					
Model 1	0.070	<0.001	Time spent (weekend)	0.189	<0.001
			Time spent (weekdays)	0.100	<0.001
			Academic performance	0.081	<0.001
			Physical activity level	−0.069	0.004
VMQ—Fantasy					
Model 1	0.110	<0.001	Time spent (weekend)	0.271	<0.001
			Time spent (weekdays)	0.081	0.003
			Academic performance	0.052	0.025
Mood repair					
Model 1	0.040	<0.001	Physical activity level	0.141	<0.001
			Academic performance	0.095	<0.001
			Time spent (weekend)	0.093	<0.001
Passion scale—Harmonious					
Model 1	0.451	<0.001	Time spent (weekend)	0.500	<0.001
			Time spent (weekdays)	0.156	<0.001
			Money spent (month)	0.086	<0.001
			Academic performance	−0.102	<0.001
Passion scale—Obsessive					
Model 1	0.472	<0.001	Time spent (weekend)	0.527	<0.001
			Time spent (weekdays)	0.153	<0.001
			Money spent (month)	0.097	<0.001
			Academic performance	−0.047	0.003
SDQ—Emotional symptoms					
Model 1	0.077	<0.001	Academic performance	−0.102	<0.001
			Physical activity level	−0.174	<0.001
			Time spent (weekend)	−0.188	<0.001
SDQ—Conduct problems					
Model 1	0.027	<0.001	Academic performance	−0.142	<0.001
SDQ—Peer relationship problems					
Model 1	0.010	<0.001	Time spent (weekdays)	0.087	0.001
			Academic performance	−0.056	0.008
SDQ—Hyperactivity/inattention					
Model 1	0.021	<0.001	Physical activity level	0.127	<0.001
			Academic performance	−0.089	<0.001
SDQ—Prosocial behavior					
Model 1	0.049	<0.001	Academic performance	0.103	<0.001
			Physical activity level	0.065	0.002
			Time spent (weekend)	−0.074	0.006
			Money spent (month)	−0.089	<0.001

4. Discussion

The first and second research questions that led to the present research were 'What factors related to video game use (playing time, game type, platform) show differences according to gender, closest environment, academic performance and physical activity level in adolescents?' and 'How are psychological variables related with video game use (playing time, game type, platform), gender, closest environment, academic performance and physical activity level in adolescents?' In order to answer both of these questions, the first aim was to determine the differences in the gaming variables and the psychological variables related to video games according to gender, the closest environment, academic performance and the level of physical activity.

4.1. Differences in the Gaming Variables According to Gender, Closest Environment, Academic Performance and Physical Activity Level

4.1.1. Differences in Video Game Use According to Gender

It was observed that males played more fighting, strategy, role playing, shooting and sports games, while females preferred casual and simulation games. These results are similar to previous research, which showed that males preferred competitive games, while females preferred social and simulation games [7]. This could be due to several reasons: (a) the design and marketing of video games has historically been associated with gender [73]; (b) gender differences in gaming motivations which would lead to different game genre choices [9,74]; (c) the barriers female face in accessing the video game industry and the gaming community, as well as in participating in the historical design and advertising processes [75]; or (d) that male and female gaming patterns are influenced by gender norms, social expectations and gender stereotypes [76,77]. These gender differences make it necessary to implement policies and campaigns that promote equal participation of males and females in this field.

Similarly, males prefer to play online with friends, while females play offline alone. This could also be related to the type of games and the platform used, as females are less oriented towards games that feature competition and three-dimensional rotation [78]. On the other hand, the fact that males prefer playing online with friends may help to foster the positive reinforcement of social connections [79]. The relevance of these findings is that social games, understood as those played with multiple individuals, either cooperatively or competitively, increase well-being [43,80]; and non-social games, those that are single-player and lack the elements of human interaction that are present in social games, are related differently to player well-being [81]. Thus, video games with social elements have been shown to have similar positive effects on players' social well-being [44,82]. Furthermore, socially oriented video games have been found to be associated with less problematic gaming symptoms compared to games with less or no social component [45].

4.1.2. Differences in Video Game Use According to the Closest Environment

Regarding the cohabitation of parents and the parental control of time spent, the results showed a relationship between adolescents whose parents live apart and the time spent playing video games during the week. No previous research is known to have analyzed this question in the area of video games, although previous studies examined the use of other technologies, showing that adolescents whose parents live apart exhibit addictive behaviors towards the Internet or mobile phones, in a more prevalent manner than adolescents who live with both parents [83,84]. One possible explanation for these results is that at the time of parental separation, adolescents are affected mentally and behaviorally, which can lead to addictive or unhealthy behaviors on their part [85]. In addition, the separation of parents leads them to live alternatively in two households, with their respective set of rules, which increases the likelihood that certain rules will be relaxed [86], so adolescents may have more freedom to choose what they do.

In terms of parental control, the most important finding was that constant parental control was related to a higher use of video games, which could be due to an adverse reaction to strict control, where adolescents develop a more conflictual and obsessive relationship with video games as a form of resistance [87]. In contrast, those with more flexible parental control tended to exhibit more balanced behavior, suggesting that a less restrictive approach might be more effective in managing video game use [87]. In addition, the greatest parental control was found in adolescents who partook in more online gaming with friends, while the least parental control was found in those who played offline alone. This could be because playing offline alone is associated with less problematic and addictive video game use, as compared to playing online with friends, with players exhibiting more addictive behaviors [47], which could result in parents being more concerned about play time in the latter case, resulting in increased monitoring.

4.1.3. Differences in Video Game Use According to Academic Performance

In terms of academic performance, the lowest-performing adolescents played more games during the week and on the weekend, mainly shooting and open-world games, on consoles and computers, and spent more money on games than the highest-performing adolescents. Regarding the day of play (weekday or weekend), studies on weekday play force the player to play at night, decreasing the time available for sleep [88], which is not the case when the player plays on weekends as they can better adjust their sleep hours [21,89]. Given that weekday play may lead to inadequate sleep compared to weekend play, and that a healthy circadian rhythm is crucial for well-being [90], it is likely that weekday play is worse for well-being, being associated with depressive and psychosomatic symptoms, which could affect academic performance [81,91]. Therefore, higher video game use may be associated with poorer academic performance, especially when playing on weekdays and, more specifically, before going to school [21]. This greater use of video games by adolescents with poorer academic performance may also reflect a compensatory use of video games as an escape mechanism from academic difficulties [92]. This behavior can contribute to a negative cycle, where increased play time interferes with academic performance, exacerbating school problems and reducing opportunities for educational success [22]. However, a noteworthy aspect of the results found is that adolescents with lower academic performance played shooting and open-world games to a greater extent, mainly on consoles and computers. No previous research is known that has analyzed different types of games or platforms in relation to academic performance, but these results may lead to future lines of research that analyze, to a greater extent, the type of video games and platforms played, and not only the time spent playing.

4.1.4. Differences in Video Game Use According to Physical Activity Level

In terms of the level of physical activity, it was observed that adolescents who were less physically active played more role playing, casual, simulation and open-world games, while those who were more physically active played more shooting and sport and racing games. These results are partially similar to those from previous research, in which ball sport simulators (e.g., FIFA or NBA) were found to be associated with more physical activity [5]. This may be because the use of sports video games may be associated with increased participation in real-life sports in the adolescent population [93]. On the other hand, the fact that shooting games were associated with increased physical activity may be due to the fact that more aggressive adolescents tend to engage in physical sporting activities that allow them to reduce or mitigate aggressive behavior [94], and shooting games are classified as violent games that are also related to aggression [95]. However, future research is needed to directly analyze the relationship between the type of video game played and physical activity.

The more active adolescents played more online with friends, while the less active adolescents played offline alone. Previous research has shown that physical activity increases adolescents' social relationships as they play mostly in teams and clubs, which is related to increased friendship attachment [96], and may also be extrapolated to other areas outside sport. Not surprisingly, previous research has pointed to the importance of the time spent by friends on both physical activity and the use of screens, and on the time spent on these two activities during adolescence [97].

In response to the first research question, the gaming variables that show significant differences are the type of platform and game used, as well as the form of gameplay in relation to gender; time spent playing and form of gameplay in relation to closest environment; time spent playing, platform and type of game and money spent in relation to academic performance; and type of game and form of gameplay in relation to level of physical activity.

4.2. Differences in the Psychological Variables According to Gender, Closest Environment, Academic Performance and Physical Activity Level

4.2.1. Differences in Psychological Variables According to Gender

The results showed that males have a higher problematic video game use as compared to females, especially on the dimensions of avoidance and negative consequence, as well as a higher total video game addiction score. This suggests that males may be more susceptible to developing problem behaviors in relation to video games, which is consistent with previous studies that indicated that males tend to engage more in competitive and high-risk games, which could increase their vulnerability to these problems [98]. However, this appears to be influenced by the type of game played, with violent video games showing more controversial results, highlighting that women tend to show greater anxiety associated with these games, possibly due to their lower familiarity with the game mechanics [99].

It is also noteworthy that emotional repair through the use of video games was higher in males than in females. However, this type of emotional repair may lead to negative consequences, as it could perpetuate problematic video game use if it is used as the main coping mechanism for difficult situations [100], and even more so when considering that males have higher scores on the passion scale. This suggests that video games occupy a central place in their lives, not only as a form of leisure, but as an activity that defines their identity and sense of achievement [101]. However, obsessive passion is associated with negative effects on psychological well-being, such as increased anxiety and reduced satisfaction of basic psychological and life needs [102]. These findings reinforce the need to promote the balanced use of video games to maximize their benefits and minimize their risks [103], with adolescent males being a particularly sensitive population that should be monitored in this regard.

4.2.2. Differences in the Psychological Variables According to the Closest Environment

In adolescents whose parents lived apart, mood repair was lower, while emotional and behavioral problems, specifically emotional symptoms, conduct problems and peer relationship problems, were larger, as compared to those whose parents lived together. These results suggest that a stable family environment may mitigate the negative effects associated with excessive video game use [41], through more effective emotional support, and helping adolescents to better manage stress and negative emotions, which in turn may reduce the need to turn to video games as an escape mechanism [104]. However, parents not living together was associated with adolescents showing more problematic video game use and greater emotional and behavioral problems, underlining the importance of the family context in adolescent mental health [105]. These findings suggest the need for interventions that address the family context as a key factor in adolescents' mental health and their relationship with video games [106].

In terms of parental control of time spent playing video games, a relationship was observed between always monitored adolescents and increased problematic use, game addiction and passion for video games. This finding is in line with previous research that showed that greater parental control may be related to engagement in deceptive gaming behaviors [107], as a reactive response to perceived parental control, where adolescents develop a more conflictual relationship with video games as a form of resistance [34,87]. However, adolescents with greater parental control also showed higher scores on motives for playing. This is consistent with previous research that alludes to the use of video games as a pastime or entertainment, or for forgetting worries or relaxation in this population [108]. On the other hand, it is noteworthy that adolescents who did not experience any type of control showed lower scores on mood repair, as well as higher scores on emotional symptoms. Previous research has found that minimal parental control is necessary and beneficial for the emotional well-being of adolescents, without falling into overprotection or a total absence of control [87].

4.2.3. Differences in the Psychological Variables According to Academic Performance

With regard to academic performance, lower-performing adolescents had higher problematic use and higher gaming addiction as compared to higher-performing adolescents, as well as greater passion for video games and greater emotional symptoms and behavioral problems. These results are consistent with previous research, in which addictive tendencies were negatively related to school performance [22]. One possible explanation for these results is that by spending too much time playing video games, adolescents may be reducing the time they spend on other activities such as studying or other educational activities [3]. Regarding the higher passion shown by adolescents with a lower academic performance, it is worth noting that the passion shown was obsessive. While harmonious passion could be beneficial and motivate adolescents to engage in activities in a balanced manner, obsessive passion is linked to an uncontrolled use of video games, which negatively affects their emotional and social well-being [98]. In addition, adolescents with a lower academic performance showed that one of their main motives for playing games was violent reward. This could be related to the fact that games that reward violent actions may increase aggressive behavior [109], which in turn is found to be related to lower academic performance [110].

4.2.4. Differences in the Psychological Variables According to the Physical Activity Level

Another relevant finding of the present research was that there were no significant differences in problematic video game use and gaming addiction as a function of the level of physical activity practiced, which is similar to previous research, in which no relationships were found between internet and gaming addiction and the level of physical activity of high school students [111]. However, differences were found in play motives, with adolescents who engaged in less physical activity showing less competitiveness, cognitive development, social interaction and violent reward as compared to those who engaged in moderate and vigorous play. These results suggest that physical activity may be related to a more balanced and less problematic use of video games, which may contribute to better social and cognitive adjustment [112]. In addition, adolescents with lower levels of physical activity showed greater emotional symptoms and peer relationship problems. This could indicate that a low level of physical activity may be associated with an increased risk of emotional and social problems, which is consistent with previous studies that found an inverse relationship between physical activity, and symptoms of anxiety and depression in adolescents [113]. On the other hand, adolescents with higher levels of physical activity showed a greater capacity for mood repair through play. This reinforces the idea that physical activity is not only beneficial for physical health, but also for emotional well-being, by providing adolescents with more effective tools to manage stress [114].

4.2.5. Differences in the Psychological Variables According to the Form of Play

In terms of the form of play, adolescents who play online, whether with friends or strangers, exhibit greater problematic video game use, with higher scores on avoidance and negative consequences, and a higher total score on the gaming addiction scale. These findings are consistent with previous research that suggested that online gaming, especially when performed with strangers, was associated with an increased risk of developing addictive behaviors and emotional problems [115]. However, these results are contrary to those found in previous research indicating that social games are associated with less problematic video game use compared to games that do not have a social component [45]. In terms of motives for playing video games, it was observed that adolescents who prefer to play online are mainly motivated by recreation, competition, cognitive development, coping, social interaction and violent reward-seeking. This contrasts with those who play offline, who show less motivation in these areas. Increased social interaction and competition are motives that are intrinsically linked to the satisfaction of emotional and social needs that may become dependent on the virtual environment in online gamers, which could be related to problematic video game use [116]. In addition, adolescents who play online also show greater emotional and behavioral problems, such as symptoms of anxiety and depression and difficulties in interpersonal relationships, as compared to those who play offline. This suggests that the online environment may exacerbate existing emotional difficulties or contribute to the development of new ones, given the anonymity and disinhibition that often characterize interaction in these environments [117].

In response to the second research question, significant differences were observed in problematic video game use, motives for playing, emotional repair and passion in relation to gender; in problematic video game use, game addiction, passion, mood repair, emotional and behavioral problems and problems in relationships with peers in relation to the closest environment; in problematic video game use, gaming addiction, passion and increased emotional and behavioral problems in relation to academic performance; in motives for gaming, mood repair and emotional and peer relationship problems according to physical activity level; and in problematic video game use, gaming addiction, motives for playing and emotional and behavioral problems according to the form of play.

4.3. *Influence of Gaming Variables, Academic Performance and Physical Activity Practice on Psychological Variables*

The third question posed for the research was 'What are the factors that determine psychological variables in adolescents: gaming habits, physical activity or academic performance?', and the second aim to respond to this was to determine which gaming variables and behavioral variables influence psychological variables in adolescents.

4.3.1. Influence of Gaming Variables on Psychological Variables

As for the time spent playing video games during the week and on the weekend, both factors showed the strongest relationship with all psychological variables. In fact, the correlation was positive and moderate in most of the variables, except for the motives for playing and social, emotional and behavioral problems, where the correlation was weak and negative in some of the variables (emotional symptoms and prosocial behavior). It is worth noting that the correlation shown for weekend play time was higher than that shown for weekday play time, probably due to the fact that it is on weekends that adolescents play for longer periods of time [118]. Regarding the linear regression analysis, time spent playing during the weekdays and on the weekend were shown to be the most predictive variables in all cases, with the exception of social, emotional and behavioral problems, where they were not the most determinant variables in the model. What these results indicate is that gaming time is related to psychological problems associated with video games among adolescents, as is the case with other variables such as depression and stress, probably because longer exposure time makes players more vulnerable to video game addictions, but also to internet-related addictions [119,120].

Money spent on video games showed weak positive correlations with video game-related experiences, gaming addiction, motives for playing video games and passion. In this respect, linear regression analysis showed the predictive ability of money spent on video game-related experiences, on gaming addiction, on some of the gaming motives such as competitiveness, cognitive development, coping, social interaction or violent reward and on passion. These results follow the line of previous research in which the more time and money invested in video games, the worse the mental state of the players, affecting variables such as depression, anxiety, stress or aggressiveness [31,121]. The relevance of the results lies in the fact that the money spent can be considered as a factor that is related to the gaming experience of the players.

4.3.2. Influence of Academic Performance on Psychological Variables

Academic performance correlated negatively with all psychological variables except mood repair and prosocial behavior. This seems to indicate that adolescents who perform better academically are those who have a better psychological state when playing video games, as they have less gaming addiction, less problematic use, lower scores on the passion scale and fewer social, emotional and behavioral problems. However, the correlations were weak between academic performance and these psychological variables analyzed. Regarding the linear regression analysis, the predictive capacity of academic performance on experiences related to video games, gaming addiction, gaming motives and passion is small; but on mood repair, emotional symptoms, behavioral problems and prosocial behavior, its influence is greater. These results add further evidence to previous research in which it was observed that addictive video game use could decrease academic performance [25], but the psychological state of video game use had not been analyzed with regard to the adolescent's academic performance. Therefore, these results are relevant because they show a relationship between better academic performance and lower psychological consequences of playing video games.

4.3.3. Influence of Physical Activity Practice on Psychological Variables

Physical activity level correlated positively, albeit weakly, with competitive play motives, cognitive development, social interaction and violent relationship, as well as with mood repair and hyperactivity/inattention, and correlated negatively with emotional symptoms. In fact, in the linear regression analysis, physical activity only appears as a predictor of the motives of recreation, competition, cognitive development, social interaction, violent reward and customization, as well as mood repair, emotional symptoms and hyperactivity/inattention, presenting a considerable influence on the model. These results add evidence to the existing scientific literature on the relationship between physical activity and psychological variables related to video games, as there seems to be a positive relationship between physical activity and motives to play and social, emotional and behavioral problems. This is highly relevant because it reinforces the beneficial role that video games can have on the psychological state of adolescents, since the previous literature had only shown benefits in those video games considered as active, but not in those played while sitting down [47], which are the ones analyzed in the present research.

In response to the third question, it was observed that there is a relationship between gaming habits, physical activity and academic performance and the psychological variables, with time spent playing video games being a variable that presents a high correlation with the psychological variables related to video games, although the level of physical activity, academic performance and money spent on video games should also be considered.

4.4. Limitations of the Present Study

Despite the novelty of the present research and the applicability of the results found, the present work is not without limitations. Firstly, the motivations for which participants decide to play video games have not been analyzed, which is a highly relevant aspect that may condition whether the behaviors with the game are adaptive or problematic, an aspect that the recent literature highlights as crucial for understanding their effects on well-being. Based on SDT [9], video games can have a positive impact on well-being when they satisfy the needs for autonomy, competence and social relatedness, being useful for coping with negative psychological states such as depression, suggesting that they may be promising for emotional regulation [12]; whereas when these needs are not met and the game is based on extrinsic or escapist motivations, the effects can be negative, reflected in higher anxiety, depression or life dissatisfaction [13,14]. Therefore, it is crucial to consider the motivations behind video game use, as psychological well-being can be positively or negatively affected [14,81,122]. Furthermore, video game use could displace other healthy activities such as exercise or meaningful social interactions, negatively affecting players' well-being [123,124]. In view of the above, this is an important point for future research. Secondly, the sample size of the comparison groups is not homogeneous in all comparisons. Thirdly, the cross-sectional design of this study prevents us from analyzing the change over time of the variables analyzed and there is a possibility of reverse causation as an explanation of the results. Future research needs to look at these issues longitudinally to address this limitation. Fourthly, the measurement of physical activity, based on self-reports, introduces a possible response bias. Although the sample is representative of Galicia, extrapolation to other populations should be made with caution. And fifthly, although gender differences are analyzed, this study does not fully address how gender dynamics influence the relationship between video game use and psychological outcomes.

4.5. Theoretical and Practical Implications

In terms of the recommendations derived from the results found, this study makes significant contributions in both theoretical and practical terms, reinforcing the understanding of the factors that influence the use of video games among adolescents. From a theoretical perspective, the results extend knowledge about the role of variables such as gender, social context, academic performance and physical activity in the relationship between video game use and psychosocial well-being. These findings support and complement conceptual frameworks such as SDT [9,11] by showing how psychological motivations and needs, together with contextual factors, can be related with video game use. In this line, correlational and linear regression analysis allow us to establish that behavioral factors (physical activity and academic performance) and game-related variables (time spent playing video games and money spent) predict psychological variables related to video game use. Furthermore, one of the main findings that can be observed in the present research is that it is not only the problematic or addictive use of video games that should be considered in the adolescent population. As has been shown, there are other psychological constructs and variables that show differences according to factors such as gender, closest environment, academic performance or physical activity level. Moreover, a high percentage of adolescents play video games without presenting problematic or addictive use, so the results of the present study are highly relevant and offer the possibility of carrying out future research in this area.

From a practical perspective, the results offer guidance for designing intervention strategies aimed at adolescents. In this respect, the promotion of video games with social and cooperative components, or those that promote physical activity, could maximize the psychological and social benefits while minimizing the risks associated with problematic use. Furthermore, the identification of gender differences suggests the need for tailored approaches that consider the specific preferences and dynamics of each group. Also noteworthy is the fact that a longer time of use, whether on weekdays or weekends, seems to predict changes in psychological variables related to video games, which should be considered to avoid possible negative effects on health, regardless of the game used. Finally, these findings can serve as a basis for developing digital education and training campaigns aimed at parents, educators and adolescents to understand the benefits that can be gained from video game use and to steer them away from a negative view of video games. Such campaigns could also help to encourage a more balanced and reasonable use of video games, promoting healthy practices and minimizing associated risks. This comprehensive approach has the potential to positively influence the design of public policies and educational tools, contributing to improving the well-being of adolescents in the context of a growing video game culture.

5. Conclusions

Males play more video games than females, mainly fighting, strategy, role playing, shooting and sports games, on both console and PC. In addition, they have a worse addictive and emotional response to video games, and they also show more passion and different motives for playing video games. Adolescents who have separated parents and who have more parental control over the use of video games play more video games and present higher addiction values. Therefore, the optimal parental control seems to be one in which there is no exhaustive control, nor is this control omitted. Adolescents with poorer academic performance play more shooting and open-world games; they have a higher problematic and addictive use of video games, and their emotional response is also worse. Adolescents who play shooting and sport and racing games are more physically active; there is a difference according to the level of physical activity in the motives for playing and mood repair. Adolescents who played online games, mainly with strangers, showed more problematic and addictive use, and a worse emotional response. As predictor variables in the changes in psychological state related to video games, the hours of play stand out mainly, regardless of whether they are on weekdays or weekends, although the latter seem to be even more decisive. Money spent on video games, physical activity and academic performance, although relevant, are not as important predictors of these psychological variables.

Author Contributions: Conceptualization, M.I.-F., J.M.F.-G. and M.D.D.-C.; methodology, M.I.-F., J.M.F.-G. and M.D.D.-C.; formal analysis, A.M.-O. and R.V.-C.; investigation, M.I.-F., J.M.F.-G. and M.D.D.-C.; data curation, M.I.-F. and A.M.-O.; writing—original draft preparation, M.I.-F., A.M.-O. and R.V.-C.; writing—review and editing, M.I.-F., A.M.-O. and R.V.-C.; supervision, M.I.-F. All authors have read and agreed to the published version of the manuscript.

Funding: This research received no external funding.

Institutional Review Board Statement: This study was conducted in accordance with the Declaration of Helsinki and approved by the Institutional Ethics Committee of University of Vigo (protocol CE-DCEC-UVIGO-2022-10-04-5109; 04-10-2022).

Informed Consent Statement: Informed consent was obtained from all subjects involved in this study.

Data Availability Statement: The database can be accessed through the corresponding author.

Conflicts of Interest: The authors declare no conflicts of interest.

References

1. Labrador, M.; Sánchez-Iglesias, I.; Bernaldo-de-Quirós, M.; Estupiñá, F.J.; Fernandez-Arias, I.; Vallejo-Achón, M.; Labrador, F.J. Video Game Playing and Internet Gaming Disorder: A Profile of Young Adolescents. *Int. J. Environ. Res. Public Health* **2023**, *20*, 7155. [CrossRef] [PubMed]
2. Purwaningsih, E.; Nurmala, I. The Impact of Online Game Addiction on Adolescent Mental Health: A Systematic Review and Meta-Analysis. *Open Access Maced. J. Med. Sci.* **2021**, *9*, 260–274. [CrossRef]
3. Ferguson, C.J. Do Angry Birds Make for Angry Children? A Meta-Analysis of Video Game Influences on Children's and Adolescents' Aggression, Mental Health, Prosocial Behavior, and Academic Performance. *Perspect. Psychol. Sci.* **2015**, *10*, 646–666. [CrossRef]
4. Díaz-Ruiz, R.; Aladro-Castañeda, M. Relación Entre Uso de Las Nuevas Tecnologías y Sobrepeso Infantil, Como Problema de Salud Pública. *RqR Enfermería Comunitaria* **2016**, *4*, 46–51.
5. Ng, K.; Karhulahti, V.-M.; Koskimaa, R.; Sokka, M.; Husu, P.; Kokko, S.P.; Koski, P. Associations between Physical Activity and Digital Gaming Activity among Finnish Adolescents. *Eur. J. Public Health* **2023**, *33*, ckad160.624. [CrossRef]
6. Martinez, L.; Gimenes, M.; Lambert, E. Entertainment Video Games for Academic Learning: A Systematic Review. *J. Educ. Comput. Res.* **2022**, *60*, 1083–1109. [CrossRef]
7. Leonhardt, M.; Overå, S. Are There Differences in Video Gaming and Use of Social Media among Boys and Girls?—A Mixed Methods Approach. *Int. J. Environ. Res. Public Health* **2021**, *18*, 6085. [CrossRef] [PubMed]
8. Ponce-Blandón, J.A.; Espejel-Hernández, I.; Romero-Martín, M.; Lomas-Campos, M.L.M.; Jiménez-Picón, N.; Gómez-Salgado, J. Videogame-Related Experiences among Regular Adolescent Gamers. *PLoS ONE* **2020**, *15*, e0235327. [CrossRef]
9. Ryan, R.M.; Rigby, C.S.; Przybylski, A. The Motivational Pull of Video Games: A Self-Determination Theory Approach. *Motiv. Emot.* **2006**, *30*, 344–360. [CrossRef]
10. Ryan, R.M.; Deci, E.L. Intrinsic and Extrinsic Motivation from a Self-Determination Theory Perspective: Definitions, Theory, Practices, and Future Directions. *Contemp. Educ. Psychol.* **2020**, *61*, 101860. [CrossRef]
11. Ryan, R.; Deci, E. Self-Determination Theory and the Facilitation of Intrinsic Motivation, Social Development, and Well-Being. *Am. Psychol.* **2000**, *55*, 68–78. [CrossRef]
12. Kühn, S.; Berna, F.; Lüdtke, T.; Gallinat, J.; Moritz, S. Fighting Depression: Action Video Game Play May Reduce Rumination and Increase Subjective and Objective Cognition in Depressed Patients. *Front. Psychol.* **2018**, *9*, 129. [CrossRef] [PubMed]
13. Goh, C.; Jones, C.; Copello, A. A Further Test of the Impact of Online Gaming on Psychological Wellbeing and the Role of Play Motivations and Problematic Use. *Psychiatr. Q.* **2019**, *90*, 747–760. [CrossRef]
14. von der Heiden, J.M.; Braun, B.; Müller, K.W.; Egloff, B. The Association Between Video Gaming and Psychological Functioning. *Front. Psychol.* **2019**, *10*, 1731. [CrossRef] [PubMed]
15. Che, T.; Peng, Y.; Zhou, Q.; Dickey, A.; Lai, F. The Impacts of Gamification Designs on Consumer Purchase: A Use and Gratification Theory Perspective. *Electron. Commer. Res. Appl.* **2023**, *59*, 101268. [CrossRef]

16. Li, Z.; Li, H.; Liu, X. Finer-Grained Understanding of Travel Livestreaming Adoption: A Synthetic Analysis from Uses and Gratifications Theory Perspective. *Tour. Manag. Perspect.* **2023**, *47*, 101130. [CrossRef]
17. Jang, S.; Kitchen, P.J.; Kim, J. The Effects of Gamified Customer Benefits and Characteristics on Behavioral Engagement and Purchase: Evidence from Mobile Exercise Application Uses. *J. Bus. Res.* **2018**, *92*, 250–259. [CrossRef]
18. Nouvanty, V.; Suryanto, T.; Faroqi, A. Evaluation of Uses and Gratificationson Online Otome Games. *Tek. J. Teknol. Inf. Dan Komun.* **2023**, *12*, 120–128.
19. Yu, H. Why Do People Use Metaverse? A Uses and Gratification Theory Perspective. *Telemat. Inform.* **2024**, *89*, 102110. [CrossRef]
20. Ramírez, S.; Gana, S.; Garcés, S.; Zúñiga, T.; Araya, R.; Gaete, J. Use of Technology and Its Association With Academic Performance and Life Satisfaction Among Children and Adolescents. *Front. Psychiatry* **2021**, *12*, 764054. [CrossRef]
21. Drummond, A.; Sauer, J.D. Timesplitters: Playing Video Games before (but Not after) School on Weekdays Is Associated with Poorer Adolescent Academic Performance. A Test of Competing Theoretical Accounts. *Comput. Educ.* **2020**, *144*, 103704. [CrossRef]
22. Skoric, M.M.; Teo, L.L.C.; Neo, R.L. Children and Video Games: Addiction, Engagement, and Scholastic Achievement. *CyberPsychol. Behav.* **2009**, *12*, 567–572. [CrossRef]
23. Bradley, B.J.; Greene, A.C. Do Health and Education Agencies in the United States Share Responsibility for Academic Achievement and Health? A Review of 25 Years of Evidence About the Relationship of Adolescents' Academic Achievement and Health Behaviors. *J. Adolesc. Health* **2013**, *52*, 523–532. [CrossRef] [PubMed]
24. Suvitha, S.; Kanimozhi, S.; Kanimozhi, S.; Kathiyayani, M.; Madhuri, K. Literature Review Related to Association between Mental Health and Academic Performance among Adolescents. *A V Pub Int. J. Nurs. Med. Res.* **2023**, *2*, 130–132. [CrossRef]
25. Musshafen, L.A.; Tyrone, R.S.; Abdelaziz, A.; Sims-Gomillia, C.E.; Pongetti, L.S.; Teng, F.; Fletcher, L.M.; Reneker, J.C. Associations between Sleep and Academic Performance in US Adolescents: A Systematic Review and Meta-Analysis. *Sleep. Med.* **2021**, *83*, 71–82. [CrossRef] [PubMed]
26. Chan, G.; Huo, Y.; Kelly, S.; Leung, J.; Tisdale, C.; Gullo, M. The Impact of ESports and Online Video Gaming on Lifestyle Behaviours in Youth: A Systematic Review. *Comput. Human. Behav.* **2022**, *126*, 106974. [CrossRef]
27. Huard Pelletier, V.; Lessard, A.; Piché, F.; Tétreau, C.; Descarreaux, M. Video Games and Their Associations with Physical Health: A Scoping Review. *BMJ Open Sport Exerc. Med.* **2020**, *6*, e000832. [CrossRef]
28. Kemel, P.N.; Porter, J.E.; Coombs, N. Improving Youth Physical, Mental and Social Health through Physical Activity: A Systematic Literature Review. *Health Promot. J. Aust.* **2021**, *33*, 590–601. [CrossRef]
29. Williams, W.M.; Ayres, C.G. Can Active Video Games Improve Physical Activity in Adolescents? A Review of RCT. *Int. J. Environ. Res. Public Health* **2020**, *17*, 669. [CrossRef] [PubMed]
30. Santos, I.K.d.; Medeiros, R.C.d.S.C.d.; Medeiros, J.A.d.; Almeida-Neto, P.F.d.; Sena, D.C.S.d.; Cobucci, R.N.; Oliveira, R.S.; Cabral, B.G.d.A.T.; Dantas, P.M.S. Active Video Games for Improving Mental Health and Physical Fitness—An Alternative for Children and Adolescents during Social Isolation: An Overview. *Int. J. Environ. Res. Public Health* **2021**, *18*, 1641. [CrossRef]
31. Moncada Jiménez, J.; Chacón Araya, Y. The Effect of Playing Videogames on Social, Psychological and Physiological Variables in Children and Adolescents. *Retos* **2015**, *21*, 43–49. [CrossRef]
32. Khan, A.; Burton, N.W. Electronic Games, Television, and Psychological Wellbeing of Adolescents: Mediating Role of Sleep and Physical Activity. *Int. J. Environ. Res. Public Health* **2021**, *18*, 8877. [CrossRef] [PubMed]
33. Krossbakken, E.; Pallesen, S.; Mentzoni, R.A.; King, D.L.; Molde, H.; Finserås, T.R.; Torsheim, T. A Cross-Lagged Study of Developmental Trajectories of Video Game Engagement, Addiction, and Mental Health. *Front. Psychol.* **2018**, *9*, 2239. [CrossRef]
34. Király, O.; Nagygyörgy, K.; Koronczai, B.; Griffiths, M.D.; Demetrovics, Z. The Psychological and Social Impacts of Online Gaming. *Curr. Opin. Psychol.* **2018**, *31*, 29–35. [CrossRef]
35. Chou, C.; Tsai, M.-J. Gender Differences in Taiwan High School Students' Computer Game Playing. *Comput. Human. Behav.* **2007**, *23*, 812–824. [CrossRef]
36. López-Fernández, F.J.; Mezquita, L.; Griffiths, M.D.; Ortet, G.; Ibáñez, M.I. The Role of Personality on Disordered Gaming and Game Genre Preferences in Adolescence: Gender Differences and Person-Environment Transactions. *Adicciones* **2021**, *33*, 263–272. [CrossRef]
37. Campbell, O.L.K.; Bann, D.; Patalay, P. The Gender Gap in Adolescent Mental Health: A Cross-National Investigation of 566,829 Adolescents across 73 Countries. *SSM Popul. Health* **2021**, *13*, 100742. [CrossRef] [PubMed]
38. Wilson, G.S.; Pritchard, M.E.; Revalee, B. Individual Differences in Adolescent Health Symptoms: The Effects of Gender and Coping. *J. Adolesc.* **2005**, *28*, 369–379. [CrossRef]
39. Desai, R.A.; Krishnan-Sarin, S.; Cavallo, D.; Potenza, M.N. Video-Gaming Among High School Students: Health Correlates, Gender Differences, and Problematic Gaming. *Pediatrics* **2010**, *126*, e1414–e1424. [CrossRef]
40. van Rooij, A.J.; Kuss, D.J.; Griffiths, M.D.; Shorter, G.W.; Schoenmakers, T.M.; van de Mheen, D. The (Co-)Occurrence of Problematic Video Gaming, Substance Use, and Psychosocial Problems in Adolescents. *J. Behav. Addict.* **2014**, *3*, 157–165. [CrossRef] [PubMed]
41. Schneider, L.A.; King, D.L.; Delfabbro, P.H. Family Factors in Adolescent Problematic Internet Gaming: A Systematic Review. *J. Behav. Addict.* **2017**, *6*, 321–333. [CrossRef] [PubMed]
42. Rapheal, J.; Paul, V. Significance of Home Environment in Adolescent Psychological Well-Being and Distress. *J. Indian Acad. Appl. Psychol.* **2015**, *41*, 199–205.

43. Halbrook, Y.J.; O'Donnell, A.T.; Msetfi, R.M. When and How Video Games Can Be Good: A Review of the Positive Effects of Video Games on Well-Being. *Perspect. Psychol. Sci.* **2019**, *14*, 1096–1104. [CrossRef] [PubMed]
44. Mandryk, R.L.; Frommel, J.; Armstrong, A.; Johnson, D. How Passion for Playing World of Warcraft Predicts In-Game Social Capital, Loneliness, and Wellbeing. *Front. Psychol.* **2020**, *11*, 2165. [CrossRef]
45. Colder Carras, M.; Van Rooij, A.J.; Van de Mheen, D.; Musci, R.; Xue, Q.-L.; Mendelson, T. Video Gaming in a Hyperconnected World: A Cross-Sectional Study of Heavy Gaming, Problematic Gaming Symptoms, and Online Socializing in Adolescents. *Comput. Human. Behav.* **2017**, *68*, 472–479. [CrossRef]
46. Bodi, G.; Maintenant, C.; Pennequin, V. The Role of Maladaptive Cognitions in Gaming Disorder: Differences between Online and Offline Gaming Types. *Addict. Behav.* **2021**, *112*, 106595. [CrossRef] [PubMed]
47. Smohai, M.; Urbán, R.; Griffiths, M.D.; Király, O.; Mirnics, Z.; Vargha, A.; Demetrovics, Z. Online and Offline Video Game Use in Adolescents: Measurement Invariance and Problem Severity. *Am. J. Drug Alcohol. Abus.* **2017**, *43*, 111–116. [CrossRef] [PubMed]
48. Verheijen, G.P.; Stoltz, S.E.M.J.; van den Berg, Y.H.M.; Cillessen, A.H.N. The Influence of Competitive and Cooperative Video Games on Behavior during Play and Friendship Quality in Adolescence. *Comput. Human. Behav.* **2019**, *91*, 297–304. [CrossRef]
49. Coyne, S.M.; Padilla-Walker, L.M.; Stockdale, L.; Day, R.D. Game On... Girls: Associations Between Co-Playing Video Games and Adolescent Behavioral and Family Outcomes. *J. Adolesc. Health* **2011**, *49*, 160–165. [CrossRef] [PubMed]
50. Shoshani, A.; Krauskopf, M. The Fortnite Social Paradox: The Effects of Violent-Cooperative Multi-Player Video Games on Children's Basic Psychological Needs and Prosocial Behavior. *Comput. Human. Behav.* **2021**, *116*, 106641. [CrossRef]
51. Stenseng, F.; Hygen, B.W.; Wichstrøm, L. Time Spent Gaming and Psychiatric Symptoms in Childhood: Cross-Sectional Associations and Longitudinal Effects. *Eur. Child. Adolesc. Psychiatry* **2020**, *29*, 839–847. [CrossRef] [PubMed]
52. Vandenbroucke, J.P.; von Elm, E.; Altman, D.G.; Gøtzsche, P.C.; Mulrow, C.D.; Pocock, S.J.; Poole, C.; Schlesselman, J.J.; Egger, M. Strengthening the Reporting of Observational Studies in Epidemiology (STROBE): Explanation and Elaboration. *Int. J. Surg.* **2014**, *12*, 1500–1524. [CrossRef]
53. Rodríguez del Águila, M.; González-Ramírez, A. Sample Size Calculation. *Allergol. Immunopathol.* **2014**, *42*, 485–492. [CrossRef]
54. Naing, L.; Nordin, R.B.; Abdul Rahman, H.; Naing, Y.T. Sample Size Calculation for Prevalence Studies Using Scalex and ScalaR Calculators. *BMC Med. Res. Methodol.* **2022**, *22*, 209. [CrossRef]
55. Michelini, Y.; Ibáñez, M.I.; Pilatti, A.; Bravo, A.J.; López-Fernández, F.J.; Ortet, G.; Mezquita, L. Motives to Play Videogames across Seven Countries: Measurement Invariance of the Videogaming Motives Questionnaire. *Addict. Behav.* **2023**, *140*, 107624. [CrossRef] [PubMed]
56. Olson, C.K.; Kutner, L.A.; Warner, D.E.; Almerigi, J.B.; Baer, L.; Nicholi, A.M.; Beresin, E.V. Factors Correlated with Violent Video Game Use by Adolescent Boys and Girls. *J. Adolesc. Health* **2007**, *41*, 77–83. [CrossRef] [PubMed]
57. Telama, R.; Yang, X.; Viikari, J.; Välimäki, I.; Wanne, O.; Raitakari, O. Physical Activity from Childhood to Adulthood: A 21-Year Tracking Study. *Am. J. Prev. Med.* **2005**, *28*, 267–273. [CrossRef]
58. Raitakan, O.T.; Porkka, K.; Taimela, S.; Telama, R.; Räsänen, L.A.; Vllkari, J.S. Effects of Persistent Physical Activity and Inactivity on Coronary Risk Factors in Children and Young Adults. The Cardiovascular Risk in Young Finns Study. *Am. J. Epidemiol.* **1994**, *140*, 195–205. [CrossRef]
59. Piéron, M. Análisis de La Práctica de Actividades Físico-Deportivas En Alumnos de ESO y ESPO de Las Provincias de Almería, Granada y Murcia, Por Un Índice Compuesto de Participación. *Fit. Perform. J.* **2008**, *7*, 52–58. [CrossRef]
60. Juan, F.R.; Bengoechea, E.G.; Montes, M.E.G.; Bush, P.L. Role of Individual and School Factors in Physical Activity Patterns of Secondary-Level Spanish Students. *J. Sch. Health* **2010**, *80*, 88–95. [CrossRef]
61. Chamarro, A.; Carbonell, X.; Manresa, J.M.; Munoz-Miralles, R.; Ortega-Gonzalez, R.; Lopez-Morron, M.R.; Batalla-Martinez, C.; Toran-Monserrat, P. El Cuestionario de Experiencias Relacionadas con los Videojuegos (CERV): Un instrumento para detectar el uso problemático de videojuegos en adolescentes españoles. *Adicciones* **2014**, *26*, 303–311. [CrossRef] [PubMed]
62. Lemmens, J.S.; Valkenburg, P.M.; Peter, J. Development and Validation of a Game Addiction Scale for Adolescents. *Media Psychol.* **2009**, *12*, 77–95. [CrossRef]
63. Lloret Irles, D.; Morell Gomis, R.; Marzo Campos, J.C.; Tirado González, S. Validación Española de La Escala de Adicción a Videojuegos Para Adolescentes (GASA). *Aten. Primaria* **2018**, *50*, 350–358. [CrossRef] [PubMed]
64. López-Fernández, F.J.; Mezquita, L.; Griffiths, M.D.; Ortet, G.; Ibáñez, M.I. The Development and Validation of the Videogaming Motives Questionnaire (VMQ). *PLoS ONE* **2020**, *15*, e0240726. [CrossRef] [PubMed]
65. Fernández-Berrocal, P.; Extremera, N.; Ramos, N. Validity and Reliability of the the Spanish Modified of the Trait Meta-Mood Scale 1, 2. *Psychol. Rep.* **2004**, *94*, 751–755. [CrossRef] [PubMed]
66. Marsh, H.; Vallerand, R.; Lafrenière, M.-A.; Parker, P.; Morin, A.; Carbonneau, N.; Jowett, S.; Bureau, J.; Fernet, C.; Guay, F.; et al. Passion: Does One Scale Fit All? Construct Validity of Two-Factor Passion Scale and Psychometric Invariance Over Different Activities and Languages. *Psychol. Assess.* **2013**, *25*, 796–809. [CrossRef] [PubMed]
67. Chamarro, A.; Penelo, E.; Fornieles, A.; Oberst, U.; Vallerand, R.J.; Fernández-Castro, J. Psychometric Properties of the Spanish Version of the Passion Scale. *Psicothema* **2015**, *27*, 402–409. [CrossRef]
68. Goodman, R. The Strengths and Difficulties Questionnaire: A Research Note. *J. Child Psychol. Psychiatry* **1997**, *38*, 581–586. [CrossRef]

69. Español-Martín, G.; Pagerols, M.; Prat, R.; Rivas, C.; Sixto, L.; Valero, S.; Artigas, M.S.; Ribasés, M.; Ramos-Quiroga, J.A.; Casas, M.; et al. Strengths and Difficulties Questionnaire: Psychometric Properties and Normative Data for Spanish 5- to 17-Year-Olds. *Assessment* **2020**, *28*, 1445–1458. [CrossRef] [PubMed]
70. Cramér, H. *Mathematical Methods of Statistics*; Princeton University Press: Princeton, NJ, USA, 1946.
71. Cohen, J. *Statistical Power Analysis for the Behavioral Sciences Second Edition*, 2nd ed.; Lawrence Erlbaum Associates: New York, NY, USA, 1988; ISBN 0-8058-0283-5.
72. Hopkins, W.G.; Marshall, S.W.; Batterham, A.M.; Hanin, J. Progressive Statistics for Studies in Sports Medicine and Exercise Science. *Med. Sci. Sports Exerc.* **2009**, *41*, 3–13. [CrossRef]
73. Cote, A.C. Writing "Gamers" the Gendered Construction of Gamer Identity in Nintendo Power (1994–1999). *Games Cult.* **2018**, *13*, 479–503. [CrossRef]
74. Yee, N. Motivations for Play in Online Games. *CyberPsychology Behav.* **2006**, *9*, 772–775. [CrossRef] [PubMed]
75. Robinson, J.A. "I Ain't No Girl": Exploring Gender Stereotypes in the Video Game Community. *West. J. Commun.* **2023**, *87*, 857–878. [CrossRef]
76. Kuss, D.J.; Kristensen, A.M.; Williams, A.J.; Lopez-Fernandez, O. To Be or Not to Be a Female Gamer: A Qualitative Exploration of Female Gamer Identity. *Int. J. Environ. Res. Public Health* **2022**, *19*, 1169. [CrossRef] [PubMed]
77. Ruvalcaba, O.; Shulze, J.; Kim, A.; Berzenski, S.R.; Otten, M.P. Women's Experiences in ESports: Gendered Differences in Peer and Spectator Feedback During Competitive Video Game Play. *J. Sport. Soc. Issues* **2018**, *42*, 295–311. [CrossRef]
78. Lucas, K.; Sherry, J.L. Sex Differences in Video Game Play: A Communication-Based Explanation. *Communic Res.* **2004**, *31*, 499–523. [CrossRef]
79. Wu, Y.-J.; Outley, C.; Matarrita-Cascante, D.; Murphrey, T.P. A Systematic Review of Recent Research on Adolescent Social Connectedness and Mental Health with Internet Technology Use. *Adolesc. Res. Rev.* **2016**, *1*, 153–162. [CrossRef]
80. Kowert, R.; Domahidi, E.; Festl, R.; Quandt, T. Social Gaming, Lonely Life? The Impact of Digital Game Play on Adolescents' Social Circles. *Comput. Human. Behav.* **2014**, *36*, 385–390. [CrossRef]
81. Hartanto, A.; Lua, V.Y.Q.; Quek, F.Y.X.; Yong, J.C.; Ng, M.H.S. A Critical Review on the Moderating Role of Contextual Factors in the Associations between Video Gaming and Well-Being. *Comput. Hum. Behav. Rep.* **2021**, *4*, 100135. [CrossRef]
82. Kaye, L.K.; Kowert, R.; Quinn, S. The Role of Social Identity and Online Social Capital on Psychosocial Outcomes in MMO Players. *Comput. Human. Behav.* **2017**, *74*, 215–223. [CrossRef]
83. Rejaän, Z.; van der Valk, I.E.; Branje, S. Adolescents' Belonging in Post-divorce Families: Examining Residential and Digital Contact with Mothers and Fathers. *J. Res. Adolesc.* **2024**, *34*, 568–583. [CrossRef]
84. Niu, H.; Wang, S.; Tao, Y.; Tang, Q.; Zhang, L.; Liu, X. The Association between Online Learning, Parents' Marital Status, and Internet Addiction among Adolescents during the COVID-19 Pandemic Period: A Cross-Lagged Panel Network Approach. *J. Affect. Disord.* **2023**, *333*, 553–561. [CrossRef]
85. Lucas, N.; Nicholson, J.M.; Erbas, B. Child Mental Health after Parental Separation: The Impact of Resident/Non-Resident Parenting, Parent Mental Health, Conflict and Socioeconomics. *J. Fam. Stud.* **2013**, *19*, 53–69. [CrossRef]
86. Dokter, G. How to Belong in More than One Home? A Geographical Perspective on a Sense of Belonging amongst Children of Divorce in Shared Residence in the Netherlands. Master's Thesis, Utrecht University, Utrecht, The Netherlands, 2021.
87. Wartberg, L.; Kriston, L.; Zieglmeier, M.; Lincoln, T.; Kammerl, R. A Longitudinal Study on Psychosocial Causes and Consequences of Internet Gaming Disorder in Adolescence. *Psychol. Med.* **2019**, *49*, 287–294. [CrossRef]
88. Mahmassani, H.S.; Chen, R.B.; Huang, Y.; Williams, D.; Contractor, N. Time to Play? *Transp. Res. Rec. J. Transp. Res. Board.* **2010**, *2157*, 129–137. [CrossRef]
89. Hartanto, A.; Toh, W.X.; Yang, H. Context Counts: The Different Implications of Weekday and Weekend Video Gaming for Academic Performance in Mathematics, Reading, and Science. *Comput. Educ.* **2018**, *120*, 51–63. [CrossRef]
90. Lemola, S.; Brand, S.; Vogler, N.; Perkinson-Gloor, N.; Allemand, M.; Grob, A. Habitual Computer Game Playing at Night Is Related to Depressive Symptoms. *Pers. Individ. Dif.* **2011**, *51*, 117–122. [CrossRef]
91. Hellström, C.; Nilsson, K.W.; Leppert, J.; Åslund, C. Effects of Adolescent Online Gaming Time and Motives on Depressive, Musculoskeletal, and Psychosomatic Symptoms. *Ups. J. Med. Sci.* **2015**, *120*, 263–275. [CrossRef] [PubMed]
92. King, D.L.; Potenza, M.N. Not Playing Around: Gaming Disorder in the International Classification of Diseases (ICD-11). *J. Adolesc. Health* **2019**, *64*, 5–7. [CrossRef]
93. Adachi, P.J.C.; Willoughby, T. Does Playing Sports Video Games Predict. Increased Involvement in Real-Life Sports Over Several Years Among Older Adolescents and Emerging Adults? *J. Youth Adolesc.* **2016**, *45*, 391–401. [CrossRef] [PubMed]
94. Zhu, Y.; Li, J.; Zhang, M.; Li, C.; Lau, E.Y.H.; Tao, S. Physical Activity Participation and Physical Aggression in Children and Adolescents: A Systematic Review and Meta-Analysis. *Psychol. Sport. Exerc.* **2022**, *63*, 102288. [CrossRef]
95. Dickmeis, A.; Roe, K. Genres Matter: Video Games as Predictors of Physical Aggression among Adolescents. *Communications* **2019**, *44*, 105–129. [CrossRef]
96. McGee, R.; Williams, S.; Howden-Chapman, P.; Martin, J.; Kawachi, I. Participation in Clubs and Groups from Childhood to Adolescence and Its Effects on Attachment and Self-esteem. *J. Adolesc.* **2006**, *29*, 1–17. [CrossRef] [PubMed]
97. Garcia, J.M.; Sirard, J.R.; Deutsch, N.L.; Weltman, A. The Influence of Friends and Psychosocial Factors on Physical Activity and Screen Time Behavior in Adolescents: A Mixed-Methods Analysis. *J. Behav. Med.* **2016**, *39*, 610–623. [CrossRef] [PubMed]

98. Király, O.; Nagygyörgy, K.; Griffiths, M.D.; Demetrovics, Z. Problematic Online Gaming. In *Behavioral Addictions: Criteria, Evidence, and Treatment*; Elsevier Academic Press: San Diego, CA, USA, 2014; pp. 61–97. ISBN 978-0-12-407724-9; 978-0-12-407858-1.
99. Ferguson, C.J.; Trigani, B.; Pilato, S.; Miller, S.; Foley, K.; Barr, H. Violent Video Games Don't Increase Hostility in Teens, but They Do Stress Girls Out. *Psychiatr. Q.* **2016**, *87*, 49–56. [CrossRef]
100. Przybylski, A.K.; Weinstein, N. Violent Video Game Engagement Is Not Associated with Adolescents' Aggressive Behaviour: Evidence from a Registered Report. *R. Soc. Open Sci.* **2019**, *6*, 171474. [CrossRef]
101. Rohlinger, D.A.; Sobieraj, S. *The Oxford Handbook of Digital Media Sociology*; Oxford University Press: Oxford, UK, 2022.
102. Stenseng, F.; Rise, J.; Kraft, P. The Dark Side of Leisure: Obsessive Passion and Its Covariates and Outcomes. *Leis. Stud.* **2011**, *30*, 49–62. [CrossRef]
103. Enwereuzor, I.K.; Ugwu, L.I.; Ugwu, D.I. Role of Smartphone Addiction in Gambling Passion and Schoolwork Engagement: A Dualistic Model of Passion Approach. *Asian J. Gambl. Issues Public Health* **2016**, *6*, 9. [CrossRef] [PubMed]
104. McLanahan, S.; Tach, L.; Schneider, D. The Causal Effects of Father Absence. *Annu. Rev. Sociol.* **2013**, *39*, 399–427. [CrossRef] [PubMed]
105. Obeid, S.; Al Karaki, G.; Haddad, C.; Sacre, H.; Soufia, M.; Hallit, R.; Salameh, P.; Hallit, S. Association between Parental Divorce and Mental Health Outcomes among Lebanese Adolescents: Results of a National Study. *BMC Pediatr.* **2021**, *21*, 455. [CrossRef] [PubMed]
106. Karhina, K.; Bøe, T.; Hysing, M.; Nilsen, S.A. Parental Separation, Negative Life Events and Mental Health Problems in Adolescence. *BMC Public Health* **2023**, *23*, 2364. [CrossRef] [PubMed]
107. Shin, W.; Huh, J. Parental Mediation of Teenagers' Video Game Playing: Antecedents and Consequences. *New Media Soc.* **2011**, *13*, 945–962. [CrossRef]
108. Wallenius, M.; Rimpelä, A.; Punamäki, R.-L.; Lintonen, T. Digital Game Playing Motives among Adolescents: Relations to Parent–Child Communication, School Performance, Sleeping Habits, and Perceived Health. *J. Appl. Dev. Psychol.* **2009**, *30*, 463–474. [CrossRef]
109. Carnagey, N.L.; Anderson, C.A. The Effects of Reward and Punishment in Violent Video Games on Aggressive Affect, Cognition, and Behavior. *Psychol. Sci.* **2005**, *16*, 882–889. [CrossRef]
110. Simpson, R. A Case Study of the Perceived Impact of Disruptive Behavior among Grades 9 and 11 Students on Their Academic Performance at a Corporate High School. *J. Educ.* **2022**, *5*, 28–42. [CrossRef]
111. Alagoz, N.; Keskinkilic, A. The Relationship between Internet and Game Addiction and the Levels of Physical Activity of the Secondary Education Students. *Med. Sci. Int. Med. J.* **2022**, *11*, 267. [CrossRef]
112. Biddle, S.J.H.; Asare, M. Physical Activity and Mental Health in Children and Adolescents: A Review of Reviews. *Br. J. Sports Med.* **2011**, *45*, 886–895. [CrossRef]
113. Lubans, D.; Richards, J.; Hillman, C.; Faulkner, G.; Beauchamp, M.; Nilsson, M.; Kelly, P.; Smith, J.; Raine, L.; Biddle, S. Physical Activity for Cognitive and Mental Health in Youth: A Systematic Review of Mechanisms. *Pediatrics* **2016**, *138*, e20161642. [CrossRef] [PubMed]
114. Ahn, S.; Fedewa, A.L. A Meta-Analysis of the Relationship Between Children's Physical Activity and Mental Health. *J. Pediatr. Psychol.* **2011**, *36*, 385–397. [CrossRef]
115. Huang, E.; Xing, Y.; Song, X. Emotional Analysis of Multiplayer Online Battle Arena Games Addiction. *Front. Psychol.* **2024**, *15*, 1347949. [CrossRef] [PubMed]
116. King, D.L.; Delfabbro, P.H. Internet Gaming Disorder Treatment: A Review of Definitions of Diagnosis and Treatment Outcome. *J. Clin. Psychol.* **2014**, *70*, 942–955. [CrossRef] [PubMed]
117. Suler, J. The Online Disinhibition Effect. *CyberPsychology Behav.* **2004**, *7*, 321–326. [CrossRef]
118. Gómez-Gonzalvo, F.; Molina, P.; Devís-Devís, J. Which Are the Patterns of Video Game Use in Spanish School Adolescents? Gender as a Key Factor. *Entertain. Comput.* **2020**, *34*, 100366. [CrossRef]
119. Guermazi, F.; Halouani, N.; Yaich, K.; Ennaoui, R.; Chouayakh, S.; Aloulou, J.; Amami, O. Video and Internet Gaming Addiction Among Young Adults. *Eur. Psychiatry* **2017**, *41*, S203–S204. [CrossRef]
120. Cudo, A.; Kopiś, N.; Stróżak, P.; Zapała, D. Problematic Video Gaming and Problematic Internet Use Among Polish Young Adults. *Cyberpsychol. Behav. Soc. Netw.* **2018**, *21*, 523–529. [CrossRef]
121. Li, L.; Abbey, C.; Wang, H.; Zhu, A.; Shao, T.; Dai, D.; Jin, S.; Rozelle, S. The Association between Video Game Time and Adolescent Mental Health: Evidence from Rural China. *Int. J. Environ. Res. Public Health* **2022**, *19*, 14815. [CrossRef] [PubMed]
122. Hartanto, A.; Quek, F.Y.X.; Tng, G.Y.Q.; Yong, J.C. Does Social Media Use Increase Depressive Symptoms? A Reverse Causation Perspective. *Front. Psychiatry* **2021**, *12*, 641934. [CrossRef]
123. Williams, D.; Yee, N.; Caplan, S.E. Who Plays, How Much, and Why? Debunking the Stereotypical Gamer Profile. *J. Comput.-Mediat. Commun.* **2008**, *13*, 993–1018. [CrossRef]
124. Przybylski, A.K.; Weinstein, N. A Large-Scale Test of the Goldilocks Hypothesis. *Psychol. Sci.* **2017**, *28*, 204–215. [CrossRef] [PubMed]

behavioral sciences

MDPI

Article

A Study of the Tennis Trust-Based System on the Psychology and Cognition of Amateur Tennis Enthusiasts

Fanghuan Yang and Yi-Sub Kwak *

DEU Exe-Physio Lab, Department of Physical Education, Dong-Eui University, 176, Eomgwangno, Busanjin-gu, Busan 47340, Republic of Korea
* Correspondence: ysk2003@deu.ac.kr; Tel.: +82-51-890-1546

Abstract: Currently, amateur tennis events are developing rapidly, and the trust system has become a common rule, integrating considerations of entertainment, fitness, and cost control. However, human-centered trust system rules still face some controversy, and there is limited specialized research on the topic. This study explores amateur tennis players' perceptions of the trust system rules. Using focus group discussions and interviews, we collected semi-structured interview data from 23 participants in tennis events. Based on grounded theory and the perceptual cycle model (PCM) framework, we developed a theoretical model of the tennis trust system and a model of the operational mechanism of the tennis trust system. Based on the grounded theory model results, four main factors influencing the tennis trust system were identified: interest orientation, information acquisition and judgment, communication and interaction, and development strategies. The operational mechanism model based on the PCM framework explains that the functioning of the tennis trust system includes five stages: foundation stage, trust-based emergence stage, monitor and detect stage, anticipate and respond stage, and development improvement stage. Among these stages, the anticipate and respond stage is crucial for the effectiveness of the trust system and is also the stage most prone to controversy. To address this, we propose targeted improvements to enhance the fairness of the tennis trust system and meet the needs of amateur tennis events.

Keywords: amateur tennis; trust-based; the grounded theory; the perceptual cycle model (PCM); psychology

1. Introduction

Since its inception in the late 19th century, tennis has rapidly gained worldwide popularity, becoming a significant event in important international competitions such as the Olympics and the four Grand Slam tournaments. This has greatly contributed to the popularization and development of the sport [1]. In recent years, with the rise of the national fitness movement and the increasing awareness of health, amateur tennis competitions have gradually emerged both domestically and internationally, attracting a large number of tennis enthusiasts to participate [2–4]. In China, tennis tournaments have gradually evolved from being considered "elite events" to "white-collar events" and are now increasingly becoming "popular events". The number of cities hosting tennis tournaments is steadily increasing, the scale of the events is expanding, the number of participants is rising, and the variety and categories of events are continuously diversifying [5]. Starting in 2009, the Beijing CRT China Open-level tournament has divided China into six regions, with each region selecting seven cities to host the competitions. This approach has not only promoted the development of local amateur tennis populations but also benefited the publicity of the events, thereby enhancing their visibility and influence [6]. According to the "2021 Global Tennis Report" published by the International Tennis Federation (ITF), approximately 20 million people in China participated in tennis (playing at least once a year) in 2020, making it the country with the second-highest number of tennis participants in the world [7]. However, ensuring fairness in these competitions remains an urgent issue that needs to be addressed.

In tennis matches, referees play a crucial role in ensuring fair play and making decisions based on the rules. One key aspect of their role is making calls on whether the ball is in or out, which is also the area most prone to disputes. At critical moments in a match, such as during an advantage, deuce, or match point, an incorrect call can result in losing a point, a game, a set, or even the entire match [8]. Such errors can also affect a player's performance [9]. However, in actual matches, referees are prone to making incorrect calls due to the inherent limitations of their cognitive and sensory abilities, as well as various potential biases that may influence their judgment [10]. Research indicates that sports referees' decisions are influenced by their individual prior knowledge and values, early experiences, training, and cognitive factors [11]. In summary, the accuracy of decisions in a match is considered crucial for the integrity of the sport. However, in many cases, human-driven judgments do not always provide reliable results [12]. Some scandals involving human referees and other negative influences have threatened the legitimacy of human officiating in sports. Although existing studies have provided interpretations of referees' decision-making in officiating, these studies primarily focus on how various factors affect the accuracy of referees' decisions [13,14]. However, there is still a lack of in-depth and systematic exploration regarding the core issue of how referees make decisions to ensure the fairness of competitions. The decision-making mechanisms of referees remain in a 'cognitive black box', and public doubts and controversies about the fairness of referees' judgments remain unresolved.

To overcome issues of subjectivity and bias in refereeing and to improve objectivity and accuracy, electronic systems assisting referees have been widely adopted in competitive sports since the mid-1990s. Currently, the application of artificial intelligence technology in the field of sports refereeing has demonstrated immense potential for development, particularly in terms of revolutionizing the precision of rule enforcement and decision-making in competitive sports. In tennis, the introduction of the challenge system using artificial intelligence began in 2006 [15]. Artificial intelligence, in the form of video assistant referee (VAR), is used in tennis just as it is in other ball sports [16]. Among these technologies, Hawk-Eye [17] has achieved an accuracy of 2.6 mm [18]. By combining this with AI software designed for high-speed sports like badminton, it can be effectively applied to tennis [19]. Such systems have the potential to bypass the limitations of human perception and cognition by combining artificial intelligence technologies to support (or even replace) human judgment. This can help counteract or eliminate biases in officiating [20]. From the spectators' perspective, using various electronic systems to reduce the impact of human factors on officiating can enhance the quality of the matches, make the game easier to understand, and provide real-time feedback that adds excitement for the audience [21]. The development and advancement of any technology have their dual nature. The integration of artificial intelligence into sports officiating not only receives praise for promoting fairness in sports and enhancing the accuracy of officiating but also sparks considerable controversy. Some even argue that intelligent officiating systems, such as VAR, are the 'killers' of sports enthusiasm [14,22]. The precision of AI has eliminated redundancies in rules, which has led to increasing rigidity of the rules themselves, becoming a point of controversy and a challenge to resolve. With AI intervention, aspects that were previously imperceptible to the human eye are now measured with millimeter-level accuracy, leaving no substantive gap between the rules and practical standards. This has resulted in a rise in calls such as fouls, invalid goals, and out-of-bounds plays. These changes have sparked discussions about the purpose of rules and prompted reflection on whether we can accept such transformations [23].

This controversy is particularly evident in professional events; however, in amateur competitions, the issues become even more complex. Most tennis events currently cater to amateur players [24]. In amateur tournaments, especially in terms of officiating and dispute resolution, the lack of professional referees and high-tech equipment means that decisions often rely on the participants' self-judgment and negotiation. This raises a critical question: How can fairness in officiating and the smooth progression of matches be ensured in amateur competitions that lack technological tools like artificial intelligence? At this point, the role of trust in sports becomes evident. The conduct of sports activities is built on trust, which is a universally present characteristic, particularly between athletes and between athletes and coaches [25]. In competitive sports, trust is an indispensable element, influenced by three main factors: interdependence, risk, and uncertainty. Trust is prevalent between athletes, between athletes and coaches, between captains and team leaders, and between teams. In the process of sports training, interpersonal trust is far more important than competition against each other [26]. In this context, tennis matches often use a system known as the "trust-based system", where each player acts as a referee for the opponent. In cases where the judgment of ball placement is inaccurate or ambiguous, the decision is based on the receiving player's opinion. Therefore, for some unclear calls, the verbal statements of the players become the basis for the ruling [27]. The core principle of the trust-based system is based on mutual trust and respect among participants, aiming to ensure fairness and justice in the match through self-management and self-discipline [28]. However, timely, accurate, and reliable decisions require more experienced officials [29]. Research shows that under time pressure, the combination of situational priors and dynamic environmental background information jointly influences athletes' judgment and decision-making [30]. Although the trust-based system has many advantages in amateur tennis tournaments, it also faces some issues and challenges in practice. Some participants may act dishonestly due to match pressure or competitive psychology, which can affect the fairness and integrity of the competition. Without a referee, the trust-based system lacks an effective dispute-resolution mechanism, which can lead to prolonged arguments and dissatisfaction during the match [31]. In summary, the trust-based system is more suitable for informal matches such as friendly games and practice sessions. Its effectiveness and feasibility in highly competitive and influential matches remain to be further validated.

Given the potential application value of the trust-based system in amateur tennis events, this study aims to explore a preliminary theoretical model. The study is based on qualitative research using grounded theory. Additionally, it addresses the issues encountered in practical operations. The goal is to provide more information on the scientific and effective application of the trust-based system in amateur tennis tournaments.

2. Methodology

2.1. Model Theory

2.1.1. Grounded Theory

The grounded theory is a qualitative research method proposed by Glaser and Strauss in 1967. It involves the systematic collection and analysis of data to generate theory. The central idea is to allow the theory to be grounded in the data [32]. Unlike traditional research methods, the grounded theory emphasizes deriving theories from actual data rather than starting with a theory and then verifying it with data. During the research process, researchers conduct detailed analysis through constant comparison and open coding, identifying initial concepts and filtering out core concepts from a large amount of data, ultimately constructing a theory [33]. The study aims to explore the mechanisms and future development directions of the trust-based system in tennis based on the grounded theory. It divides the coding process into three levels: open coding, axial coding, and selective coding. Open coding requires researchers to approach the collected raw data without any subjective bias or theoretical preconceptions and, with an open mind, conduct preliminary coding to identify concepts and categories that reflect social phenomena in the investigation [34]. Axial coding, through inductive and deductive analysis, involves constant comparative analysis to deeply explore relationships between categories, leading to more abstract insights and identifying core categories [35]. Selective coding is the final phase of data analysis, where the relationships between core categories and main categories are determined through integration and refinement, thus organizing the storyline between core categories and constructing the theoretical framework [36].

2.1.2. Perceptual Cycle Model

The perceptual cycle model (PCM) is a cognitive model developed by Ulric Neisser in 1976 to explain how perception, action, and the environment interact dynamically in human cognition [37]. The model illustrates how individuals actively seek information from their environment to guide their actions and how these actions, in turn, influence their perception. The PCM emphasizes the cyclical and continuous nature of this process, where perception and action are interdependent and constantly influence each other. The PCM emphasizes the dynamic interaction between perception, action, and the environment, which is closely related to the decision-making mechanisms of amateur tennis referees in complex and uncertain match situations. Referees' decisions not only rely on current perceptual information but also involve drawing on past experiences and anticipating future situations. These characteristics align well with the research objective, which is to explore how referees make quick judgments and responses through a trust-based system during matches.

2.1.3. Theoretical Framework

This study combines grounded theory and the PCM to explore the operational mechanisms of the trust-based refereeing system in amateur tennis matches. The trust-based refereeing system refers to situations where, in the case of ambiguous ball placement, the receiving player's judgment becomes the final ruling. The purpose of this research is to reveal how athletes make decisions based on mutual trust within this system.

Through the continuous comparative analysis of grounded theory, this study identifies the core factors of trust from athletes' actual match data, uncovering how they establish, maintain, and adjust trust in their opponents throughout the game. Meanwhile, the perceptual cycle model provides a cognitive framework for explaining the dynamic nature of trust, showing how athletes make quick judgments and take action based on environmental perception, past experiences, and trust in their opponents in ever-changing match situations.

The grounded theory and the PCM model form a complementary relationship in explaining trust-based systems (Figure 1). Grounded theory employs a bottom-up data analysis approach to reveal how participants build trust through interaction and negotiation during competitions. In contrast, the PCM model offers a cognitive-level explanation, demonstrating how participants adapt to the dynamic nature of the competition through continuous perception, feedback, and response. While grounded theory emphasizes the induction of behaviors and experiences, the PCM model supplements this by elucidating the cognitive mechanisms underlying those behaviors, helping to explain how participants make judgments, adjustments, and responses within a trust framework. In this refereeing system, trust is not just a static judgment criterion; it is a dynamic process that evolves throughout the game, influenced by multiple factors such as the match stage, score differences, and interactions between athletes. By integrating these two theories, this study not only reveals the crucial role of trust in ambiguous officiating decisions but also explores how this trust-based refereeing system impacts the fairness of amateur tennis matches and athletes' behavioral responses.

2.2. Participants

The essence of the grounded theory research model is that theory is directly extracted from actual data rather than relying on a priori assumptions. This method typically employs semi-structured interviews using sampling techniques, and there is no strict requirement for the sample size. However, research indicates that a sample size of 20 to 30 interviewees is generally reasonable [38]. Therefore, based on the research objective of the tennis trust-based system, this study employed purposive sampling and randomly selected 23 amateur tennis enthusiasts from various tennis event venues in Fuzhou, China, for interviews and focus group discussions. The participants included a diverse group of individuals, including members from various industries' elite groups. When discussing their socioeconomic status and its impact on their sports participation, opportunities, and experiences, the athletes expressed different viewpoints. Among them, the average age was 45.6 years, encompassing a variety of professions. Specific details are available in Table 1. Each participant signed an informed consent form and received a CNY 10 reward.

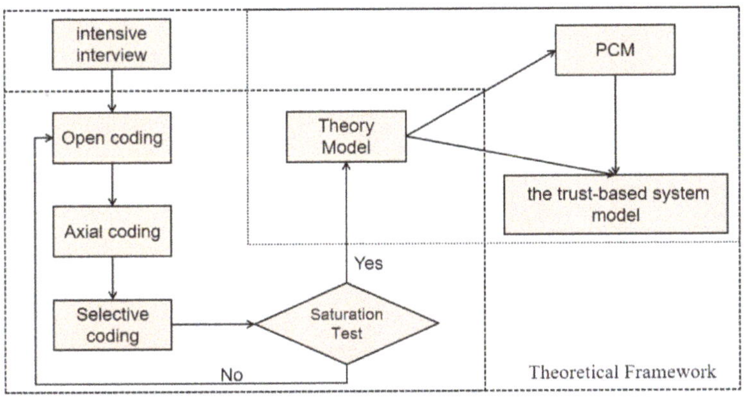

Figure 1. Theoretical framework.

Table 1. Summary statistics of demographic variables.

Variables	N	%
Gender		
Male	18	78.3
Female	5	21.7
Age		
18–30	2	8.7
31–40	6	26.1
41–50	10	43.5
50–65	5	21.7
Tennis experience		
3–5 years	2	8.7
6–10 years	15	65.2
10–20 years	6	26.1
Occupation		
Professor	6	26.1
PE teacher	5	21.7
Administrative agent	3	13.1
National tennis umpire	1	4.3
Others	8	34.8

2.3. Interview Design and Data Collection

To ensure the validity of the survey results, preliminary interviews were conducted before formal interviews, and the interview outline was modified based on the effectiveness of these preliminary discussions. During the formal interviews, all participants underwent concentrated semi-structured interviews, which relied on open-ended questions as a technique, emphasizing participants' experiences and their understanding of the tennis trust-based system [39]. Each participant's interview lasted between half an hour and one hour, totaling 23 interviews conducted. Additionally, considering the iterative nature of the coding process in the grounded theory, further exploration was conducted in subsequent stages to understand participants' social status and other background factors. This included aspects such as participants' professions, family perspectives on tennis, and phenomena related to parent–child tennis activities. The final interview outline can be found in Table 2.

Table 2. Semi-structured interview outline.

No.	Question
1	How did you get into the sport of tennis?
2	Do you think you're playing tennis to get something?
3	Have you ever played in an amateur tennis tournament? What are some of the things that matter to you during a tournament?
4	Have there been any disputes with opponents or referees during a match? What was the reason for each dispute, and did it affect your pace of play?
5	Tell us your thoughts or knowledge about the Tennis Trust-based System.
6	What do you think of rules like the Tennis Trust-based System?
7	Under the rules of the Tennis Trust-based System, describe your entire playing experience, including movements and mental swings.
8	Any other suggestions for the future of the Tennis Trust-based System?

We conducted semi-structured 1-on-1 interviews, recording all interview conversations through audio and transcribing them verbatim into textual materials. The final textual materials were uploaded into NVivo 13 software for analysis and coding [40].

2.4. Model Development

We employed a constructivist grounded theory approach and utilized multiple analytical tools during the model development process [41]. Firstly, we conducted an in-depth analysis of the 23 interviews using primary coding and focused coding. Primary coding was used to explore concise and direct initial concepts, while focused coding further deepened the theory by comparing and contrasting differences between various codes and identifying directions for further exploration. The constant comparison technique was applied throughout the coding process. This technique helped identify similarities and differences between data codes. It included comparisons among participants as well as between the researchers' and participants' viewpoints [42].

Secondly, theoretical sampling was used to support the development of the theory. This method does not aim to increase the number of participants but rather to refine and develop theoretical concepts through iterative interviews and a literature review, redirecting, developing, and refining theoretical concepts [43]. In addition, memos played a crucial role in the category establishment and concept extraction stages, helping to describe the characteristics and conditions of categories and allowing for comparisons between categories. The use of theoretical sampling detailed and refined the developing categories, explored new theoretical interpretations through further interviews, and ultimately formed coherent theoretical models. For example, in this study, concerns about the tennis trust-based system were reported by participants. At this stage, theoretical sampling could be employed to select participants who have expressed controversies related to the trust-based system for inclusion in the investigation. These methods together form a flexible research framework that emphasizes deep theoretical development and interaction between participants and researchers [44].

Finally, using the three-level coding process of the grounded theory, we analyzed the logical relationships between primary categories and core categories. Through saturation testing (checking for the presence of new concepts or categories), we constructed the initial theoretical model of the tennis trust-based system, represented the developed theory using diagrams and charts [44]. Based on the coding derived from the grounded theory, we used the PCM to construct a trust mechanism model, explaining the reciprocal relationship between perception and action in the trust-based system. This approach highlights how humans actively construct their understanding of the world through continuous interaction with their environment.

3. Results

In the analysis of the results, we focused on the theoretical model constructed using the three-level coding of the grounded theory. Additionally, we developed a stage model based on the operational process of the tennis trust-based system rules to illustrate the influencing factors and mechanisms of operation of these rules.

3.1. Encoding Results

We systematically analyzed the interview transcripts to summarize new concepts and categories related to the trust-based system in tennis, using participants' responses as the basis for open coding. For instance, one participant's statement, "I have loved watching tennis matches since I was a child; tennis has always been my favorite sport, and I play almost every week", reflects a long-standing passion for tennis and ongoing engagement with the sport as a hobby. Therefore, this response was categorized as a passion for tennis. By repeating this process, we identified a total of 28 concepts through open coding. We conducted an in-depth analysis of the differences and similarities among these concepts, restructured initial concepts, and developed relationships between concepts. This process yielded eight axial codes representing secondary categories. Building upon the secondary concepts, this study conducted an internal analysis of the eight core concepts, refining them into four primary core categories that reflect the characteristics of the tennis trust-based system.

The development of the tennis trust-based system was primarily characterized by interest-driven, information acquisition and judgment, interactive communication, and development strategy. Interest-driven formed the fundamental premise for amateur tennis enthusiasts adopting the trust-based system, involving the enjoyment derived from recreational hobbies and competitive entertainment. The assessment of subjective and objective information in tennis competitions constituted the core content of the trust-based system, specifically in terms of information acquisition and judgment. This directly influenced the rationality and contentiousness of rule application, while interactive communication involved feedback and acceptance, encompassing psychological aspects and stress. The introduction of the trust-based system concept was a form of communication between opponents in competitive matches characterized by psychological and social dimensions.

Finally, we summarized the strategies for the development of the trust-based system, highlighting its advantages, such as cost reduction and efficiency improvement. However, we also acknowledged its potential for controversy and identified certain limitations. To validate the coherence of the grounded theory model results, we conducted theoretical saturation testing on 3 out of the 23 transcripts. No new concepts or categories were identified, confirming the model's inclusiveness and enhancing its credibility. The final conceptual model is presented in Table 3.

Table 3. The three-stage coding results for grounded theory.

Open Coding	Axial Coding	Selective Coding
Like to watch professional tennis matches	Recreational hobbies	Interest-driven
Passion for tennis		
Enjoy the competition	Competitive entertainment	
Gain a sense of accomplishment		
Monitoring of the playing field	Objective information	Information acquisition and judgment
Observe where the tennis ball lands		
Observe the opponent's movements		
Observe the referee's hand signals	Subjective information	
Subjective judgment of where the ball lands		

Table 3. *Cont.*

Open Coding	Axial Coding	Selective Coding
Communicating penalties with opponents	Feedback and acceptance	Interactive communication
Negotiation of the disputed ball		
Acceptance of opponent's penalty		
Communication and interpretation of penalties		
Strengthening trust among players		
Dissatisfaction with or challenge of penalties		
Increased interaction between players		
Eliminates subjective misjudgments by referees		
Athletic ethics	Psychology and stress	
Psychological factors (tension, stress)		
Penalties at key moments of the game		
Reducing the cost of competition	Dominance	Development strategy
Improving the efficiency of the game		
Promotion and popularization of tennis		
Favorable to exploring innovative approaches		
Lack of credibility and seriousness	Technology standard	
Lack of harmonized implementation standards		
Lack of technical support		
Unclear rules		
Easy to misjudge		

3.2. *A Mechanistic Model of the Trust-Based System*

Based on the coding results from grounded theory and integrating the PCM perception–action process, we constructed a tennis trust-based system model. This model outlined the understanding mechanism of the tennis trust-based system across five stages (Figure 2), including the foundation stage, trust-based emergence stage, monitor and detect stage, anticipate and respond stage, and development improvement stage.

3.2.1. Foundation Stage

The rise of any sports event is closely tied to its professionalization, which attracts more amateur enthusiasts to participate in the sport [45]. The emergence of the trust-based system in tennis indeed addresses the challenges of officiating in amateur events. It relies on the collective agreement of a sufficient number of participants to gain recognition for these new rules. This principle mirrors the collaborative spirit seen in various community-driven projects where consensus and widespread participation are crucial for success, much like your approach to involving diverse perspectives in your projects. In focus groups and discussions, participants have expressed their interest in tennis, highlighting how their passion drives them to participate in amateur events. This interest-driven forms a solid foundation for the emergence of the tennis trust-based system rules in competitive settings.

Interest-driven primarily encompasses two aspects: recreational hobbies and competitive entertainment. At the recreational hobbies level, tennis is seen as an activity that promotes health and social interaction. Participants typically engage in it to enjoy the pleasure of the game and to relax both mentally and physically. During this stage, players cultivate a fundamental understanding of tennis rules and skills through informal matches and friendly competition. Simultaneously, they build confidence in their abilities and trust in fair competition among others. At the competitive entertainment level, while participants still prioritize enjoyment, the competitive nature of the matches and the demand for skill gradually increase. During this stage, players begin participating in club tournaments and local events, aiming to enhance their technical skills and mental resilience through more challenging competitions. They experience a sense of achievement and team spirit within the competitive environment. Some participants expressed, *"I often follow professional tennis tournaments such as Grand Slams, ATP, and WTA tours. By watching top players' matches, I can learn their techniques and tactics, gaining deeper insights into the strategies and mental battles behind the game. This not only helps me improve my own game level but also increases my passion and dedication to the sport."* (P1). The development of professional tournaments has sparked enthusiasm among amateur players. Similarly, the evolution of amateur competition has also heightened everyone's interest in tennis. *"Participating in tournaments is a significant challenge and opportunity for me. Each match not only tests my skills and strategies but also allows me to continually improve in competition. Regardless of the outcome, every experience brings a sense of achievement and satisfaction, motivating me to love and dedicate myself more to this sport."* (P3).

Therefore, tennis, as both a recreational hobby and a competitive sport, forms the foundation stage of the development of the tennis trust-based system. This lays a solid groundwork for further promoting and advancing the sport.

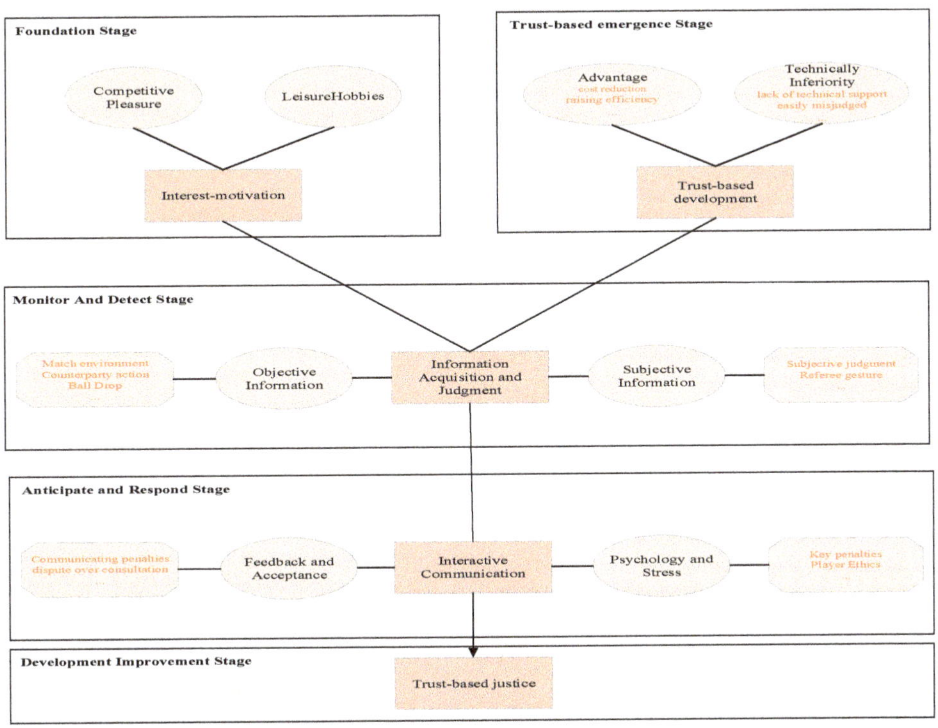

Figure 2. A mechanistic model of the trust-based system.

3.2.2. Trust-Based Emergence Stage

The trust-based emergence stage primarily explains the surge in amateur tennis events due to the increasing number of tennis enthusiasts. However, due to factors such as costs and facility technology, advanced AI technologies like Hawk-Eye used in professional tournaments may not be available. This could lead to contested calls, potentially influencing match outcomes. We analyzed the advantages and some disadvantages of the emergence of the trust-based system at this stage.

The emergence of the tennis trust-based system can reduce competition costs and improve efficiency, thereby addressing, to some extent, the adjudication issues in most non-professional tennis events. Amateur players discussed the advantages of the trust-based system in tennis matches, which are crucial for promoting this rule and even the sport itself. *"In many amateur matches, we rely on self-regulation and integrity to abide by the rules, which not only simplifies the adjudication process but also strengthens mutual trust."* (P11). With the gradual implementation of the trust-based system in tennis matches, players have experienced a more challenging way of competing. This model not only promotes the development of tennis but also provides new ideas and insights for other sports. Through innovative practices in trust-based tennis competition models, it is possible to explore and discover more innovative ways to further enrich and improve competition formats. *"I believe that the rules of the tennis trust-based system not only ensure fair competition and sportsmanship but also provide opportunities to explore innovative ways. Through self-regulation and fair play, we can simplify management procedures and improve the efficiency of competitions. At the same time, this trust-based system encourages us to try new strategies and techniques during matches, promoting continuous progress and innovation both individually and across the sport."* (P16).

It is worth noting that despite the many benefits of the tennis trust-based system for amateur events, it also faces certain issues, such as ambiguous rules, susceptibility to errors in judgment, and the potential for subjective bias in rulings. *"Due to the lack of official referees, there is a tendency for errors and disputes to arise during matches. As players, we may sometimes disagree due to differing perspectives."* (P12). *"Some rules of the trust-based system may be somewhat ambiguous, leading to inconsistency in their enforcement. This can easily affect the fairness of the competition and our overall tournament experience."* (P19).

Participants' reports explain that the emergence of the tennis trust-based system has, to some extent, resolved controversies in amateur tournaments, but they have also raised some objections and expressed concerns about the trust-based system. By continuously refining and adjusting the trust-based system, we can gradually reduce these issues and enhance the overall fairness and enjoyment of the matches.

3.2.3. Monitor and Detect Stage

We define the "monitor and detect stage" as the phase where players in tennis matches observe their opponents' strokes, referee gestures, and the court environment. This stage precedes the implementation of the tennis trust-based system and involves players gathering anticipatory information about officiating decisions. Monitor refers to the monitoring of the entire court environment, while detect focuses on observing the action of the ball touching the ground.

When applying the trust-based system, players rely on their own experience in sports practice to judge the landing point of the tennis ball. *"During the match, I pay attention to observing the surrounding environment, especially conditions like wind speed and lighting, which directly affect my judgment of the ball's landing point."* (P10). Especially in non-professional matches without referees, participants are very concerned about whether the ball is out of bounds, particularly regarding the trajectory of the ball. *"In our matches, referees are often absent, so we have to rely on our own observations to quickly judge the ball's trajectory to maintain fairness in the game."* (P19). The monitor and detect stage explains how trust-based tennis rules affect players' judgment during implementation. It elucidates how players rely on self-monitoring and detection in matches to uphold fairness and the spirit of competition.

3.2.4. Anticipate and Respond Stage

The "anticipate and respond stage" occurs during the implementation of the trust-based tennis rules, where players anticipate the tennis ball about to land on the court and react to whether the ball stays within the boundaries, revealing the interactive nature of the trust-based tennis rules.

In this study, amateur tennis enthusiasts reported on their responses and feedback during the implementation of trust-based rules, including the psychological pressures and stress, controversies over critical judgment moments, the role of players' ethical standards, and the acceptance or questioning of opponents' judgment outcomes. *"Indeed, in trust-based tennis, disputes can arise at times. Without referees present, we rely on our own eyes and integrity to judge whether the ball is out or in the valid area. In such situations, disagreements may occur due to differing perspectives, especially at crucial moments determining the outcome."* (P20). If trust-based systems are not applied effectively, they can also have adverse effects on the players. *"This system also brings us quite a bit of psychological fluctuations. We tend to favor rulings in our own favor. Sometimes, even though the ball clearly landed within the court boundaries, opponents claim it's out. It really affects my mood, and it's frustrating. I hope there will be more auxiliary technologies to solve this problem."* (P13).

Additionally, at this stage, the impact of the trust-based system is more reflected in the interaction between the players. At this point, mutual trust, values, and familiarity levels become crucial, and the acceptance of each other's rulings will directly reflect this interaction. *"In this trust-based tennis competition, I prefer to compete with friends whom I know rather than trusting strangers. After all, people tend to have their own interests, especially when dealing with someone unfamiliar."* (P7). A more critical point is that existing amateur competitions, especially youth tournaments, may involve interests and honors, which can make such rules more biased. *"I have previously served as a referee in youth tournaments and have encountered some disputes among players, especially in qualification and group stages where there are no referees. Under the trust-based rules, everyone tends to favor themselves, even arguing over each point with their opponents because it involves their own interests. This is an inevitable phenomenon in these rules."* (P5).

In tennis matches, it is understandable that both players seek their own interests, leading to occasional disputes. In the anticipate and respond stage of tennis matches, participants continuously engage in communication and negotiate the outcomes of rulings with their opponents. While participants express a desire for friendly exchanges and hope for better technology to assist in making rulings, the trust-based system persists in the long term due to cost considerations and other factors. Thus, interactive feedback and communication between both sides remain inevitable in tennis competitions.

3.2.5. Development Improvement Stage

The trust-based system in tennis has a significant impact and challenge on the fairness of the game. This system emphasizes self-monitoring and integrity among players, motivating them to maintain high levels of focus and responsibility during matches, ensuring that every decision aligns with the rules of the competition. However, the lack of formal referees can lead to biases and disputes in judgment, especially in crucial moments. Therefore, players need to possess excellent judgment skills and maintain a calm demeanor to address these challenges, ensuring the fairness of the game and upholding the spirit of fair competition.

We focused on a professional tennis referee, aiming to understand the development trends of the tennis trust-based system through his years of adjudication experience. *"There is indeed room for improvement in the rules of the tennis trust-based system. To enhance its fairness and operational clarity, clearer and more specific game rules and standards could be established, especially regarding criteria for determining whether a ball is out of bounds. Additionally, systematic participant training and education can improve players' judgment and discipline. Utilizing technological tools such as video replays can reduce errors and disputes. Importantly, fostering a positive competitive culture and community atmosphere that emphasizes integrity and fair play will encourage players to conscientiously adhere to the trust-based system. These improvement measures can enhance the tennis trust-based system, making it more robust and sustainable, thereby providing better support for the conduct of matches and the experience of participants."* (P5, National Tennis umpire). Some participants also expressed concerns, *"In tense score situations, opponents often tend to favor their own judgments, which is truly infuriating."* (P14).

The trust-based system fundamentally relies on human judgment, transitioning from third-party referees to mutual adjudication between the players themselves, inevitably leading to some controversy. Both professional referees and amateur tennis enthusiasts have voiced concerns about this rule. Moving forward, improvements to the trust-based system rules will need to address ethical, psychological, and educational aspects.

4. Discussion

4.1. Implications for Theory

The 'trust-based system', derived from a culture of mutual respect, equality, and sportsmanship in tennis, evoked deep admiration. In these rules, players completely delegated the responsibility of determining whether their shots were in or out to their opponents, maintaining 'absolute trust' in them. This practice not only distinguished tennis from other sports but also highlighted its unique emphasis on gentlemanly conduct. The trust-based system was not just a 'code of conduct'; it also carried an expectation that compared to winning or losing, 'sportsmanship' and 'integrity' were more significant. This study conducted interviews and analyzed focus group discussions with 23 amateur tennis enthusiasts to explore their understanding and opinions on the tennis trust-based system rules. Participants included university professors, professional tennis referees, government officials, and sports teachers, reflecting on the operational mechanisms of the trust-based system in various amateur settings.

Firstly, based on the grounded theory, we analyzed four key factors of the tennis trust-based system rules: interest-driven, information acquisition and judgment, interactive communication, and development strategy. The open-ended results of grounded theory demonstrated that interest-driven factors have facilitated the development of amateur tennis, especially in economically developed regions. Tennis, once seen as an exclusive sport, has become more accessible due to its simplicity and health benefits. This accessibility has made tennis attractive and encourages competition across different ages, genders, and skill levels, transforming it into a comprehensive sport [46]. As amateur tennis competitions continue to evolve, the trust-based system is gradually taking the lead [24]. This required participants to exert greater effort, akin to the information acquisition and judgment categories outlined by grounded theory. They need to pay closer attention to the court environment to effectively implement this system and ensure fairness. Despite this, the trust-based system can reduce the cost of organizing competitions and improve efficiency [28]. However, the core of the trust-based system remains the interaction between the players themselves, representing a human-centric adjudication rule similar to referee judgments. Due to various human biases and factors, human-based judgments are prone to errors [47]. Additionally, the vulnerability of the trust system can lead to difficulty in decision-making for participants in complex situations. When faced with high levels of uncertainty or emotional pressure, participants may exhibit biases in their trust judgments, which can affect their behavior and decision-making. In a competitive environment, particularly for players with a strong desire to win, relying on a trust-based system for officiating presented a psychological challenge. Such a system required players to remain calm during tense moments and respect their opponents' judgments, which had varying effects on players from different backgrounds. Experienced players, especially those with considerable competitive experience, had higher expectations regarding the fairness of the officiating system, making them more likely to doubt or distrust it during critical moments. This psychological state weakened their adherence to the trust-based system, especially when decisions went against them; they were more inclined to question their opponents' judgments, potentially leading to disputes. In contrast, less experienced amateur players might have been more inclined to adhere to the trust-based system. For them, maintaining trust and sportsmanship was often more important in their competition experiences, and the pressure of winning was relatively lower. As a result, these players were generally more accepting of their opponents' judgments, even if there were occasional misjudgments. This differing emphasis on competition could have significantly influenced how players perceived and committed to the trust-based system.

Secondly, based on the coding results of the grounded theory, we adapted the basic framework of PCM, constructing a model of the operational mechanisms of the tennis trust-based system. This model aimed to capture the environmental conditions of specific scenarios and suggests how participants can interpret them to inform their actions and decisions [48]. We divided the tennis trust-based system into five stages. The first stage was the foundational stage, where amateur tennis enthusiasts joined the sport due to interests, hobbies, leisure, and other means. The next stage was the emergence of the trust-based system, where the increasing number of participants and objective conditions facilitated the effective resolution of issues through this system. Following that was the monitoring and detection stage. During matches, participants needed to continuously adjust their relationship with the external environment before applying these rules to ensure proper implementation and fairness. Furthermore, there was the anticipation and response stage. During the operation of the trust-based system, constant communication between both participants was necessary. Differences of opinion between them were inevitable at this stage, leading to disputes that required careful attention. Lastly, there was the development and improvement stage. Every rule had its limitations, and the fairness of the trust-based system fundamentally depended on human judgment. It was essential to continuously improve the regulatory aspects of the tennis trust-based system from ethical and other human-centered perspectives [49].

The model of the operational mechanisms of the tennis trust-based system, based on grounded theory research, captures the social context in which behaviors occur [50]. By mapping this model onto the PCM framework, our approach centered on amateur tennis participants, effectively addressing concerns regarding human factors in the tennis trust-based system. It explained the theoretical framework of trust in amateur tennis competitions and laid a foundation for further enhancing the trust-based system.

4.2. Recommendations

The operational mechanism model of the tennis trust-based system we proposed explains the application scenarios and interaction processes within tennis competitions. However, we also identified some concerns from participants regarding this system. To address these concerns, we offer the following policy development suggestions:

Firstly, establish an integrity management system. The effective implementation of the tennis trust-based system in competition mode is closely related to the ethical foundation of participating players [51]. Therefore, sports integrity is crucial. Establishing an integrity management system that includes strict screening and assessment of participating players is essential to ensure fair competition. For example, implementing a credit rating mechanism to rank and score players and imposing penalties or bans on players who are dishonest or make erroneous judgments can enhance players' awareness of integrity. Additionally, establishing a disciplinary notice board and setting up channels for reporting and appeals can enhance player self-discipline and oversight mechanisms, ensuring that matches are conducted in a fair and honest manner. In the selection and review of players, strict selection criteria should be established and publicly disclosed so that both players and spectators can understand and accept them, thereby enhancing the transparency and credibility of the competition.

Secondly, establish unified standards and processes. Event organizers should ensure that competition rules are easily understood and implemented through standardized rule training and process design. This includes detailed rule training courses, standardized processes, establishment of rule interpretation mechanisms, and ongoing management supervision to enhance the fairness of the competition and participant satisfaction. For example, establish oversight teams such as event supervision and data analytics groups, clearly defining responsibilities and divisions of labor. These teams would be collectively responsible for managing and guiding the trust-based system in tennis competitions, overseeing and managing the entire competition process. Additionally, there should be strengthened education and training for participants, which is crucial to ensuring the effective implementation of the rules [52].

4.3. Limitations

The study reveals the tensions and conflicts that arise with the application of tennis trust-based system rules. Despite these contributions, it also has its limitations. The study population selected for this paper, although comprising 23 tennis players from all walks of life, is not representative of all tennis participants' perceptions of the trust-based system and may need to consider expanding the sample in the future. Testing the trust-based system in more competitive or professional environments is essential. Research could consider conducting studies at different levels of competition (such as youth, adult, or professional leagues) to further validate the effectiveness and adaptability of the trust system. In addition, the construction of the trust theory system model is based on self-reporting, which is somewhat subjective, and in this case, not everyone may truthfully report their true thoughts, which is a reflection of social expectations that cannot be completely avoided [53]. Future research could adopt a broader range of quantitative methods, such as surveys, to encompass a larger population of amateur tennis participants, ensuring the representativeness of the results. Additionally, using mixed methods (combining qualitative and quantitative approaches) could provide a more comprehensive perspective. For instance, alongside interviews, incorporating observational methods could offer deeper insights into the operation of the trust system in actual matches. Furthermore, long-term tracking studies (longitudinal research) could help us understand the dynamic processes of how the trust system evolves over time.

5. Conclusions

The study proposes a human-centered trust theory framework model based on grounded theory. Through focus group discussions and interviews and using a three-stage coding process, it identifies 28 main factors influencing the rules of the tennis trust-based system. These factors are categorized into four major groups: interest orientation, information acquisition and judgment, interactive communication, and development strategies. Furthermore, building upon this foundation, a PCM framework was used to construct a model of the operational mechanisms of the tennis trust-based system. This model encompasses five stages: foundation stage, trust-based emergence stage, monitor and detect stage, anticipate and respond stage, and development improvement stage.

In the context of introducing more technologically assisted officiating systems (such as Hawk-Eye and VAR), the establishment of a trust-based system provides a new perspective on interpersonal interactions and self-refereeing in competitions. In the absence of technological support, a trust system can operate effectively; however, it requires standardized management mechanisms and processes to reduce disputes and enhance fairness. By implementing clear guidelines and protocols, players can engage in a more collaborative and respectful environment, which reinforces the principles of trust and sportsmanship, ultimately contributing to a smoother and more equitable competitive experience. Within the operational process of the trust system, the anticipate and respond stage is the most likely to generate controversy. To address the shortcomings of the trust system, we can establish integrity management systems and standardized processes. This study effectively explains the formation mechanism and process of the tennis trust-based system, providing a theoretical foundation for the development of amateur tennis trust-based competitions. Future research can further explore how trust-based systems can adapt to other amateur sports events and various participant groups. By establishing new rule mechanisms for more amateur sports, such studies could promote fair competition and enhance officiating efficiency. Additionally, this exploration can provide new directions for future research on technology and trust systems, highlighting the importance of fostering trust and collaboration in diverse sporting contexts. Such investigations could lead to a deeper understanding of how these systems function across different environments, ultimately contributing to the development of more effective and equitable officiating practices in amateur sports.

Author Contributions: F.Y. and Y.-S.K. conceptualized the original idea and the study design and analyzed and interpreted the data; F.Y. drafted the main manuscript; and Y.-S.K. critically revised the manuscript. All authors have read and agreed to the published version of the manuscript.

Funding: This research received no external funding.

Institutional Review Board Statement: The study was conducted in accordance with the Declaration of Helsinki. According to the "Implementation of Ethical Review Measures for Human-Related Life Science and Medical Research" issued by the Chinese government, research conducted in China using anonymized data can be exempt from ethical review (Article 32). Our research is based on interviews and utilizes anonymized data. Therefore, it qualifies for exemption from ethical review in China.

Informed Consent Statement: Informed consent was obtained from all subjects involved in the study.

Data Availability Statement: The data that support the findings of this study are available from the corresponding author upon reasonable request.

Conflicts of Interest: The authors declare no conflicts of interest.

References

1. Taymazov, V.; Bakulev, S.; Pavlenko, A.; Simakov, A.; Chistyakov, V. To a question of electronic refereeing systems application in taekwondo (VTF). *Uchenye Zap. Univ. Im. PF Lesgafta* **2013**, *98*, 155–160. [CrossRef]
2. Hwang, Y.S.; Yoo, H.J. Relations among Sport-for-All Tennis Instructors' Coaching Behavior, Class Satisfaction and Intention of Re-registration. *J. Sport Leis. Stud.* **2014**, *58*, 643–652. [CrossRef]
3. Li, Y.; Li, L.; Shen, P. Probability-based visual comfort assessment and optimization in national fitness halls under sports behavior uncertainty. *Build. Environ.* **2023**, *242*, 110596. [CrossRef]
4. Yoo, H.-J. Pedagogical Content Knowledge of Sport for All Tennis Instructors and the Intention to Participate Continuously. Ph.D. Thesis, Pusan National University, Busan, Republic of Korea, 2015.
5. Su, X. Trends of and expectations for the development of amateur tennis games in China. *J. Phys. Educ.* **2012**, *19*, 69–71. [CrossRef]
6. Sun, J. A Study on the Operational Model of Amateur Tennis Events in Beijing: A Case Study of the CRT China Open Level League. *Sport* **2017**, 38–39. [CrossRef]
7. *ITF Global Tennis Report 2021*; International Tennis Federation: London, UK, 2021.
8. Abramitzky, R.; Einav, L.; Kolkowitz, S.; Mill, R. On the optimality of line call challenges in professional tennis. *Int. Econ. Rev.* **2012**, *53*, 939–964. [CrossRef]
9. Anbarci, N.; Lee, J.; Ulker, A. Win at all costs or lose gracefully in high-stakes competition? Gender differences in professional tennis. *J. Sports Econ.* **2016**, *17*, 323–353. [CrossRef]
10. Mazurova, E.; Standaert, W.; Penttinen, E.; Tan, F.T.C. Paradoxical tensions related to AI-powered evaluation systems in competitive sports. *Inf. Syst. Front.* **2022**, *24*, 897–922. [CrossRef]
11. Plessner, H.; Haar, T. Sports performance judgments from a social cognitive perspective. *Psychol. Sport Exerc.* **2006**, *7*, 555–575. [CrossRef]
12. Kerr, R. Technologies for judging, umpiring and refereeing. In *Sport and Technology*; Manchester University Press: Manchester, UK, 2016; pp. 114–134.
13. Dufner, A.-L.; Schütz, L.-M.; Hill, Y. The introduction of the Video Assistant Referee supports the fairness of the game–An analysis of the home advantage in the German Bundesliga. *Psychol. Sport Exerc.* **2023**, *66*, 102386. [CrossRef]
14. Spitz, J.; Wagemans, J.; Memmert, D.; Williams, A.M.; Helsen, W.F. Video assistant referees (VAR): The impact of technology on decision making in association football referees. *J. Sports Sci.* **2021**, *39*, 147–153. [CrossRef] [PubMed]
15. Kovalchik, S.A.; Sackmann, J.; Reid, M. Player, official or machine? Uses of the challenge system in professional tennis. *Int. J. Perform. Anal. Sport* **2017**, *17*, 961–969. [CrossRef]
16. Araújo, D.; Couceiro, M.; Seifert, L.; Sarmento, H.; Davids, K. *Artificial Intelligence in Sport Performance Analysis*; Routledge: London, UK, 2021.
17. Kolbinger, O.; Lames, M. Scientific approaches to technological officiating aids in game sports. *Curr. Issues Sport Sci. (CISS)* **2017**, *2*, 1. [CrossRef]
18. Mlakar, M.; Kovalchik, S.A. Analysing time pressure in professional tennis. *J. Sports Anal.* **2020**, *6*, 147–154. [CrossRef]
19. Kopania, M.; Nowisz, J.; Przelaskowski, A. Automatic Shuttlecock Fall Detection System in or out of a Court in Badminton Games—Challenges, Problems, and Solutions from a Practical Point of View. *Sensors* **2022**, *22*, 8098. [CrossRef]
20. Benbya, H.; Pachidi, S.; Jarvenpaa, S. Special issue editorial: Artificial intelligence in organizations: Implications for information systems research. *J. Assoc. Inf. Syst.* **2021**, *22*, 10. [CrossRef]
21. Ferger, K.; Hackbarth, M. New way of determining horizontal displacement in competitive trampolining. *Sci. Gymnast. J.* **2017**, *9*, 303–310.
22. Dadı, M.M.; Yıldız, O. Opinions of football referees on the VAR system and VAR training. *Turk. J. Sport Exerc.* **2022**, *24*, 52–65.

23. Collins, H.; Evans, R. You cannot be serious! Public understanding of technology with special reference to "Hawk-Eye". *Public Underst. Sci.* **2008**, *17*, 283–308. [CrossRef]
24. Liu, L. Research and Survey on Development of Qingdao Amateur Tennis Matches. *Asian Soc. Sci.* **2014**, *10*, 196. [CrossRef]
25. Suk, J.; Andělová, K. The Power of the Powerless and Further Havelian Paradoxes in the Stream of Time. *East Eur. Politics Soc.* **2018**, *32*, 214–231. [CrossRef]
26. Kramer, R.M. Trust and distrust in organizations: Emerging perspectives, enduring questions. *Annu. Rev. Psychol.* **1999**, *50*, 569–598. [CrossRef] [PubMed]
27. Kang, P. A research on the value of the tennis trust system in developing the quality of integrity in adolescents. *Tennis World* **2023**, *1*, 81–83.
28. Zhang, W. Guidelines on the Confidence-Building System. *Tennis World* **1997**, *2*, 29–30. (In Chinese)
29. Harding, J.W.; James, D.A. Performance assessment innovations for elite snowboarding. *Procedia Eng.* **2010**, *2*, 2919–2924. [CrossRef]
30. Gredin, N.V.; Bishop, D.T.; Broadbent, D.P.; Tucker, A.; Williams, A.M. Experts integrate explicit contextual priors and environmental information to improve anticipation efficiency. *J. Exp. Psychol. Appl.* **2018**, *24*, 509. [CrossRef]
31. Wenli, W. SWOT Analysis and lmplementation Strategy Research of the Trust-Based Tennis Match Mode. *Contemp. Sports Technol.* **2023**, *13*, 157–161. [CrossRef]
32. Glaser, B.G.; Strauss, A.L. *The Discovery of Grounded Theory: Strategies for Qualitative Research*; Aldine: Chicago, IL, USA, 1967.
33. Safari Jafarloo, H.R.; Mohamadi Turkmani, E.; Ghorbani, M.H. Lessons learned from the Glaserian grounded theory approach: Professionalizing as a basic social process in elite athletes' lifestyle. *Int. J. Qual. Methods* **2022**, *21*, 16094069221103070. [CrossRef]
34. Bamkin, M.; Maynard, S.; Goulding, A. Grounded theory and ethnography combined: A methodology to study children's interactions on children's mobile libraries. *J. Doc.* **2016**, *72*, 214–231. [CrossRef]
35. McCallin, A.M. Designing a grounded theory study: Some practicalities. *Nurs. Crit. Care* **2003**, *8*, 203–208. [CrossRef]
36. Glaser, B.G. Conceptualization: On theory and theorizing using grounded theory. *Int. J. Qual. Methods* **2002**, *1*, 23–38. [CrossRef]
37. Niesser, U. *Cognition and Reality: Principles and Implications of Cognitive Psychology*; W. H. Freeman and Company: New York, NY, USA, 1976.
38. Fassinger, R.E. Paradigms, praxis, problems, and promise: Grounded theory in counseling psychology research. *J. Couns. Psychol.* **2005**, *52*, 156. [CrossRef]
39. Charmaz, K. *Constructing Grounded Theory*; Sage: San Jose, CA, USA, 2014.
40. Dhakal, K. NVivo. *J. Med. Libr. Assoc. JMLA* **2022**, *110*, 270. [CrossRef] [PubMed]
41. Thrower, S.N.; Harwood, C.G.; Spray, C.M. Educating and supporting tennis parents: A grounded theory of parents' needs during childhood and early adolescence. *Sport Exerc. Perform. Psychol.* **2016**, *5*, 107. [CrossRef]
42. Pennock, K.; Tamminen, K.A.; McKenzie, B.; Mainwaring, L. A grounded theory of youth athlete concussion under-reporting decisions. *Psychol. Sport Exerc.* **2024**, *73*, 102646. [CrossRef]
43. Holt, N.L.; Tamminen, K.A. Moving forward with grounded theory in sport and exercise psychology. *Psychol. Sport Exerc.* **2010**, *11*, 419–422. [CrossRef]
44. Corbin, J.; Strauss, A. *Basics of Qualitative Research: Techniques and Procedures for Developing Grounded Theory*; Sage Publications: San Jose, CA, USA, 2014.
45. Yi, Q.; Liu, Z.; Liu, X.; Wang, Y.; Li, R. The development strategies of amateur table tennis matches in China based on the SWOT-AHP model: A case study in Shanghai. *Sci. Rep.* **2024**, *14*, 12060. [CrossRef]
46. Musa, R.M.; Hassan, I.; Abdullah, M.R.; Latiff Azmi, M.N.; Abdul Majeed, A.P.; Abu Osman, N.A. A longitudinal analysis of injury characteristics among elite and amateur tennis players at different tournaments from electronic newspaper reports. *Front. Public Health* **2022**, *10*, 835119. [CrossRef]
47. Perederij, V. The problem of the quality of judging in rhythmic gymnastics. *Pedagog. Psychol. Med.-Biol. Probl. Phys. Train. Sports* **2013**, *3*, 43–46.
48. Parnell, K.J.; Wynne, R.A.; Griffin, T.G.; Plant, K.L.; Stanton, N.A. Generating design requirements for flight deck applications: Applying the perceptual cycle model to engine failures on take-off. *Int. J. Hum.–Comput. Interact.* **2021**, *37*, 611–629. [CrossRef]
49. Lucidi, F.; Zelli, A.; Mallia, L.; Nicolais, G.; Lazuras, L.; Hagger, M.S. Moral attitudes predict cheating and gamesmanship behaviors among competitive tennis players. *Front. Psychol.* **2017**, *8*, 571. [CrossRef] [PubMed]
50. Ungar, M. Qualitative contributions to resilience research. *Qual. Soc. Work* **2003**, *2*, 85–102. [CrossRef]
51. Wright, B.; Rodenberg, M.R.; Sackmann, J. Incentives in best of N contests: Quasi-Simpson's paradox in tennis. *Int. J. Perform. Anal. Sport* **2013**, *13*, 790–802. [CrossRef]
52. Soltani, P.; Morice, A.H. Augmented reality tools for sports education and training. *Comput. Educ.* **2020**, *155*, 103923. [CrossRef]
53. Fischer, D.G.; Fick, C. Measuring social desirability: Short forms of the Marlowe-Crowne social desirability scale. *Educ. Psychol. Meas.* **1993**, *53*, 417–424. [CrossRef]

behavioral sciences

MDPI

Article

Problematic Use of Video Games in Schooled Adolescents: The Role of Passion

José María Faílde Garrido, María Dolores Dapía Conde *, Manuel Isorna Folgar and Fátima Braña Rey

Faculty of Education and Social Work, University of Vigo, 32004 Ourense, Spain; jfailde@uvigo.es (J.M.F.G.); isorna.catoira@uvigo.gal (M.I.F.); fatimab@uvigo.gal (F.B.R.)
* Correspondence: ddapia@uvigo.es

Abstract: The present study aims to determine the predictive value of sociodemographic, academic, educational clinical psychological variables—ADHD diagnosis, emotional self-regulation, passion and emotional and behavioural symptoms—and modality of use of video games in adolescents who either make potentially problematic or severely problematic use of video games. This is a descriptive cross-sectional study in which 2.533 Galician students (region located in the northwest of Spain) aged between 11 and 20 years participated, who were selected through multistage random sampling. The mean age was 14.78 years (SD = 1.76). The analysis of the data seems to indicate that in the prediction of the problematic use of video games, different variables are combined, among which passion plays a capital role. In addition, the problematic use of video games is related to poor parental control, poor academic performance, use of addictive substances or to an earlier onset, as well as with the diagnosis of ADHD and with greater negative emotional and behavioural symptoms. The results of this study may be of interest for the design and implementation of preventive and corrective actions aimed at reducing the problematic or addictive use of video games.

Keywords: video games; problematic use; addiction; adolescents; obsessive passion; harmonious passion

1. Introduction

Video games have become a widespread leisure activity. According to the latest report by DFC Intelligence more than three billion people are regular consumers of video games, which represents almost 40% of the world's population [1]. In Europe, according to the latest report by Europe's video games industry [2], 51% of the population aged 6 to 64 play video games, with young people aged 11 to 14 doing so the most (with 84%), followed by the group aged 15 to 24 (with 75%), while in the group of 6 to 10 years also do so in a very prevalent way (with 73%). The data in this report indicate that as age increases, the use of video games decreases, with the age group of 45 to 64 years being the that which uses them the least (34%).

Spain follows a similar trend, as it can be seen in recent years. A recent study on digital entertainment among young people aged 15 to 29 shows that approximately 90% consume content related to video games [3]. This trend is like that observed in the ESTUDES survey, which reflects that 85.1% of students aged 14 to 18 have used video games during the last 12 months [4].

According to these data, we can affirm that video games are a playful practice that characterises the leisure of adolescents and young people. This extension of the use of video games not only refers to the fact that it is an activity mostly practised in this age group but also that it is carried out with great intensity given the time dedicated to it. Thus, according to the Spanish Observatory of Drugs and Addictions [4], almost half of the students aged 14 to 18 spend approximately two hours a day playing video games. Focusing on the group that makes potentially problematic use of video games, they dedicate 5 or more hours a day to gaming. In a similar way, Calderón and Gómez indicate that students dedicate 4.3 h per day to gaming [3].

For the vast majority of video game users, gaming constitutes a mode of entertainment without negative consequences [5]; however, the intensity in the involvement of young people—excessive use of video games—has caused significant concern and is becoming considered a behavioural addiction [6]. In this sense, the DSM-V of the American Psychiatric Association [7] has expanded and modified the category "substance-related disorders" to "substance use and addictive disorders", in which it integrates the internet gaming disorder and defines it as "persistent and recurrent use of video games on the Internet, usually with other players, resulting in a clinical disorder or anguish, with five (or more) of the following symptoms, in a period of twelve months: worry, withdrawal syndrome, loss of control, loss of interest in previous hobbies, continued use despite having knowledge of their psychosocial problems, disappointment, avoidance and conflict in personal, work or academic environments" [7].

The prevalence of video game addiction is variable according to studies [8], being influenced by different factors and methodological issues, such as age, characteristics of the participants, country, game mode or instruments used. A recent meta-analysis places the global prevalence at 3.05% and 1.96%, being stricter in the selection of studies [9]. Similar values are confirmed in a meta-analytic study that quantifies the prevalence rates reported worldwide; it establishes the global prevalence grouped at 3.3% (8.5% in men and 3.5% in women), reducing to 2.4% in studies with representative samples, placing the adjusted prevalence at 1.4% through the application of stricter methodological calculation criteria [10].

In Spain, according to data from the Spanish Observatory of Drugs and Addictions [4], 7.1% of students aged 14 to 18 would present a possible disorder due to the use of video games (according to DSM-V criteria).

In recent years, research on video game addiction has increased, with interest in identifying what factors can predict this addiction. Different studies have associated sociodemographic, academic, parental control, playing manners, substance use or clinical variables (ADHD diagnosis, emotional self-regulation or emotional symptoms) with this behavioural addiction [11]. In line with a bibliographic review of existing scientific production until mid-2019, groups the different predictors of addiction to video games or problem gambling into the following: demographic, game characteristics, family influence, social influence, school environment, psychological and behavioural predictors and physiological indicators [11]. The conclusions of this study result in a majority profile characterised by being male, playing online, with low parental control and interest, little social interaction, negative school experience and low levels of emotional regulation.

The problems with the use of video games have been repeatedly associated in the scientific literature with the male gender, although it is not considered one of the most relevant factors. Thus, in a study using regression analysis conducted by Bernaldo de Quirós et al. [12], general mental health, gender and age only explain 1.3% of the total variance, while commitment to the game and cognitive distortions explain 59.3% of the variance of problematic video game use.

Other research suggests that passionate involvement in the use of video games can influence the development of problematic behaviours, although it depends on the type of passion that the player presents. Taking as a reference the dual model of passion (DMP) proposed by Vallerand et al. [13,14], harmonious passion (HP) and obsessive passion (OP) are distinguished. Regardless of the type of passion, it is defined by the authors as "a strong inclination towards an activity that people like, that seems important and in which they invest time and energy" [14], becoming, therefore, a meaningful, highly valued and self-defined activity that implies dedication and that causes satisfaction of basic psychological needs. Although at the level of functioning both types of passion follow the same scheme, HP is compatible with adaptive behaviours and individuals are able to maintain control in the execution of the activity that they are passionate about, not interfering with other responsibilities. On the contrary, OP causes individuals to lose control, causing a dependency that leads them to abandon other responsibilities. Some studies find that high levels of HP are associated with higher school engagement/success, while high OP is associated with low school engagement [15].

In a similar way, other studies have identified PH as protective and OP as a predictor of problematic behaviours and higher levels of abusive use of video games [16,17], associating low levels of satisfaction of needs in life with an OP for video games [18]. As a vicious circle, an intense OP towards gaming predicts and, in turn, is reinforced by a high frustration of needs [19], which in turn can generate OP and lead to problematic use of video games [20]. In short, playing video games with obsessive involvement can be interpreted as an escape route for a frustrated life that can favour problem gambling. In this sense, some authors consider the problematic use of video games as an emotional coping strategy [21].

The excessive use of video games is a complex and multifaceted phenomenon resulting from the interaction of various factors, including attention deficit hyperactivity disorder (ADHD), academic performance, parental control, gaming modality and substance use.

ADHD has been linked to a higher risk of developing video game addiction. Individuals with ADHD often struggle to control their impulses and maintain attention, which predisposes them to engage in activities that provide immediate gratification, such as video games. A recent study by Boer et al. [22] confirms that adolescents with ADHD are significantly more likely to engage in problematic video game use, using these games as a means to regulate their emotional state and avoid the frustration of academic or everyday tasks.

Additionally, academic performance is another factor that has shown a significant relationship with problematic video game use. Students who face difficulties in academics may use video games as a form of escape, which in turn exacerbates their academic performance. Recent research, such as that by Anjum et al. [23], has highlighted that excessive video game use is associated with a decline in academic achievement.

Parental control and supervision also play a crucial role in preventing problematic video game use. Krossbakken et al. [24] pointed out that adolescents with parents who implement screen time controls are less likely to develop video game addiction. However, when parents lack clear rules or are overly permissive, the risk of problematic use increases significantly.

The gaming modality is noted as another important factor related to video game use. In this regard, online video games, especially those with social components such as MMORPGs and battle royale games (e.g., Fortnite and League of Legends) have proven to be highly addictive. Montag et al. [25] indicated that features of these games, such as variable reward cycles, competitive social environments and the endless nature of gameplay, are factors that promote addiction. These games provide constant positive feedback and a sense of achievement, which can make it difficult for players to interrupt their sessions.

Finally, substance use has also been linked to problematic video game use. Individuals experiencing substance abuse tend to have a greater predisposition to other forms of addictive behaviour, such as excessive video game use. In a recent study [26] found that adolescents who reported excessive video game use also had a higher likelihood of engaging in performance-enhancing drug consumption.

In a literature review, we detected that few studies focused on analysing the joint influence of different variables with problematic use or addiction to video games. Thus, the objective of this study is to determine the predictive value of sociodemographic, academic, educational, clinical psychological variables—ADHD diagnosis, emotional self-regulation, passion and emotional and behavioural symptoms—and modality of video game use in adolescents who make potentially problematic use or severely problematic use of video games. To this end, a rigorous statistical methodology was used with a novel approach such as the Classification and Regression Tree (CART).

2. Methods

2.1. Participants

A total of 2533 participants took part in the study, after excluding 57 cases for exceeding 20 years or for not having completed any of the evaluation instruments. The mean age was 14.78 years (SD = 1.76), with a range between 11 and 20 years; all of the students were enrolled in secondary education (compulsory secondary education, high school and vocational and training cycles). Of these, 58.8% were male and 48.2% female.

For empirical contrast purposes, participants were classified into three groups based on the scores obtained in the Questionnaire of Experiences Related to Video Games [27]: (i) non-problematic use of video games (NPUVG); potentially problematic video game use (PPUVG); and severe or possibly addictive problematic use of video games (AUVG). A more detailed description of the characteristics of the participants can be seen in Table 1.

Table 1. Characteristics of the participants (gender, academic performance, ADHD diagnosis, hours of video game use and parental control) depending on the type of players (chi square).

Variables	NPUVG N = 1357 F(%)	PPUVG N = 829 F(%)	AUVG N = 124 F(%)	X^2	p
Gender					
Males	445 (38.6)	607 (74.1)	101 (82.8)	403.08	0.000
Females	911 (67.2)	212 (25.9)	21 (17.2)		
Repeat course					
No	1095 (80.8)	659 (79.5)	98 (79.7)	9.47	0.050
Yes. One Course	190 (14.0)	111 (13.4)	23 (18.7)		
Yes. 2 or more	70 (5.2)	59 (7.1)	2 (1.6)		
Number of failures					
4 or more	173 (12.9)	154 (18.8)	39 (32.0)	64.20	0.000
From 1 to 3	381 (28.4)	269 (32.9)	41 (33.6)		
Average performance	152 (11.3)	105 (12.8)	14 (11.5)		
Superior performance	634 (47.3)	290 (35.5)	28 (23.0)		
Diagnosis ADHD					
Yes	56 (4.2)	58 (7.2)	18 (15.1)	27.74	0.000
No	1273 (95.8)	745 (92.8)	101 (84.9)		
ADHD medication					
Yes	27 (47.4)	36 (62.1)	10 (58.8)	2.61	0.271
No	30 (52.6)	22 (37.9)	7 (41.2)		
Play over 18 games					
Yes	253 (21.3)	371 (45.4)	57 (47.5)	222.02	0.000
No	472 (39.7)	121 (14.8)	10 (8.3)		
I do not care	463 (39.0)	325 (39.8)	53 (44.2)		
Game mode					
Online	612 (45.0)	620 (74.7)	99 (78.9)	213.26	0.000
Offline	749 (55.0)	210 (25.3)	25 (20.2)		
Game time per week					
0 to 2 h per week	1193 (87.7)	458 (55.2)	35 (28.2)	495.34	0.000
3 to 5 h per week	136 (10.0%)	219 (26.4)	30 (24.8)		
6 or more hours per week	32 (2.4)	153 (18.4)	59 (47.6)		
Parents control game					
Yes. Always	895 (65.8)	404 (48.7)	63 (50.8)	146.13	0.000
Yes. sometimes	251 (18.4)	110 (13.3)	16 (12.9)		
Nope. Never	215 (15.8)	316 (38.1)	45 (36.3)		
Parental interest in game					
Yes. Always	727 (53.4)	311 (37.5)	52 (41.9)	69.03	0.000
Sometimes	208 (15.3)	119 (14.3)	17 (13.7)		
No. never	426 (31.3)	400 (48.2)	55 (44.4)		

Note: NPUVG: non-problematic use of video games; PPUVG: potentially problematic use of video games; AUVG: severe or possibly addictive problematic use of video games.

2.2. Instruments

For data collection, a set composed of the following instruments was administered:

Video Game Experiences Questionnaire (CERV) [27]. Instrument composed of 17 items, with a 4-point Likert response format (never/almost never, sometimes, quite often and almost always) that allows evaluating the problematic and abusive use of video games on any platform. It allows to obtain a total score and two subscales: evasion (8 items) and negative consequences (9 items). Likewise, cluster analyses offer a three-group solution based on the following cut-off points: no problems with the use of video games (scores between 17 and 25 points); potential problems (between 26 and 38 points); and severe problems (between 39 and 68 points). Cronbach's alpha coefficients for the subscales are considered acceptable for the two subscales: negative consequences ($\alpha = 0.87$) and evasion ($\alpha = 0.86$). In this study, McDonald's omega coefficients were 0.73 and 0.82 for each of the scales, respectively, and 0.89 for the global scale.

Emotional Repair Subscale of the Spanish version of the Trait Meta-Mood Scale (TMMS-249) [28]. It is composed of 8 items that evaluate metaknowledge for the regulation of emotions, with a 5-point Likert-type response format (from 1 strongly disagree to 5 strongly agree). The psychometric properties show adequate internal consistency ($\alpha = 0.86$) for the emotional repair subscale; in this study, McDonald's omega coefficient was also adequate ($\omega = 0.86$).

Spanish version of the Strengths and Difficulties Questionnaire (SDQ) [29]. It is an instrument for clinical screening of mental disorders in childhood and adolescence, taking as a criterion the last 6 months. It is composed of 25 items, with a response format of three options (not true, a little true and absolutely true) grouped into 5 subscales (with 5 items each): emotional symptoms, behavioural problems, hyperactivity, relationship problems with peers and prosocial behaviour. A difficulty score can also be obtained, which is the sum of the previous subscales, except prosocial behaviour. The levels of reliability and validity for use in adolescents are adequate [29]. For this study, the McDonald's omega coefficient obtained was 0.71 for the total difficulties scale and 0.72 for the prosocial behaviour scale.

Spanish version of the Escala da Pasión (adapted to video games) [30]. Passion is one of the elements of psychological processes present in various activities such as sports, leisure, work, interpersonal relationships or video games. This scale consists of 17 items, with seven answer options (strongly agree, fairly agree, agree, neither agree nor disagree, disagree, strongly disagree and strongly disagree). It allows us to obtain three dimensions: OP (6 items) and HP (6 items) and passion criteria (5 items). The internal consistency levels of the scale are adequate, with $\alpha = 0.81$ for HP and $\alpha = 0.87$ for OP. The values of the McDonald's omega coefficient in the present study were suitable for both HP ($\omega = 0.73$) and OP ($\omega = 0.75$).

In addition to the above instruments, a questionnaire was administered, designed ad hoc, in which sociodemographic information was collected and on certain aspects related to the use of video games, parental control and the consumption of psychoactive substances.

2.3. Procedure

The selection of participants was carried out via multistage random sampling. First, from the list of centres of the Ministry of Culture, Education and University of the Xunta de Galicia (Government of Galicia, Spain), the number of students and centres in each province was determined and the number of centres (public and private/subsidised) per province in each of the educational levels (first stage) was selected. Secondly, the ratio of urban to rural centres by province (second stage) was established. Finally, we proceeded to select the class unit (third stage). Prior to the administration of the evaluation instruments to the participants, pertinent permission was requested from the parents through the direction of the educational centres.

The study was approved by the ethics committee of (masked for review purposes). This authorisation guarantees that the study complies with the ethical principles included in the Declaration of Helsinki for studies with human beings. All participants were informed of the purpose of the research and their written informed consent was obtained.

Data collection was carried out in groups in the presence of the researchers. The average time participants spent completing the instruments was 25 to 30 min.

2.4. Design

This is a descriptive study using cross-sectional surveys in which the independent variable was the type of player based on the cut-off scores of the Questionnaire of Experiences Related to Video Games (CERV) with three levels [27]: non-problematic use (NPUVG); potentially problematic use (PPUVG); and severe or possibly addictive problematic use (AUVG). The dependent variables were emotional self-regulation, symptomatology of emotional and behavioural problems, passion, sociodemographic characteristics, aspects related to the use of video games, parental control and consumption of psychoactive substances.

2.5. Data Analysis

After obtaining the data set and its subsequent digitisation, we proceeded to the treatment and analysis of the same.

First, the data were cleaned and coded for further analysis. Then, descriptive and exploratory analyses were carried out to determine the characteristics of the sample by calculating the measures of position, dispersion and shape, thus being able to establish the first results of homogeneity and presence of anomalous elements that could produce incoherent results. Next, a normality test was performed using the Kolmogorov–Smirnov statistic. Considering that the sample was not normally distributed, the Kruskal–Wallis test (non-parametric alternative to ANOVA) and the Mann–Whitney U test were used to perform post hoc contrasts (two to two). Likewise, the effect size was calculated using the Hedges g statistic.

To determine the levels of internal consistency of the instruments, we opted for McDonald's omega coefficient, as it provides a more accurate estimate than Cronbach's alpha. To do this, we followed the procedure indicated by [31].

In the final stage of the analysis, given that the dependent variable encompasses both quantitative and qualitative elements (once grouped), the decision was made to apply the classification and regression Tree (CART) statistical technique due to its ability to produce clear and understandable interpretations. The analysis included the following calculations:

- Error rate of the classification model: assessed to measure model accuracy.
- Classification rules for each observation: each observation enters the tree at the root and follows a descending path based on the values of its variables. At the terminal node, the classification percentage for each category of the dependent variable is determined.
- Variable importance in predicting the player type: the importance of each variable is evaluated based on its position in the tree, where variables located at higher levels carry more weight in the classification rules.
- Percentage probability of classifying a participant into a player category: the highest and lowest probabilities were analysed to identify the profiles of participants with the highest likelihood of belonging to a specific group or type of player.

The analysis process using classification trees was iterative. Based on an initial analysis of the influence of variables, various trees were developed using the complete set of independent variables, narrowing them down to those most representative for classification.

All analyses were performed using the statistical software SPSS 24.0 (IBM Corp., 2020).

3. Results

First, the results of the descriptive and influence analyses will be presented. Next, the classification and regression tree (CART) will be introduced.

3.1. Descriptive and Influence Analysis

The results of this section have been structured in three blocks: (1) Characteristics of the participants and patterns of use of video games; (2) consumption of psychoactive substances; and (3) psychological variables—passion and emotional and behavioural symptoms. For empirical contrast purposes, all variables were analysed based on the type of player (NPUVG, PPUVG and AUVG).

3.2. Participant Characteristics and Video Game Usage Patterns

As it can be seen in Table 1, a statistically significant association was detected between the variable type of player, with different variables that have been grouped into gender, academic performance, ADHD diagnosis, video game use and parental control, and that we describe as follows:

Gender (X^2 = 403.08; p = 0.000)

The percentages of problematic and addictive use of video games are clearly higher in males, with 74.1% and 82.8, respectively. On the other hand, females mostly make non-problematic use of video games (67.2%).

Repeat course (X^2 = 9.47; p = 0.050)

The participants of the AUVG group are those with the highest percentages of repeating a course (18.7%), while the PPUVG participants are the those who repeated two or more courses to a greater extent (7.1%). However, these data should be carefully observed, since the association between the repeats course variable and type of player is at the limit of statistical significance.

Number of failed subjects (X^2 = 64.20; p = 0.000)

In line with the above, there is a clear statistically significant association between the number of failed subjects and the type of use made by the video game player. Thus, we identified that academic performance is worse in the PPUVG and AUVG groups compared to the NPUVG group.

ADHD diagnosis (X^2 = 27.74; p = 0.000)

The data reflect a clear statistically significant association between the diagnosis of ADHD and the type of player. Thus, 7.2% of the PPUVG group have an ADHD diagnosis established by the national health system, a percentage that rises to 15.1% for the AUVG group.

Games for over 18 years (X^2 = 222.02; p = 0.000)

The data show that those adolescents who deliberately opt for games for over 18 years (despite being minors) accumulate higher percentages of potentially problematic use or with severely problematic use.

Game mode (X^2 = 213.26; p = 0.000)

The game mode (online versus offline) was significantly associated with the type of player. The online gambling modality accumulated a higher percentage of potentially problematic players (74.7%) and severely problematic players (78.9%).

Weekly play time (X^2 = 495.34; p = 0.000)

We observed that the PPUVG and AUVG groups invest a greater number of hours of video game use. If we take a deeper look at the study of this variable, we observe the existence of statistically significant differences (Kruskal–Wallis test and post hoc contrasts, two by two, with the Mann–Whitney U statistic), depending on the type of player, in the number of weekly hours dedicated to the use of video games (X^2 = 930.31; p = 0.000). The PPUVG (p = 0.000; g_+ = 1.46) and AUVG (p = 0.000; g_+ = −2.73) groups invested significantly more hours of play than the NPUVG group. Likewise, the AUVG group reported playing more weekly hours than the UPPVG, these differences being statistically significant (p = 0.000; g_+ = −0.96).

Game parental controls (X^2 = 146.13; p = 0.000)

Regarding the relationship between the type of player and parental control, we observed that the lack of parental control is related to higher percentages of potentially problematic (38.1%) or severe problematic (36.3%) use. Systematic parental control was also associated with moderate levels of potentially problematic (48.7%) and severely problematic (50.8%) use. On the other hand, partial (discretionary) parental control was associated with lower percentages of potentially problematic (13.3%) or severely problematic (11.5%) (12.9%) use.

Parental interest in play ($X^2 = 69.03$; $p = 0.000$)

In a similar line to that observed in relation to the parental control variable, it is observed that the non-systematic or discretionary interest of parents in their children's gambling was associated with lower rates of potentially problematic use (14.3%) or severely problematic use (13.7%).

3.3. *Use of Psychoactive Substances*

On the other hand, if we focus on the consumption of addictive substances in the last six months (see Table 2), we observe that alcohol consumption is more prevalent in the NPUVG typology ($X^2 = 7.06$; $p = 0.029$). Regarding tobacco, the AUVG and NPUVG groups reported consuming alcohol more frequently ($X^2 = 8.67$; $p = 0.013$), while the AUVG and PPUVG groups reported a higher consumption of energy drinks ($X^2 = 13.19$; $p = 0.001$).

Table 2. Substance use in the past 6 months (chi square) and ages of onset in substance use (Kruskal–Wallis test).

Have You Consumed in the Last 6 Months...?	NPUVG N = 1357 F(%)	PPUVG N = 829 F(%)	AUVG N = 124 F(%)	X^2	p
Alcohol					
No	220 (28.6)	159 (35.8)	23 (34.3)	7.06	0.029
YES	549 (71.4)	285 (64.2)	44 (65.7)		
Tobacco					
No	124 (32.2)	89 (44.3)	8 (30.8)	8.67	0.013
YES	261 (66.8)	112 (55.7)	18 (69.2)		
Cannabis					
Yes	74 (40.0)	43 (43.9)	5 (38.5)	0.44	0.802
NO	111 (60.0)	55 (56.1)	8 (61.5)		
Energy drinks					
No	273 (34.3)	138 (25.6)	21 (24.1)	13.19	0.001
YES	523 (65.7)	401 (74.4)	66 (75.9)		
Psychotropic drugs					
No	80 (32.5)	30 (24.6)	6 (23.1)	3.01	0.222
YES	166 (67.5)	92 (75.4)	20 (76.9)		
Age of onset of consumption of...	**NPUVG Media (SD) N = 1361**	**PPUVG Media (SD) N = 830**	**AUVG Media (SD) N = 124**	X^2	p
Alcohol	13.67 (2.07)	13.21 (2.60)	12.19 (3.23)	15.16	0.001
Energy drinks	12.80 (2.35)	12.58 (2.16)	11.60 (2.36)	21.84	0.001
Tobacco	14.20 (1.77)	13.85 (2.22)	13.96 (1.58)	3.38	0.184
Cannabis	14.99 (2.01)	14.89 (2.06)	14.30 (1.97)	3.15	0.207
Psychopharmaceuticals	14.25 (4.32)	13.39 (3.90)	11.88 (2.55)	14.77	0.001

Note: NPUVG: non-problematic use of video games; PPUVG: potentially problematic use of video games; AUVG: severe or possibly addictive problematic use of video games.

Statistically significant differences were also detected in the initiation of psychoactive substance use. Potentially problematic and addictive gambling are associated with earlier initiation of substance use (Table 2). Specifically, statistically significant differences were detected (Kruskal–Wallis test) between the type of player and the early onset of the following substances:

Alcohol ($X^2 = 15.16$; $p = 0.001$)

Post hoc, two-to-two analyses with the Mann–Whitney U statistic show that players belonging to the NPUVG group have a significantly later onset of alcohol use. These differences were statistically significant with respect to the PPUVG ($p = 0.038$; $g_+ = -0.22$ and AUVG ($p = 0.000$; $g_+ = -0.77$) groups. Likewise, differences were detected between the ages of onset of PPUVG and AUVG ($p = 0.013$; $g_+ = -0.45$), the latter being those with an earlier onset of alcohol.

Energy drinks (X^2 = 21.84; p = 0.001)

NPUVG players start consuming energy drinks later, with a posteriori analysis showing that there are statistically significant differences only with respect to the AUVG group (p = 0.000; g_+ = −0.37). Also, statistically significant differences were detected between the ages of onset of PPUVG and AUVG (p = 0.000; g_+ = −0.45), the latter being those with an earlier onset in the consumption of energy drinks.

Psychotropic drugs (X^2 = 14.77; p = 0.001)

In a similar line to what happened with alcohol, the post hoc contrasts reveal that NPUVG players have a significantly later start of the use of psychotropic drugs, reflecting the existence of statistically significant differences with respect to the PPUVG (p = 0.044; g_+ = −0.21) and AUVG (p = 0.000; g_+ = −0.67) groups. On the other hand, differences were detected between the PPUVG and AUVG groups (p = 0.009; g_+ = −0.67); once again, it is the latter that starts earlier in the consumption of psychotropic drugs.

Psychological variables

On the other hand, as can be seen in Table 3, statistically significant differences were detected, depending on the variable type of player, in the levels of passion towards video games and in the emotional and behavioural symptoms.

Table 3. Passion, emotional self-regulation and emotional and behavioural symptoms depending on the type of player (Kruskal–Wallis test).

Variables	NPUVG Mean (SD) N = 1361	PPUVG Mean (SD) N = 830	AUVG Mean (SD) N = 124	X^2	p
Harmonious passion	6.78 (1.04)	10.49 (1.95)	15.00 (2.84)	1539.98	0.000
Obsessive passion	7.21 (1.22)	11.22 (1.92)	16.35 (2.63)	1563.16	0.000
Emotional repair	24.37 (7.24)	24.92 (6.93)	25.03 (7.88)	4.19	0.123
Emotional symptoms	14.52 (4.82)	13.70 (4.72)	14.88 (4.75)	19.54	0.000
Behavioural problems	11.94 (2.86)	12.62 (2.93)	13.39 (3.34)	50.23	0.000
Relationship problems	15.42 (2.48)	15.72 (2.46)	16.04 (3.51)	13.36	0.001
Hyperactivity	16.08 (2.89)	16.31 (2.97)	16.40 (3.99)	5.17	0.076
Prosocial	21.53 (2.97)	20.68 (3.31)	19.62 (4.44)	52.03	0.000
Total score difficulties	57.98 (9.11)	58.37 (8.58)	60.73 (11.35)	16.42	0.000

Note: NPUVG: non-problematic use of video games; PPUVG: potentially problematic use of video games; AUVG: severe or possibly addictive problematic use of video games.

In relation to the passion towards video games, statistically significant differences were detected depending on the variable type of player for both HP (X^2 = 1539.98; p = 0.000) and for OP (X^2 = 1563.16; p = 0.000). A posteriori analyses indicated statistically significant differences between the NPUV and PPUVG groups (p = 0.000; g_+ = 2.55) and the AUVG group (p = 0.000; g_+ = −6.37) in HP, the latter being the ones that referred to higher levels. Likewise, statistically significant differences were detected between the PPUVG and AUVG groups (p = 0.000; g_+ = −2.15), the latter being the ones with the highest scores in HP. With regard to OP, the post hoc contrasts reflected the existence of statistically significant differences between the NPUVG and PPUVG groups (p = 0.000; g_+ = 2.63) and the AUVG group (p = 0.000; g_+ = 6.56). OP levels were also significantly higher in the AUVG group compared to PPUVG players (p = 0.000; g_+ = 2.53).

Regarding emotional and behavioural symptoms (see Table 3), statistically significant differences were detected, depending on the type of player, in the following subscales of the Strengths and Difficulties Questionnaire (SDQ):

Emotional symptoms (X^2 = 19.54; p = 0.000)

The AUVG and NPUVG typologies have the highest scores on this scale. Regarding the NPUVG group, their scores were significantly higher than those of the PPUVG (p = 0.000; g_+ = −0.17). On the other hand, the AUVG group presented significantly higher scores than the PPUVG group (p = 0.005; g_+ = 0.25).

Behavioural problems (X^2 = 50.23; p = 0.000)

The AUVG group exhibited the highest scores on this scale, being statistically significant with respect to the NPUVG (p = 0.000; g_+ = −0.47) and PPUVG (p = 0.005; g_+ = 0.26) groups. Likewise, the PPUVG group had significantly higher scores than the NPUVG group (p = 0.000; g_+ = 0.23).

Relationship problems (X^2 = 13.36; p = 0.000)

Once again, the AUVG group obtained higher scores on this scale, being statistically significant with respect to the NPUVG group (p = 0.007; g_+ = 0.24). The PPUVG group scored significantly higher than the NPUVG group (p = 0.004; g_+ = 0.12).

Prosocial (X^2 = 52.03; p = 0.001)

Unlike what happened in the previous scales, the NPUVG group obtained the highest scores in this dimension, with the differences with respect to the PPUVG (p = 0.000; g_+ = −0.27) and AUVG (p = 0.000; g_+ = −0.61) groups being statistically significant. Finally, the post hoc contrasts indicate the existence of statistically significant differences between the PPUVG and AUVG groups (p = 0.047; g_+ = −0.30).

Classification and regression trees (CART)

After processing the data and completing the descriptive and influence analyses, the first analysis was conducted using classification trees. To evaluate the differentiated contribution of the variables to the model, they were incorporated into three sequential blocks. Due to space limitations, only the trees corresponding to step 3 are displayed.

In the first step, sociodemographic, academic, video game use and parental control variables were introduced as independent. At this stage, the model provided an overall percentage of classification that reached 70.2%; however, the model was not able to classify any case of the type of player belonging to the AUVG group.

In the second step, variables related to substance use, emotional self-regulation and emotional and behavioural symptomatology (the five dimensions of the Strengths and Difficulties Questionnaire) and ADHD diagnosis were introduced into the model. At this stage, the model remained at 70.2% of global classification and was not able to classify any case of the type of player belonging to the AUVG group.

In the last step, the variables related to passion towards video games (HP and OP) were introduced. The classification analysis, once all the variables were introduced (step 3), resulted in a model that significantly improved the percentage of correct classification, reaching 87.5% (See Figure 1). In this model, the risk estimate for a case is 0.125, which means that 12.5% of the cases were incorrectly classified (typical error = 0.007). In addition, the percentage of correct classification for each group was adequate: 89.6% for the NPUVG group; 90.4% for the PPUVG group; and 46.1% for the AUVG group.

It is important to bear in mind that, inside the error, the model errs in classifying only the adjacent classes, not in classifying any participant of the AUVG group in the category of NPUVG; similarly, no NPUVG was classified in the AUVG category.

In this model, it is observed that the variables related to the passion towards video games reached 87.5% (See Figure 1). In this model, the risk estimate for a case is 0.125, which means that 12.5% of the cases were incorrectly classified (typical error = 0.007). Video games are those that contribute relevant information. Therefore, the most important variables for the classification are OP and PH (see Figure 1). The main results obtained when analysing the tree are the following:

- The variable that matters most within the categorisation was the OP, presented at the first level.
- The most probable case of being a member of the NPUVG group can be extracted with a probability of 99.5%, defining a profile of adolescents who have low OP scores, located in quartile 1, and parental control, systematic or partial.
- The highest probability of belonging to the PPUVG group was set at 98.0%. It describes a type of player with OP scores located in quartile 3 and HP scores located in quartile 4.
- For the AUVG group, the most likely case was extracted with 50.4%, describing video game users with OP scores located in quartile 4, with HP scores located in quartile 4 and who play 6 or more hours.

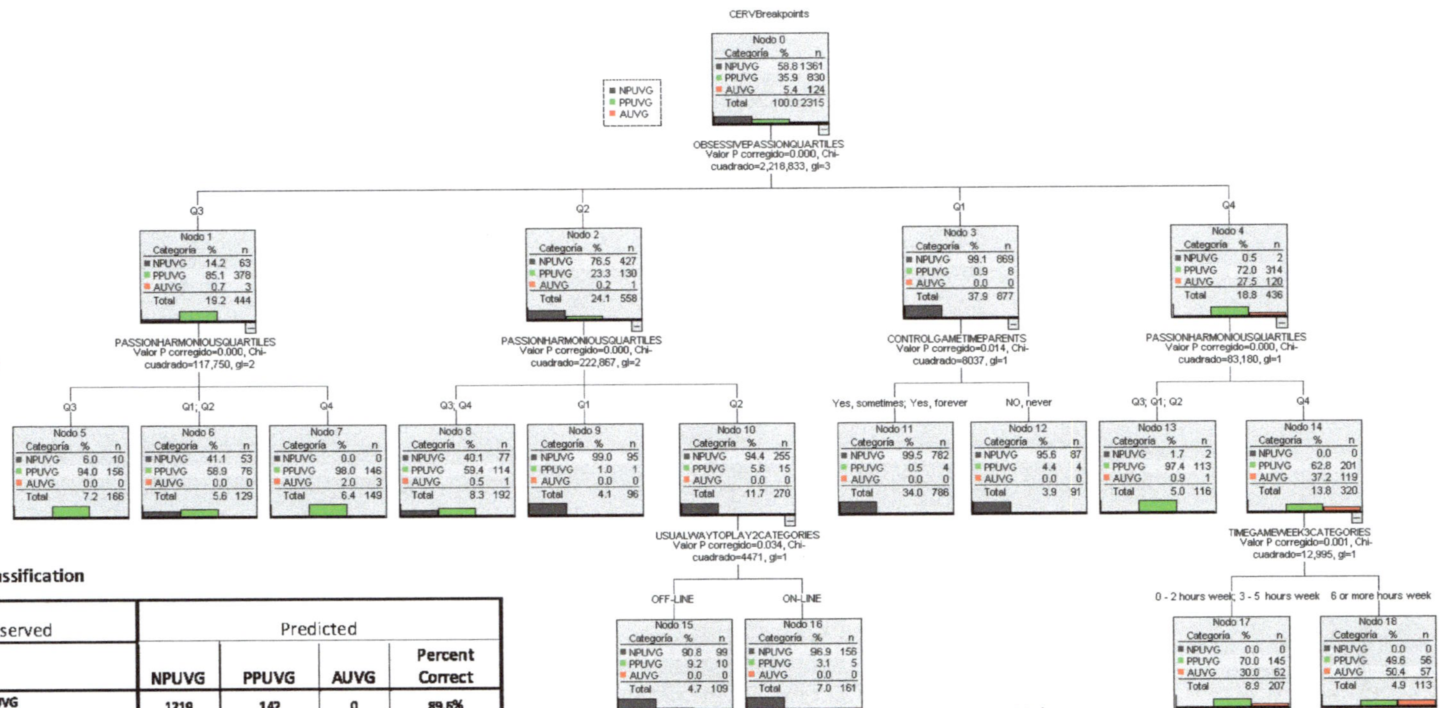

Classification

Observed	Predicted			
	NPUVG	PPUVG	AUVG	Percent Correct
NPUVG	1219	142	0	89.6%
PPUVG	24	750	56	90.4%
AUVG	0	67	57	46.0%
Overall percentage	53.7%	41.4%	4.9%	87.5%

Growing Method: CHAID
Dependent Variable: CERVBreakpoints

Risk

Method	Estimate	Typical error
Replacement	0.125	0.007
Cross-validation	0.130	0.007

Figure 1. Classification and regression trees (CART) by type of video game player.

4. Discussion

New technologies have caused changes in everyday behaviours, also modifying our leisure practices, particularly among younger generations. It is not possible to approach the leisure patterns of minors, adolescents and young people without taking into account digital leisure. A type of leisure that occupies a large part of the time and that presents different manifestations "allows to carry out traditional activities of the offline environment, but renewed or reformulated—listen to music, watch series or play video games, although, on the other hand, it allows to carry out activities that can only be carried out through the online medium—connect to virtual social networks or participate in virtual communities in a broad sense-. . ." [3]. In addition, such technologies allow their enjoyment at any time and anywhere. Internet access, therefore, opens a new field towards social, cooperative and competitive games, allowing users to interact with each other through so-called massively multiplayer online games [16].

In the scientific literature, there is no unanimous agreement on the terminology used to define players based on their mode of use of video games, using terms such as excessive use, problematic use, pathological use [32] or even addictive use [33]. In this study, we classified the players based on the cut-off scores of the CERV questionnaire [27], which establishes three types of players based on the following scores: (1) Non-problematic use; (2) potentially problematic use; and (3) severely problematic use.

The results of this study show that of the total number of participants who report playing video games, 46.0% make potentially problematic use, while 7% make severely problematic use, data that are in line with what has been reported in other studies [4].

In addition, consistent with what has been reported in the literature, problematic and addictive use of video games is more prevalent in males [12]. In this study, male adolescents are three times more prevalent in the PPUVG group than girls, while AUVG is five times more prevalent. This is something commonly reported in the scientific literature regarding addictive behaviours linked to substances, where use and abuse is more prevalent in males, with the exception of the use and abuse of hypnosedants [34,35]. Moreover, in terms of content preference, video games that promote competition, aggression and personal achievement tend to be more appealing to men. Additionally, men show a greater inclination toward action games and online multiplayer games, which tend to be more addictive due to their reward structures, intermittent reinforcements and competitive environments [36].

We have also observed that problematic and potentially addictive use is more prevalent among those participants diagnosed with ADHD [37]. This link can be explained by the difficulties individuals with ADHD have in regulating attention and impulses, as well as their tendency to seek rapid stimulation. In this regard, Nuyens et al. [38] indicated that adolescents with ADHD tend to prefer video games that provide immediate gratification and high levels of activation—such as action and multiplayer games—because they offer quick reward cycles and constant reinforcement. Additionally, Boer et al. [39] identified that problematic video game use in adolescents with ADHD may be influenced by the fact that video games provide a structured environment that these adolescents can control, unlike other areas of their lives that they often perceive as chaotic or difficult to manage. Video games provide a way to achieve success and control.

In addition, participants belonging to the PPUVG and AUVG groups have worse academic performance [40,41], lower parental control [42], a lack of concern for gambling recommendations based on their age and a greater predilection for online gambling [43].

Moreover, PPUVG and AUVG are associated with a higher prevalence of energy drink consumption [44]. Likewise, UPPVG and AUVG are associated with the earlier onset of certain addictive substances (alcohol, energy drinks and psychotropic drugs), which is consistent with studies that found a link between problematic video game use with consumption and earlier use of addictive substances [45,46]. Likewise, and in the same line, as has been reported in some studies, in terms of tobacco and video game use, it was found that other variables such as impulsivity may be common personality factors connecting both behaviors. Individuals with high impulsivity tend to be more likely to engage in both tobacco use and problematic video game use [47].

Regarding mental health, several studies have established the relationship between the problematic use of video games and its deterioration [48]. In this research, we found that PPUVG and AUVG present significantly higher scores than NPUVG, in most of the negative emotional and behavioural symptoms (emotional symptoms, behavioural problems, relationship problems) and lower scores in prosocial behaviour, data that are consistent with what was reported in studies such as García-Gil et al. [48].

Taking the type of player as a dependent variable, based on the criteria defined above, the CART analysis reflects that passion behaves as a factor of great relevance in the prediction and classification of the type of player. According to the dual model of passion [14], passion has a strong implication in identity, making exciting activities part of the player's identity. PH predicts high levels of involvement in the use of video games; however, such individuals are able to reconcile the game with the optimal performance of other activities, allowing them to stop or moderate gaming if it were to have negative repercussions or cause serious interference with other important activities in their lives. On the contrary, OP causes serious interference with activities of daily living of such individuals, decreasing time to the detriment of these. Persistence is a consequence of this process, which becomes rigid and occurs, although the activity does not provide positive sensations and entails significant personal costs, such as the deterioration of relationships or less involvement in other tasks [13].

Although passion and addiction are different concepts, high levels of passion, especially OP, become compatible with potentially problematic or addictive behaviours. In our study, CART analyses indicated that AUVG was related to high levels of OP and PH, with the number of weekly hours spent playing a relevant role [49].

On the other hand, the model identified that the best ranking of players who make PPUVG corresponded to those who had moderate levels of OP and high levels of harmonious passion. The fact that both types of passion, OP and HP, are present in the prediction of potentially problematic use and, also, with severely problematic use, contradicts, in some way, the results of those studies that indicate that high levels of harmonious passion are linked to positive gaming behaviours and experiences (Fuster et al., 2014 [49]). However, this is consistent with what has been reported in recent studies that relate passion and the risk of addiction to video games. Thus, Szabo et al. [50] report high levels of OP and HP in people with exercise addiction, concluding that PH and OP could coexist as a single passion.

This study highlights that high levels of passion are related to problematic video game use [15]. Most likely, this is enhanced by marketing and the design of video games that make them highly attractive, with platforms, images and sounds of high quality. An aspect that can act on the ability to control the game, which, together with other personal and environmental factors, would facilitate the abusive and inappropriate use of these [24].

Although there is not much research related to the prevention of this problem [51], some initiatives, such as carrying out surveillance actions, prevention and treatment of internet addiction or legislating limited use in minors or controlling the time of use, could be effective in minimizing the negative impact of video game abuse [52].

In summary, the results of this study seem to indicate that in predicting problematic use of video games, different variables are combined, among which passion plays a capital role. In addition, the problematic use of video games is related to poor parental control, poor academic performance, ADHD diagnosis, time spent and game mode, consumption of addictive substances or with earlier initiations of consumption, as well as with greater negative emotional and behavioural symptoms [11,43,48]. The results of this study may be useful for the design and implementation of preventive measures, which should pay special attention to the passion variable, which when high (especially OP), in light of the results of this study, can be considered as a predictor variable of the risk of potentially problematic use of video games.

The strength of this study is in analysing the use of video games from a of multivariate analysis perspective, considering sociodemographic and academic factors, parental control, aspects related to the use of video games, substance use, passion and other clinical psychological variables. We also used a relatively large and representative sample of the population under study. However, it has several limitations that must be taken into consideration.

First, this study involved a cross-sectional design, which limits the ability to examine these issues from a more extended temporal perspective. Additionally, although the instruments used demonstrated good levels of internal consistency, this does not rule out the possibility that participants may have been influenced by social desirability bias. Therefore, future research should consider including additional measures to assess the impact of this bias. However, it is important to note that we made every effort to ensure that participants felt comfortable and free to express their responses, and that they perceived their anonymity to be fully guaranteed.

Author Contributions: Conceptualization, J.M.F.G., M.D.D.C., M.I.F. and F.B.R.; Methodology, J.M.F.G., M.I.F. and F.B.R.; Software, J.M.F.G. and M.D.D.C.; Validation, J.M.F.G., M.D.D.C., M.I.F. and F.B.R.; Formal analysis, J.M.F.G. and M.D.D.C.; Investigation, J.M.F.G., M.D.D.C., M.I.F. and F.B.R.; Resources, J.M.F.G. and M.D.D.C.; Data curation, J.M.F.G., M.D.D.C., M.I.F. and F.B.R.; Writing – original draft, J.M.F.G., M.D.D.C. and M.I.F.; Writing – review & editing, J.M.F.G. and M.I.F.; Visualization, M.D.D.C., M.I.F. and F.B.R.; Supervision, J.M.F.G., M.D.D.C. and M.I.F.; Project administration, J.M.F.G., M.D.D.C., M.I.F. and F.B.R.; Funding acquisition, J.M.F.G., M.D.D.C., M.I.F. and F.B.R. All authors have read and agreed to the published version of the manuscript.

Funding: The authors of this work are grateful for the funding received through the Ourense Provincial Council through INOU2021 to carry out this study.

Institutional Review Board Statement: The study was conducted in accordance with the Declaration of Helsinki, and approved by the Sciences Education Faculty, University of Vigo (protocol code CE-DCEC-UVIGO-2022-10-04-5109; 5 May 2023).

Informed Consent Statement: Informed consent was obtained from all subjects involved in the study.

Data Availability Statement: The original contributions presented in the study are included in the article, further inquiries can be directed to the corresponding author.

Conflicts of Interest: The authors declare no conflicts of interest.

References

1. DFC Intelligence. Global Video Game. Consumer Segmentation. DFC Inteligence. 2020. Available online: https://www.dfcint.com/product/global-video-game-consumer-segmentation/ (accessed on 29 July 2024).
2. ISFE. Key Facts 2020. 2020. Available online: https://www.isfe.eu/wp-content/uploads/2021/10/2021-ISFE-EGDF-Key-Facts-European-video-games-sector-FINAL.pdf (accessed on 26 August 2024).
3. Calderón Gómez, D.; Gómez Miguel, A. *Consumir, Crear, Jugar. Panorámica del ocio Digital de la Juventud*; Centro Reina Sofía sobre Adolescencia y Juventud, Fundación FAD Juventud: Madrid, Spain, 2022; Available online: https://www.centroreinasofia.org/publicacion/investigacion_ocio_digital/ (accessed on 2 September 2024).
4. Observatorio Español de las Drogas y las Adicciones. *Informe 2022. Alcohol, Tabaco y Drogas Ilegales en España*; Ministerio de Sanidad. Delegación del Gobierno para el Plan Nacional sobre Drogas: Madrid, Spain, 2022; Available online: https://pnsd.sanidad.gob.es/en/profesionales/sistemasInformacion/sistemaInformacion/pdf/ESTUDES_2022_Informe.pdf (accessed on 1 July 2024).
5. Brunborg, G.S.; Mentzoni, R.A.; Frøyland, L.R. Is video gaming, or video game addiction, associated with depression, academic achievement, heavy episodic drinking, or conduct problems? *J. Behav. Addict.* **2014**, *3*, 27–32. Available online: https://www.ncbi.nlm.nih.gov/pmc/articles/PMC4117274/ (accessed on 2 September 2024). [CrossRef] [PubMed]
6. Carbonell, J. El diagnóstico de adicción a videojuegos en el dsm-5 y la cie-11: Retos y oportunidades para clínicos. *Papeles Del Psicólogo* **2020**, *41*, 211–218. [CrossRef]
7. APA. *Diagnostic and Statistical Manual of Mental Disorders DSM-5*, 5th ed.; American Psychiatric Association: Washington, DC, USA, 2013.
8. Fam, J.Y. Prevalence of internet gaming disorder in adolescents: A meta-analysis across three decades. *Scand. J. Psychol.* **2018**, *59*, 524–531. [CrossRef] [PubMed]
9. Stevens, M.W.; Dorstyn, D.; Delfabbro, P.H.; King, D.L. Global prevalence of gaming disorder: A systematic review and meta-analysis. *Aust. N. Z. J. Psychiatry* **2021**, *55*, 553–568. [CrossRef] [PubMed]

10. Kim, H.S.; Son, G.; Roh, E.B.; Ahn, W.Y.; Kim, J.; Shin, S.H.; Chey, J.; Choi, K.H. Prevalence of gaming disorder: A meta-analysis. *Addict. Behav.* **2022**, *126*, 107183. [CrossRef]
11. Rodríguez, M.; García, F.M. El uso de videojuegos en adolescentes. Un problema de Salud Pública. *Enfermería Glob.* **2021**, *20*, 557–591. [CrossRef]
12. Bernaldo-de-Quirós, M.; Sánchez-Iglesias, I.; González-Alvarez, M.; Labrador, F.; Estupiña, F.; Fernández-Arias, I.; Labrador, M. Factors Associated with the Problematic Use of Video Games in Adolescents and Young People. *Int. J. Ment. Health Addict.* **2022**, *20*, 2706–2717. [CrossRef]
13. Vallerand, R.J. *The Psychology of Passion: A Dualistic Model*; Oxford University Press: Oxford, UK, 2015. [CrossRef]
14. Vallerand, R.J.; Blanchard, C.; Mageau, G.A.; Koestner, R.; Ratelle, C.; Léonard, M.; Gagné, M.; Marsolais, J. Les passions de l'âme: On obsessive and harmonious passion. *J. Personal. Soc. Psychol.* **2003**, *85*, 756–767. [CrossRef]
15. Lotar Rihtarić, M.; Vrselja, I.; Löw, A. Relationship between passion for playing video games and behavioral school engagement: Mediation through time spent playing. *Cyberpsychology J. Psychosoc. Res. Cyberspace* **2022**, *16*, 7. [CrossRef]
16. Bertran, E.; Chamarro, A. Videojugadores del League of Legends: El papel de la pasión en el uso abusivo y en el rendimiento. *Adicciones* **2016**, *28*, 28–34. [CrossRef]
17. Mandryk, R.L.; Frommel, J.; Armstrong, A.; Johnson, D. How Passion for Playing World of Warcraft Predicts In-Game Social Capital, Loneliness, and Wellbeing. *Front. Psychol.* **2020**, *11*, 2165. [CrossRef] [PubMed]
18. Johnson, D.; Formosa, J.; Perry, R.; Lalande, D.; Türkay, S.; Obst, P.; Mandryk, R. Unsatisfied needs as a predictor of obsessive passion for videogame play. *Psychol. Pop. Media* **2022**, *11*, 47–55. [CrossRef]
19. Mills, D.J.; Milyavskaya, M.; Mettler, J.; Heath, N.L.; Derevensky, J.L. How do passion for video games and needs frustration explain time spent gaming? *Br. J. Soc. Psychol.* **2018**, *57*, 461–481. [CrossRef] [PubMed]
20. Sibilla, F.; Musetti, A.; Mancini, T. Harmonious and obsessive involvement, self-esteem, and well-being. A longitudinal study on MMORPG players. *Cyberpsychology J. Psychosoc. Res. Cyberspace* **2021**, *15*, 1. [CrossRef]
21. Blasi, M.D.; Giardina, A.; Giordano, C.; Coco, G.L.; Tosto, C.; Billieux, J.; Schimmenti, A. Problematic video game use as an emotional coping strategy: Evidence from a sample of MMORPG gamers. *J. Behav. Addict.* **2019**, *8*, 25–34. [CrossRef]
22. Boer, M.; van den Eijnden, R.J.; Boniel-Nissim, M.; Wong, S.L.; Mathews, C.; Morrell, H.; Molle, J. Video game addiction, ADHD symptomatology, and video game reinforcement. *Am. J. Drug Alcohol Abus.* **2019**, *45*, 67–76. [CrossRef]
23. Anjum, R.; Nodi, N.H.; Das, P.R.; Roknuzzaman, A.S.M.; Sarker, R.; Islam, M.R. Exploring the association between online gaming addiction and academic performance among the school-going adolescents in Bangladesh: A cross-sectional study. *Health Sci. Rep.* **2024**, *7*, e70043. [CrossRef]
24. Krossbakken, E.; Torsheim, T.; Mentzoni, R.A.; King, D.L.; Bjorvatn, B.; Lorvik, I.M.; Pallesen, S. The effectiveness of a parental guide for prevention of problematic video gaming in children: A public health randomized controlled intervention study. *J. Behav. Addict.* **2018**, *7*, 52–61. [CrossRef] [PubMed]
25. Montag, C.; Lachmann, B.; Herrlich, M.; Zweig, K. Addictive features of social media/messenger platforms and freemium games against the background of psychological and economic theories. *Int. J. Environ. Res. Public Health* **2019**, *16*, 2612. [CrossRef]
26. Ip, E.J.; Urbano, E.P.T.; Jacobs, R.J.; Lau, W.B.; Clauson, K.A.; Torn, R.A.; Palisoc, A.J.L.; Barnett, M.J. The video gamer 500: Performance-enhancing drug use and Internet Gaming Disorder among adult video gamers. *Comput. Hum. Behav.* **2021**, *123*, 106890. [CrossRef]
27. Chamarro, A.; Carbonell, X.; Manresa, J.M.; Munoz- Miralles, R.; Ortega Gonzalez, R.; Lopez-Morrón, M.R.; Batalla-Martínez, C.; Toran, P. El Cuestionario de Experiencias Relacionadas con los Videojuegos (CERV): Un instrumento para detectar el uso problemático de videojuegos en adolescentes españoles. *Addicciones* **2014**, *26*, 303–311. [CrossRef]
28. Fernández-Berrocal, P.; Extremera-Pacheco, N.; Ramos, N. Validity and reliability of the Spanish modified version of the Trait Meta-Mood Scale. *Psychol. Rep.* **2004**, *94*, 751–755. [CrossRef] [PubMed]
29. Ortuño-Sierra, J.; Fonseca-Pedrero, E.; Paino, M.; Sastre i Riba, S.; Muñiz, J. Screening mental health problems during adolescence: Psychometric properties of the Spanish version of the Strengths and Difficulties Questionnaire. *J. Adolesc.* **2015**, *38*, 49–56. [CrossRef] [PubMed]
30. Chamarro, A.; Penelo, E.; Fornieles, A.; Oberst, U.; Vallerand, R.J.; Fernández-Castro, J. Psychometric properties of the Spanish version of the Passion Scale. *Psicothema* **2015**, *27*, 402–409. [CrossRef]
31. Hayes, A.F.; Coutts, J.J. Use Omega rather than Cronbach's Alpha for estimating reliability. But. . . . *Commun. Methods Meas.* **2020**, *14*, 1–24. [CrossRef]
32. Bailin, A.; Milanaik, R.; Adesman, A. Health implications of new age technologies for adolescents: A review of the research. *Curr. Opin. Pediatr.* **2014**, *26*, 605–619. [CrossRef]
33. Del Castillo, J.A.G. Adicciones tecnológicas: El auge de las redes sociales. *Health Addict.* **2013**, *13*, 5–14. Available online: https://www.redalyc.org/pdf/839/83928046001.pdf (accessed on 26 August 2024).
34. Fonseca, F.; Robles-Martínez, M.; Tirado-Muñoz, J.; Alías-Ferri, M.; Mestre-Pintó, J.I.; Coratu, A.M.; Torres, M. A Gender Perspective of Addictive Disorders. *Curr. Addict. Rep.* **2021**, *8*, 89–99. [CrossRef] [PubMed]
35. UNODC. *Drug Use and Health Consequences. World Drug Report 2020*; United Nations Publication: New York, NY, USA, 2020; Available online: https://wdr.unodc.org/wdr2020/field/WDR20_Booklet_2.pdf (accessed on 26 August 2024).
36. Männikkö, N.; Billieux, J.; Kääriäinen, M. Problematic gaming behavior in Finnish adolescents and young adults: Relation to game genres, gaming motives and self-awareness. *J. Behav. Addict.* **2020**, *9*, 256–266. [CrossRef]

37. Feng, W.; Ramo, D.E.; Chan, S.R.; Bourgeois, J.A. Internet gaming disorder-Trends in prevalence 1998–2016. *Addict. Behav.* **2017**, *75*, 17–24. [CrossRef]
38. Nuyens, F.; Deleuze, J.; Maurage, P.; Billieux, J. Problematic gaming in adolescents with ADHD: The roles of impulsivity, game genres, and parental control. *J. Behav. Addict.* **2022**, *11*, 38–49. [CrossRef]
39. Boer, M.; Stevens, G.; Finkenauer, C.; van den Eijnden, R. Attention Deficit Hyperactivity Disorder-Symptoms, Social Media Use Intensity, and Social Media Use Problems in Adolescents: Investigating Directionality. *Child Dev.* **2020**, *91*, e853–e865. [CrossRef] [PubMed]
40. Chung, T.; Sum, S.; Chan, M. Time to call for a global public health approach in prevention of the onset and progression of problematic gaming. *J. Behav. Addict.* **2018**, *7*, 548–552. [CrossRef] [PubMed]
41. Lobel, A.; Engels, R.C.; Stone, L.L.; Burk, W.J.; Granic, I. Video gaming and children's psychosocial wellbeing: A longitudinal study. *J. Youth Adolesc.* **2017**, *46*, 884–897. [CrossRef] [PubMed]
42. Vallejos, M.; Capa, W. Video juegos: Adicción y factores predictores. *Av. En Psicol.* **2010**, *18*, 103–110. Available online: https://www.unife.edu.pe/publicaciones/revistas/psicologia/2010/miguelvallejos.pdf (accessed on 1 July 2024). [CrossRef]
43. Lee, C.; Kim, O. Predictors of online game addiction among Korean adolescents. *Addict. Res. Theory* **2017**, *25*, 58–66. [CrossRef]
44. Visram, S.; Crossley, S.J.; Cheetham, M.; Lake, A. Children and Young People's Perceptions of Energy Drinks: A Qualitative Study. *PLoS ONE* **2017**, *12*, e0188668. [CrossRef]
45. Armstrong, K.E.; Bush, H.M.; Jones, J. Television and video game viewing and its association with substance use by Kentucky elementary school students, 2006. *Public Health Rep.* **2010**, *125*, 433–440. [CrossRef]
46. Coëffec, A.; Romo, L.; Cheze, N.; Riazuelo, H.; Plantey, S.; Kotbagi, G.; Kern, L. Early substance consumption and problematic use of video games in adolescence. *Front. Psychol.* **2015**, *6*, 501. [CrossRef]
47. Walther, B.; Morgenstern, M.; Hanewinkel, R. Co-occurrence of addictive behaviours: Personality factors related to substance use, gambling and computer gaming. *Eur. Addictive. Res.* **2012**, *18*, 167–174. [CrossRef]
48. García-Gil M, Á.; Fajardo-Bullón, F.; Rasskin-Gutman, I.; Sánchez-Casado, I. Problematic Video Game Use and Mental Health among Spanish Adolescents. *Int. J. Environ. Res. Public Health* **2022**, *20*, 349. [CrossRef] [PubMed]
49. Fuster, H.; Chamarro, A.; Carbonell, X.; Vallerand, R.J. Relationship between passion and motivation for gaming in players of massively multiplayer online role-playing games. *Cyberpsychology Behav. Soc. Netw.* **2014**, *17*, 292–297. [CrossRef] [PubMed]
50. Szabo, A.; de la Vega, R.; Kovácsik, R.; Jiménez Almendros, L.; Ruíz-Barquín, R.; Demetrovics, Z.; Boros, S.; Köteles, F. Dimensions of passion and their relationship to the risk of exercise addiction: Cultural and gender differences. *Addict. Behav. Rep.* **2022**, *16*, 100451. [CrossRef] [PubMed]
51. Pontes, H.M.; Griffiths, M.D. A new era for gaming disorder research: Time to shift from consensus to consistency. *Addict. Behav.* **2020**, *103*, 106059. [CrossRef]
52. Saunders, J.B.; Hao, W.; Long, J.; King, D.L.; Mann, K.; Fauth-Bülher, M.; Rumpf, H.J.; Bowden-Jones, H.; Rahimi-Movaghar, A.; Chung, T.; et al. Gaming disorder: Its delineation as an important condition for diagnosis, management, and prevention. *J. Behav. Addict.* **2017**, *6*, 271–279. [CrossRef]

behavioral sciences

MDPI

Article

Longitudinal Effects of Moderate to Vigorous Physical Activity in Physical Education Classes on Attention and Academic Achievement

Kyulee Shin [1], Sukkyung You [2,*] and Mihye Kim [3]

[1] Department of Sports Sciences, Seoul National University of Science & Technology, 232 Gongneung-ro, Nowon-gu, Seoul 01811, Republic of Korea; kyuleeshin@seoultech.ac.kr
[2] College of Education, Hankuk University of Foreign Studies, 107 Imun-dong, Dongdaemun-gu, Seoul 02450, Republic of Korea
[3] Korea Institute of Sport Science, Olympic Cultural Center, 424 Olympic-ro, Songpa-gu, Seoul 05540, Republic of Korea; mihyekim0912@gmail.com
* Correspondence: skyou@hufs.ac.kr; Tel.: +82-2-2173-2338

Abstract: Previous studies showed moderate to vigorous physical activity (MVPA) and aerobic fitness in adolescents are significant factors for cognitive and academic performance. Most previous studies have employed a cross-sectional design; consequently, the evidence on the longitudinal effect of physical education classes (PECs) on cognitive performance and academic achievement is limited. Therefore, the current study utilized a longitudinal design to examine the longstanding effect of MVPA during PECs on cognitive and academic performance across gender groups. Structural equation modeling analyses were employed to understand how MVPA influences youth academic achievement in a nationally representative sample (n = 2092). Study findings indicated that (a) MVPA exerted a direct effect on initial academic achievement as well as an indirect effect, which is mediated by middle school students' attention in both gender groups; (b) MVPA had both long-term direct effects on academic achievement as well as indirect effects on attention, which ultimately affected the subsequent academic achievements of female middle school students.

Keywords: moderate to vigorous physical activity; physical education classes; academic achievement; attention; KCYPS2010

1. Introduction

Cognition is the psychological activity of gaining knowledge and using it [1]. The main cognitive processes consist of attention, memory, learning, reasoning, decision making, problem-solving, and creativity [2]. Attention is classified as focusing on one thing while ignoring other stimuli and distractions [3]. Attention plays a central role in self-regulation [4] and memory [5] for children and adolescents and contributes academic development [6].

In the distant past, most cognitive scientists viewed cognition as a product of the brain. However, since the 1990s, a new perspective has emerged that cognitive is not only produced in the brain but also through bodily interaction with its environment [7]. The embodied cognition theory (ECT) has been adopted as a theoretical explanatory model of how the human body and brain work together in neuroscience and psychology [8]. According to the ECT, physical and visual bodily stimuli, as well as auditory tasks, can improve attention and academic achievement [9–11].

Recently, sports scientists have been actively discussing ECT, and it has emerged as a hot topic among sports researchers [12,13]. Empirical evidence now exists that physical activity (PA) has a positive effect on attention. For example, moderate-to-vigorous physical activity (MVPA) improved tasked-related attention in adolescents [14]. During periods of MVPA, neurotransmitters such as dopamine and norepinephrine are released [15,16].

These chemicals play important roles in improving attention [17]. Furthermore, MVPA has shown to improve academic achievement such as reading, mathematics, and science in children and adolescents [18–21].

Physical education classes (PECs) offer the inducement of MVPA and can therefore be a critical means to the above [22–24]. It is of interest that academic achievement was significantly associated with MVPA in PECs [25–27], although not with PECs alone [22,25], as MVPA must be included.

For Korean middle school students, the primary participants of this study, PECs offer a universal opportunity for participation in MVPA. Middle schools provide after-school sports activities, but there is a high probability that they will not be selected because they are no longer mandatory [28]. The college admittance process starts to take precedence at this age in Korean society, and Korean parents do not enroll their children in non-scholastic extra-curricular activities [29].

Gender, age, and puberty status are important factors related to adolescents' physical, cognitive, and academic performance [30]. Gender, of the above, impacts PA participation the most [31]. Male students are more involved and perform better in sports and exercise than their female counterparts. Considering boys and girls have different psychological values over physical activity and their relative importance varies, there are gender differences that exist in the influence of physical activity on cognitive performance [32].

In short, previous studies concluded a positive association between MVPA in PECs and attention [14,17] and between MVPA in PECs and academic performance [18–21]. However, they lacked larger sample sizes that took gender differences into account. Furthermore, most previous studies employed a cross-sectional design [11,20,21]; thus, the evidence on the long-term effects of MVPA in PECs on attention and academic performance is limited [30].

Therefore, based on the embodied cognition model, the current study utilized a longitudinal design to examine the longitudinal effect of MVPA in PECs on cognitive and academic performance across gender groups. The aim of this study was to identify the long-term impact of adolescents' PA on academic achievement using latent growth modeling. Specifically, we examined the influence of MVPA in PECs on academic achievement in reading, mathematics, and science from the 7th grade through to the 9th grade in Korean middle schools.

2. Methods

2.1. Participants and Procedure

We utilized a longitudinal sample of 2092 middle school students from the Korean Children and Youth Panel Survey (KCYPS) data. The KCYPS is a six-year longitudinal study conducted by the National Youth Policy Institute, funded by the Korean national government. The survey design includes a clustered, stratified national probability sample from approximately 85 elementary schools. This survey was initially completed in 2010 when all students were in their fourth year of elementary school; their mean age was ten. Students then re-took the survey every last quarter of the year until 2016. The current study utilized secondary data; therefore, ethical approval was not required.

The current study samples are drawn from the last three years of the panel data (i.e., 2013 to 2015) when the students were in the 7th to 9th grades. The data used for study analyses comprised a longitudinal panel of 2092 participants who were the same students evaluated three times across the 7th to 9th grades. This sample included 992 (47.4%) girls and 1100 (52.5%) boys, whose ages ranged from 13 to 15 years (M = 14.01; SD = 0.82).

2.2. Measures

2.2.1. Attention

We used the Korean Adolescent Behavior Checklist (K-ABCL) to measure students' attention levels [33]. We used seven items from K-ABCL to measure attention (e.g., When I need to concentrate and solve a problem, I have trouble focusing my attention). All items were coded so that higher scores indicated a higher level of attention during the class. Cronbach's alpha coefficient for this measure was 0.79 in this sample.

Several studies used this scale with South Korean adolescents [34–37]. The results of the studies showed that adolescents' emotional and behavioral problems were significantly related to their attention. For instance, attention was found to be related to study habits and future goals [34], school adjustment [37], and depression [37]. Furthermore, adolescents' self-control and attention were found to impact cell phone dependency significantly [36]. The Cronbach alphas in these studies ranged from 0.79 to 0.84, indicating satisfactory reliability. These findings support the validity of the instrument for use with this population.

2.2.2. Academic Achievement

We used the nationwide achievement test, i.e., the Korean Scholastic Achievement Test (KSAT). This test was designed for the accurate measurement of the ability of individuals at a given time point and of their achievement growth over time. This test was vertically equated with offering a measurement of gain across time. The outcome variable measuring academic achievement was constructed on three assessment scores: the item response theory (IRT) theta scores of readings, math, and science when students were 7th graders (i.e., in their first year in middle school).

2.2.3. Physical Activity

We used students' self-evaluations of MVPA during a week of PECs. The students were asked to compare exercise time to the extent of sweating during PECs. Students answered on a five-point Likert scale for this item (0 = not at all, 4 = 4 h or more). The higher the score, the longer the time spent engaging in MVPA.

2.3. Statistical Analysis

Study analyses were conducted in three stages. In stage one, we conducted t-tests and intercorrelations among variables. In the second stage, we conducted a univariate linear latent growth model (LGM) to test the measurement model for the three subjects. In the third stage, we conducted structural equation modeling (SEM) analysis (see Figure 1) to test the hypothesized models.

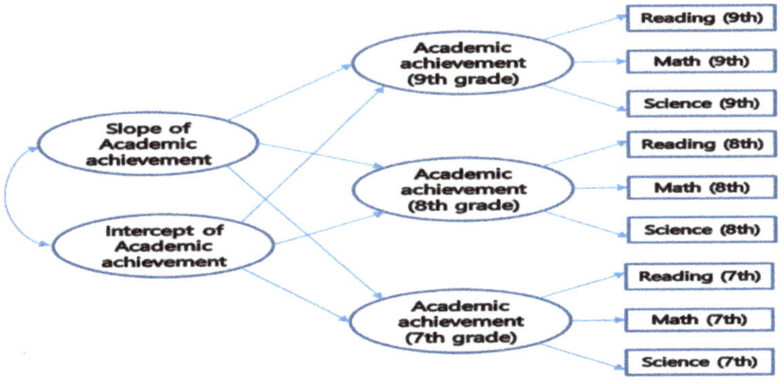

Figure 1. Unconditional latent growth model of academic achievement.

Model Evaluation

Model fit was decided based on several criteria: comparative fit index (CFI; [38]), root mean square error of approximation (RMSEA; [39]), and non-normed fit index (NNFI; [40]). Values smaller than 0.08 for the RMSEA and close to 0.95 for the NNFI and CFI were used to decide on a better fitting model. Analyses were performed using Mplus [41].

We used the nonparametric bootstrapping method [42,43] to assess the significance of mediating effects. This approach repeatedly employs sampling from the given data and assesses the indirect influence in each resampled dataset.

3. Results

3.1. Descriptive Statistics

We used *t*-tests to examine gender differences (see Table 1). Male students participated longer in PA than females, and female students showed a higher level of attention than male students. The findings showed that adolescents' PA, attention, and academic achievement scores were significantly correlated for both gender groups.

Table 1. Correlation and descriptive statistics for study variables by gender.

	1	2	3
1. MVPA in PEC $^{\alpha}$	-	0.07 *	0.11 *
2. Attention $^{\alpha}$	0.10 *	-	0.30 *
3. Academic achievement $^{\alpha}$	0.14 *	0.20 *	-
Means (SD)			
Male	3.68 (1.17)	2.77 (0.54)	4.58 (2.36)
Female	2.92 (1.33)	2.82 (0.52)	3.99 (2.12)

Note. Correlations for female students are diagonal; $^{\alpha}$ Gender difference is significant at * $p < 0.05$.

3.2. Stage I: Latent Growth Model Analysis

We conducted a univariate linear LGM (see path diagram in Figure 1) to see if academic achievement was stable or changed during adolescence. The intercept factor loadings were set to 1.0, representing the initial starting point of the growth curve at Time 1. The slope factor loadings were set to 0, 1, and 2 for three time points representing the linear growth function. The univariate linear models were acceptable based on fit indices. The value of CFI was 0.981, and the value of RMSEA was 0.066.

3.3. Stage II: Testing the Hypothesized Models

We examined two models. The initial structural model (model 1) was a model with direct and indirect paths from PA to academic achievement through a mediating variable. The second structural model (model 2) was a model without a direct path from PA to academic achievement. For boys, model 1 produced an overall χ^2 (107) value of 664.69, with CFI = 0.951, NNFI = 0.955, and RMSEA = 0.065, and model 2 produced an overall $\chi^2(108)$ value of 702.84, with CFI = 0.937, NNFI = 0.910, and RMSEA = 0.071. For girls, model 1 produced an overall χ^2 (107) value of 540.04, with CFI = 0.953, NNFI = 0.954, and RMSEA = 0.064, and model 2 yielded an overall $\chi^2(108)$ value of 595.41, with CFI = 0.938, NNFI = 0.913, and RMSEA = 0.070. A chi-square difference test endorsed model 2. Thus, we selected model 2 as the final theoretical model (see Figure 2). The results showed that there were gender differences in the two paths. Specifically, for the path from MVPA and attention to slope of academic achievement, the effects were significant for girls only ($\beta = 0.06$ and $\beta = 0.18$, $p < 0.05$, respectively). Paths from MVPA to attention and MVPA and attention to intercepts of academic achievement were significant for both gender groups. Standardized beta coefficients for these paths are shown in Figure 2.

Concerning the mediating effects, the bootstrap test outcomes specify that the indirect effects of PA on the intercept of academic achievement through attention ($\beta = 0.03$, and $\beta = 0.02$, $p < 0.05$, for girls and boys, correspondingly) and on the slope of academic achievement for girls ($\beta = 0.02$, $p < 0.05$) were significant.

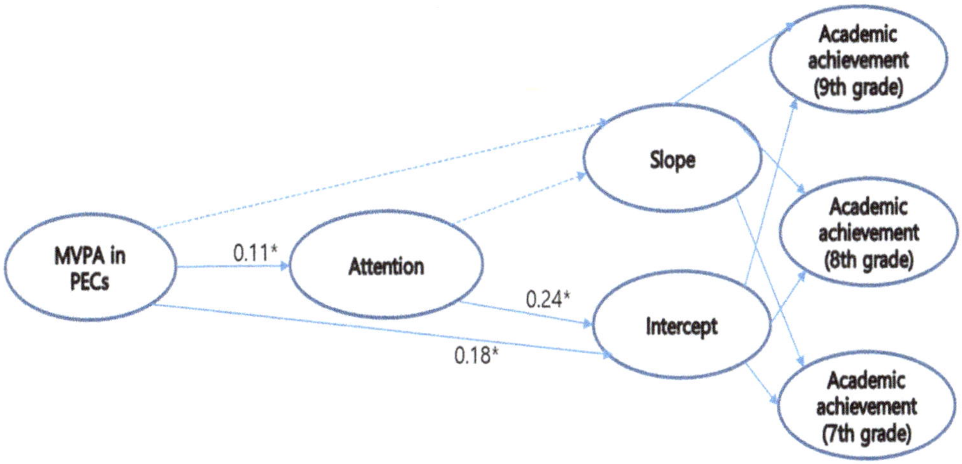

(**a**) Male group (N = 1100)

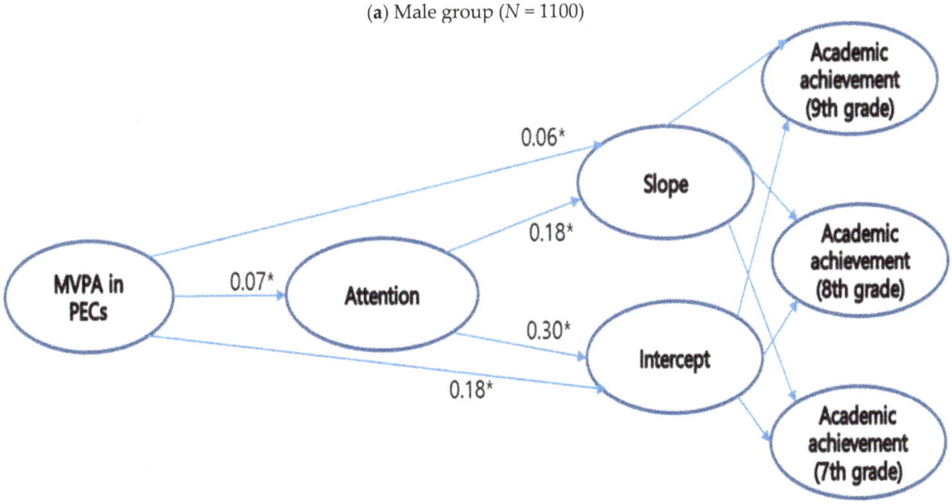

(**b**) Female group (N = 992)

Figure 2. Final model estimation with standardized beta coefficients (N = 2092) for the (**a**) male group and (**b**) female group. Note. * $p < 0.05$; Significant path coefficients are shown with a bold line; dotted line = non-significant.

4. Discussion

This study sought to identify the long-term impact of adolescents' PA on academic achievement using latent growth modeling. Specifically, we examined the influence of MVPA in PECs on academic achievement in reading, math, and science from the 7th grade through to the 9th grade in Korean middle schools.

First, the findings of the current study showed that MVPA in PECs directly and indirectly affects academic achievement by mediating variable attention for both gender groups. Such outcomes can be explained by the embodied cognition theory (ECT) [8], which emphasizes the connection between better fitness and higher cognitive performance. These findings align with previous findings in that PECs did not have detrimental effects on academic achievement; instead, it exerted a favorable effect on achievement in classroom settings [44,45]. Physical activity aids in excluding all other thoughts and emotions by immersing them in a particular activity [46]. This is frequently mentioned in studies on flow experience in sports [46]. Mainly, in exercise, a clear goal for a task is posted, and a sports instructor provides an individual with a challenging task of difficulty that can only be performed beyond the person's average capacity to perform the task. In such a situation, the individual cannot focus on any external distracting thoughts but concentrates solely on the task by organizing and analyzing the collected information [3]. Therefore, exercise provides a sense of control over the activity and encourages pursuing the activity again by rewarding pleasure [47]. The results imply the value of PE since PA positively affects adolescents' cognitive development, which may improve their academic achievement [48].

Second, study findings showed that there are gender differences. For boys, MVPA in PECs has exerted direct and indirect effects only on initial academic achievement (7th grade) through attention. These results corroborate previous research. The long-term effect of PA on academic achievement was confirmed significantly for girls only, not for boys [44,49]. The gender difference in our findings is in accordance with previous research in that girls experience more significant effects of physical fitness on academic achievement measures than boys. Since boys are generally more physically robust than girls, the stimulus gained during co-ed PE classes may not be satisfactory for boys. Therefore, there is a need to offer the optimal level of PA for boys, which may result in improved cognitive and academic performance in boys.

Third, for girls, study findings showed that MVPA in PECs had both direct and indirect effects on initial academic achievement (7th grade) through attention and on the slope of academic achievement (7th through 9th grade). These findings align with previous studies in that the greater intensity of PA leads to higher academic achievement for girls and not for boys [50,51]. The difference in our findings between genders may be explained by physiological and psychological mechanisms. Adolescent girls have lower fitness levels [52,53] and lower self-esteem than adolescent boys [54,55]. Therefore, these variables can cause differences in the relationship between PA and academic achievement. This might explain that MVPA in PEC can positively influence educational outcomes and psychological domains, and these effects may vary across gender groups. Extant research suggests that psychological factors (i.e., self-esteem and depression) are associated with PA and academic achievement [56,57]. Therefore, these potential confounding variables should be considered in future studies so that gender-specific prevention programming can be implemented in school settings.

5. Limitations

This study has several limitations. First, this study utilized a secondary dataset. Because the PE class information could not be obtained, it is impossible to know which type of class content and which teaching methods effectively increased attention and academic achievement. More research is needed to consider the content of PE. Second, this study relied on self-reported measures. Future research is needed to include more various measures, including observational data. Third, students' PA was measured based on self-reporting. Future researchers should record students' PA using more objective measures (e.g., accelerometers, pedometers). Fourth, adolescents' PA can vary depending on their physiological background and possible confounding variables (e.g., self-esteem, depression, perceived puberty status). Therefore, future research needs to address a more comprehensive understanding of PE and cognitive and academic development across gender groups.

6. Conclusions

In conclusion, the current study findings have filled the gaps in extant research that contribute to our understanding of the mechanisms of MVPA on academic achievement by investigating adolescents' attention as an internal mediating factor across gender groups. The current study findings are valuable in that the results are based on nationally representative longitudinal panel data along with the utilization of advanced statistical methods. Empirical studies examining the longitudinal relationship among PA, attention, and academic achievement using a non-Western sample are very scarce. Thus, our study is significant because it has prepared primary data for follow-up studies by verifying the relationship among these variables for adolescents.

In this study, we found that more time spent in MVPA helped adolescents function better cognitively and perform better academically. Outcomes were more favorable for girls. The outcome of the current study confirmed the argument proposed by the embodied cognition theory that improved attention through PA leads to enhanced academic achievement. It emphasizes the need to develop distinct support for a viable brain/body educational intervention based on the embodied cognition model. Previous studies report that a motivational environment constructed by a PE teacher, that is, task-oriented and mastery-oriented rather than performance-oriented, plays a vital role in students' cognitive activity [58]. In addition, PE teachers are reported to promote cognitive activity in PE classes by supporting students to create their performance routines and participate in self-directed classes rather than dedicating class time to teaching students perfect forms [59]. This study could not confirm teachers' class curricula because panel data were used. However, it can be suggested that the PE teachers' class contents are a significant factor in cognitive development [60,61]. Schools should offer PE programs for their many beneficial influences on students' cognitive and academic development. Furthermore, school administrators and teachers strive to provide gender-sensitive PE programs that reflect gender differences in physical fitness. Therefore, promoting MVPA can be a crucial educational intervention strategy in school settings.

Author Contributions: Conceptualization, K.S. and S.Y.; methodology, S.Y.; validation, S.Y.; formal analysis, S.Y.; data curation, K.S.; writing—original draft preparation, K.S., S.Y. and M.K.; writing—review and editing, S.Y., K.S. and M.K.; supervision, K.S. and S.Y. All authors have read and agreed to the published version of the manuscript.

Funding: This work was partially supported by the Hankuk University of Foreign Studies, Seoul, Korea. Research Grant Fund 2024.

Institutional Review Board Statement: The study was conducted in accordance with the Declaration of Helsinki. Ethical review and approval were waived for this study as the data used were secondary panel data.

Informed Consent Statement: Not applicable.

Data Availability Statement: Data are available from NYPI Youth and Children Data Archive form https://www.nypi.re.kr/archive/board?menuId=MENU00329 (accessed on 13 January 2024) with the permission of National Youth Policy Institute.

Conflicts of Interest: The authors declare no conflicts of interest.

References

1. Bayne, T.; Brainard, D.; Byrne, R.W.; Chittka, L.; Clayton, N.; Heyes, C.; Webb, B. What is cognition? *Curr. Biol.* **2019**, *29*, 608–615. [CrossRef] [PubMed]
2. Sreena, S.; Ilankumaran, M. Developing productive skills through receptive skills—A cognitive approach. *Int. J. Eng. Technol.* **2018**, *7*, 669–673. [CrossRef]
3. Moran, A. Concentration: Attention and performance. In *The Oxford Handbook of Sport and Performance Psychology*; Oxford Academic: Oxford, UK, 2012; pp. 117–130.
4. Luszczynska, A.; Diehl, M.; Gutiérrez-Doña, B.; Kuusinen, P.; Schwarzer, R. Measuring one component of dispositional self-regulation: Attention control in goal pursuit. *Pers. Individ. Differ.* **2004**, *37*, 555–566. [CrossRef]
5. Hannula, D.E. Attention and long-term memory: Bidirectional interactions and their effects on behavior. In *Psychology of Learning and Motivation*; Academic Press: New York, NY, USA, 2018; Volume 69, pp. 285–323.
6. Rueda, M.R.; Checa, P.; Rothbart, M.K. Contributions of attentional control to socioemotional and academic development. *Early Educ. Dev.* **2010**, *21*, 744–764. [CrossRef]
7. Lakoff, G.; Johnson, M.; Sowa, J.F. Review of Philosophy in the Flesh: The embodied mind and its challenge to Western thought. *Comput. Linguist.* **1999**, *25*, 631–634.
8. Varela, F.J.; Thompson, E.; Rosch, E. *The Embodied Mind: Cognitive Science and Human Experience*; MIT Press: Cambridge, CA, USA, 1991.

9. McClelland, E.; Pitt, A.; Stein, J. Enhanced academic performance using a novel classroom physical activity intervention to increase awareness, attention and self-control: Putting embodied cognition into practice. *Imprv. Sch.* **2015**, *18*, 83–100. [CrossRef]
10. Ma, C. The influence of college physical education teaching on students' mental health and skill improvement under the embodied cognition theory. *Rev. Psicol. Deporte (J. Sport Psychol.)* **2024**, *33*, 366–375.
11. Schmidt, M.; Benzing, V.; Wallman-Jones, A.; Mavilidi, M.F.; Lubans, D.R.; Paas, F. Embodied learning in the classroom: Effects on primary school children's attention and foreign language vocabulary learning. *Psychol. Sport Exerc.* **2019**, *43*, 45–54. [CrossRef]
12. Cappuccio, M.L. (Ed.) *Handbook of Embodied Cognition and Sport Psychology*; MIT Press: Cambridge, CA, USA, 2019.
13. Tomporowski, P.D.; Pesce, C. Exercise, sports, and performance arts benefit cognition via a common process. *Psychol. Bull.* **2019**, *145*, 929–951. [CrossRef]
14. Vanhels, J.; Béghin, L.; Duhamel, A.; Manios, Y.; Molnar, D.; De Henauw, S.; Petraki, I. Physical activity is associated with attention capacity in adolescents. *J. Pediatr.* **2016**, *168*, 126–131. [CrossRef]
15. Ng, Q.X.; Ho, C.Y.X.; Chan, H.W.; Yong, B.Z.J.; Yeo, W.S. Managing childhood and adolescent attention-deficit/hyperactivity disorder (ADHD) with exercise: A systematic review. *Complement. Ther. Med.* **2017**, *34*, 123–128. [CrossRef] [PubMed]
16. Xie, Y.; Gao, X.; Song, Y.; Zhu, X.; Chen, M.; Yang, L.; Ren, Y. Effectiveness of physical activity intervention on ADHD symptoms: A systematic review and meta-analysis. *Front. Psychiatry* **2021**, *12*, 706625. [CrossRef] [PubMed]
17. Dang, L.C.; O'Neil, J.P.; Jagust, W.J. Dopamine supports coupling of attention-related networks. *J. Neurosci.* **2012**, *32*, 9582–9587. [CrossRef] [PubMed]
18. Bueno, M.R.D.O.; Zambrin, L.F.; Panchoni, C.; Werneck, A.O.; Fernandes, R.A.; Serassuelo, H., Jr.; Ronque, E.R.V. Association between device-measured moderate-to-vigorous physical activity and academic performance in adolescents. *Health Educ. Behav.* **2021**, *48*, 54–62. [CrossRef]
19. Jenkyns, J.A. The Relationship between the Type of Physical Education Program and Student's Academic Achievement, Leisure Time Activity and Perceived Competence. Master's Thesis, University of Alberta, Edmonton, AB, Canada, 2001.
20. Visier-Alfonso, M.E.; Álvarez-Bueno, C.; Sánchez-López, M.; Cavero-Redondo, I.; Martínez-Hortelano, J.A.; Nieto-López, M.; Martínez-Vizcaíno, V. Fitness and executive function as mediators between physical activity and academic achievement: Mediators between physical activity and academic achievement. *J. Sports Sci.* **2021**, *39*, 1576–1584. [CrossRef]
21. Zhang, D.; Hong, J.; Chen, S.; Liu, Y. Associations of physical activity with academic achievement and academic burden in Chinese children and adolescents: Do gender and school grade matter? *BMC Public Health* **2022**, *22*, 1496. [CrossRef]
22. Ardoy, D.N.; Fernández-Rodríguez, J.M.; Jiménez-Pavón, D.; Castillo, R.; Ruiz, J.R.; Ortega, F.B. A physical education trial improves adolescents' cognitive performance and academic achievement: The EDUFIT study. *Scand. J. Med. Sci. Sports* **2014**, *24*, e52–e61. [CrossRef]
23. Beebe, S.L. The Impact of Content Integration in Physical Education Academic Achievement. Ph.D. Dissertation, Northcentral University, Scottsdale, AZ, USA, 2011.
24. Kulinna, P.H.; Stylianou, M.; Dyson, B.; Banville, D.; Dryden, C.; Colby, R. The effect of an authentic acute physical education session of dance on elementary students' selective attention. *Biomed. Res. Int.* **2018**, *2018*, 8790283. [CrossRef]
25. Coe, D.P.; Pivarnik, J.M.; Womack, C.J.; Reeves, M.J.; Malina, R.M. Effect of physical education and activity levels on academic achievement in children. *Med. Sci. Sports Exerc.* **2006**, *38*, 1515–1519. [CrossRef]
26. Travlos, A.K. High intensity physical education classes and cognitive performance in eighth-grade students: An applied study. *Int. J. Sport. Exerc. Psychol.* **2010**, *8*, 302–311. [CrossRef]
27. Wassenaar, T.M.; Wheatley, C.M.; Beale, N.; Salvan, P.; Meaney, A.; Possee, J.B.; Johansen-Berg, H. Effects of a program of vigorous physical activity during secondary school physical education on academic performance, fitness, cognition, mental health and the brain of adolescents (Fit to Study): Study protocol for a cluster-randomized trial. *Trials* **2019**, *20*, 189. [CrossRef] [PubMed]
28. You, S.; Shin, K.; Kim, M. Long-term effect of physical activity on internalizing and externalizing problems and life satisfaction. *Sustainability* **2021**, *13*, 2322. [CrossRef]
29. Kim, M.; Shin, K.; Park, S. Academic helplessness and life satisfaction in Korean adolescents: The moderated mediation effects of leisure time physical activity. *Healthcare* **2023**, *11*, 298. [CrossRef] [PubMed]
30. Donnelly, J.E.; Hillman, C.H.; Castelli, D.; Etnier, J.L.; Lee, S.; Tomporowski, P.; Szabo-Reed, A.N. Physical activity, fitness, cognitive function, and academic achievement in children: A systematic review. *Med. Sci. Sports Exerc.* **2016**, *48*, 1197–1222. [CrossRef]
31. Adriyani, R.; Iskandar, D.; Camelia, L. Gender differences in motor coordination and physical activity. *Adv. Health Sci. Res.* **2020**, *21*, 122–126.
32. Gao, Z.; Lee, A.M.; Harrison, L. Understanding students' motivation in sport and physical education: From the expectancy-value model and self-efficacy theory perspectives. *Quest* **2008**, *60*, 236–254. [CrossRef]
33. Cho, B.H.; Lim, K.H. Development and validation of emotional or behavioral problems scale. *Korean J. Couns. Psycholther.* **2003**, *15*, 729–746.
34. Bae, J. The Effect of Parenting Style, Attention Concentration, Future Goal on Study Habits of Adolescents. Ph.D. Dissertation, University of Brain Education, Chungcheongnam-do, Republic of Korea, 2017.
35. Choi, J. Gender differences in effects of attention deficit/hyperactivity on depression in early adolescence. *J. Korea Contents Assoc.* **2014**, *14*, 285–297. [CrossRef]

36. Heo, G. A study on the structural relationship among cell phone dependency, self-control ability, and attention with higher-order Latent Growth Modeling. *J. Educ. Media* **2013**, *19*, 861–879.
37. Kim, J.; Song, S. The moderating effect of depression on the relationship between attention problems and school adjustment levels in middle school students. *Stud. Korean Youth* **2014**, *25*, 5–27.
38. Bentler, P.M. Comparative fit indexes in structural models. *Psychol. Bull.* **1990**, *107*, 238. [CrossRef] [PubMed]
39. Steiger, J.H.; Lind, J.C. Statistically based tests for the number of common factors. In *the Annual Meeting of the Psychometric Society*; Springer Science + Business Media: Iowa City, IA, USA, 1980.
40. Bentler, P.M.; Bonett, D.G. Significance tests and goodness of fit in the analysis of covariance structures. *Psychol. Bull.* **1980**, *88*, 588. [CrossRef]
41. Muthén, L.K.; Muthén, B.O. *Mplus: User's Guide. [Software Manual]*; Muthen & Muthen: Los Angeles, CA, USA, 2006.
42. Preacher, K.J.; Hayes, A.F. Asymptotic and resampling strategies for assessing and comparing indirect effects in multiple mediator models. *Behav. Res. Methods* **2008**, *40*, 879–891. [CrossRef]
43. Shrout, P.E.; Bolger, N. Mediation in experimental and nonexperimental studies: New procedures and recommendations. *Psychol. Methods* **2002**, *7*, 422–445. [CrossRef]
44. Carlson, S.A.; Fulton, J.E.; Lee, S.M.; Maynard, L.M.; Brown, D.R.; Kohl III, H.W.; Dietz, W.H. Physical education and academic achievement in elementary school: Data from the early childhood longitudinal study. *Am. J. Public. Health* **2008**, *98*, 721–727. [CrossRef]
45. Wilkins, J.; Graham, G.; Parker, S.; Westfall, S.; Fraser, R.; Tembo, M. Time in the arts and physical education and school achievement. *J. Curric. Stud.* **2003**, *35*, 721–734. [CrossRef]
46. Nakamura, J.; Csikszentmihalyi, M. The concept of flow. In *Flow and the Foundations of Positive Psychology*; Springer: Dordrecht, The Netherlands, 2014; pp. 239–263.
47. Swann, C.; Keegan, R.J.; Piggott, D.; Crust, L. A systematic review of the experience, occurrence, and controllability of flow states in elite sport. *Psychol. Sport. Exerc.* **2012**, *13*, 807–819. [CrossRef]
48. Álvarez-Bueno, C.; Pesce, C.; Cavero-Redondo, I.; Sánchez-López, M.; Garrido-Miguel, M.; Martínez-Vizcaíno, V. Academic achievement and physical activity: A meta-analysis. *Pediatrics* **2017**, *140*, e20171498. [CrossRef]
49. Liao, P.A.; Chang, H.H.; Wang, J.H.; Wu, M.C. Physical fitness and academic performance: Empirical evidence from the national administrative senior high school student data in Taiwan. *Health Educ. Res.* **2013**, *28*, 512–522. [CrossRef]
50. Fox, C.K.; Barr-Anderson, D.; Neumark-Sztainer, D.; Wall, M. Physical activity and sports team participation: Associations with academic outcomes in middle school and high school students. *J. Sch. Health* **2010**, *80*, 31–37. [CrossRef]
51. Kwak, L.; Kremers, S.P.; Bergman, P.; Ruiz, J.R.; Rizzo, N.S.; Sjöström, M. Associations between physical activity, fitness, and academic achievement. *J. Pediatr.* **2009**, *155*, 914–918. [CrossRef] [PubMed]
52. Lee, S.; Ko, B.G.; Park, S. Physical fitness levels in Korean adolescents: The national fitness award project. *J. Obes. Metab. Syndr.* **2017**, *26*, 61. [CrossRef] [PubMed]
53. Pojskic, H.; Eslami, B. Relationship between obesity, physical activity, and cardiorespiratory fitness levels in children and adolescents in Bosnia and Herzegovina: An analysis of gender differences. *Front. Physiol.* **2018**, *9*, 1734. [CrossRef] [PubMed]
54. Gomez-Baya, D.; Mendoza, R.; Paino, S. Emotional basis of gender differences in adolescent self-esteem. *Psicologia* **2016**, *30*, 1. [CrossRef]
55. Kayani, S.; Kiyani, T.; Wang, J.; Zagalaz Sánchez, M.L.; Kayani, S.; Qurban, H. Physical activity and academic performance: The mediating effect of self-esteem and depression. *Sustainability* **2018**, *10*, 3633. [CrossRef]
56. Esteban-Cornejo, I.; Tejero-Gonzalez, C.M.; Sallis, J.F.; Veiga, O.L. Physical activity and cognition in adolescents: A systematic review. *J. Sci. Med. Sport* **2015**, *18*, 534–539. [CrossRef]
57. Van Dijk, M.L.; De Groot, R.H.; Van Acker, F.; Savelberg, H.H.; Kirschner, P.A. Active commuting to school, cognitive performance, and academic achievement: An observational study in Dutch adolescents using accelerometers. *BMC Public Health* **2014**, *14*, 799. [CrossRef]
58. Theodosiou, A.; Papaioannou, A. Motivational climate, achievement goals and metacognitive activity in physical education and exercise involvement in out-of-school settings. *Psychol. Sport Exerc.* **2006**, *7*, 361–379. [CrossRef]
59. Papaioannou, A.; Theodosiou, A.; Pashali, M.; Digelidis, N. Advancing task involvement, intrinsic motivation and metacognitive regulation in physical education classes: The self-check style of teaching makes a difference. *Adv. Physiol. Educ.* **2012**, *2*, 110–118. [CrossRef]
60. Mura, G.; Vellante, M.; Egidio Nardi, A.; Machado, S.; Giovanni Carta, M. Effects of school-based physical activity interventions on cognition and academic achievement: A systematic review. *CNS Neurol. Disord. Drug Targets* **2015**, *14*, 1194–1208. [CrossRef]
61. Stevens-Smith, D.A. Active bodies/active brains: The relationship between physical engagement and children's brain development. *Phys. Educ.* **2016**, *73*, 719–732. [CrossRef]

behavioral sciences

MDPI

Article

Intensity of Physical Activity in Young People: Focus on Emotional, Cognitive, and Healthy Lifestyle-Related Variables

Adrián S. Elliott [1], Román D. Moreno-Fernández [2,*], Ana Cordellat-Marzal [3] and Patricia Sampedro-Piquero [1,*]

1 Departamento de Psicología Biológica y de la Salud, Facultad de Psicología, Universidad Autónoma de Madrid, 28049 Madrid, Spain; adrian.sancheze@uam.es
2 Facultad de Educación y Psicología, Universidad Francisco de Vitoria, 29223 Madrid, Spain
3 Departamento de Educación Física y Deportiva, Universitat de València, 46010 Valencia, Spain; ana.cordellat@uv.es
* Correspondence: romandario.moreno@ufv.es (R.D.M.-F.); patricia.sampedro@uam.es (P.S.-P.)

Abstract: The college years represent a crucial developmental period in which unhealthy behaviors, including smoking, alcohol consumption, inadequate physical activity (PA), poor sleep quality, and unhealthy nutrition habits are often acquired, influencing the onset or exacerbation of pre-existing mental disturbances such as anxiety, depression, or difficulties in emotion regulation. Our aim was to analyze the effect of the intensity of physical activity (PA) on the emotional, behavioral, and cognitive variables in a sample of young people. We recruited 103 participants (19.85 $\pm$ 0.25) who completed several online questionnaires (IPAQ-SF, STAI-t, DERS, UPPS-P, ISP-20, and Mini-IPIP). Subsequently, face-to-face sessions were conducted to assess the cognitive variables and to collect more details about their lifestyle habits, including drug use, sleep quality, and leisure activities. Based on the IPAQ-SF results, we categorized the sample into three groups: light PA (n = 47), moderate PA (n = 29), and vigorous PA (n = 27). Vigorous PA group showed better emotional regulation, lower impulsivity, fewer prefrontal symptoms and unhealthy behaviors, better sleep quality, and more leisure activities. No significant cognitive differences were found. It seems that young people are a vulnerable group with emotional and impulsivity traits and engaging in intense PA appears to be a promising avenue for managing these symptoms. In conclusion, our study suggests that young people are a vulnerable group with emotional and impulsivity traits that may precipitate in future mental disorders. Nevertheless, engaging in PA, particularly at high intensity, appears to be a promising avenue for reducing and managing these symptoms during this critical period of life.

Keywords: cognition; emotion; lifestyle; physical activity; youth

1. Introduction

The university years are a crucial period during which students transition from late adolescence to emerging adulthood [1]: a critical phase of personal development and in the building and reinforcement of self-esteem [2,3]. Epidemiological studies suggest that 12–50% of university students meet the criteria for one or more common mental disorders [4,5]. Studies have found that psychological disorders, such as anxiety or depression, are typically more prevalent among those aged 18–34 years than those aged 35–49 [6,7]. Additionally, mental disorders in early adulthood are associated with long-term adverse outcomes in later life, including persistent emotional and physical health problems [8] or relational disorders [9], where emotional dysfunction impairs the use of appropriate emotion regulation strategies [10]. However, research into emotional dysregulation among young people remains comparatively limited, especially in Spain, which may be due to the limited number of available measurement tools for this sample [11]. Another important trait associated with psychopathology and high-risk behavior among young people is impulsivity [12]. However, a few studies have examined the association between impulsivity, often evaluated using the UPPS-P questionnaire, and healthy behaviors during this period of life [13,14]. Thus, prevention or intervention strategies focused on reducing mental distress, improving behavior control, and encouraging healthy lifestyle habits are necessary, and the university environment could be an ideal scenario for this purpose.

It is well known that the difficulties and challenges of daily life may partially explain the onset or worsening of psychological distress and mental illness. This is a period when most students move to another city, state, or province, often leaving home for the first time and taking responsibility for themselves. In addition, university students face academic, social, and employment pressures, [15] and, with the increased time spent on studies and extracurricular activities, leisure time is often restricted [16]. Furthermore, unhealthy habits (including smoking, alcohol consumption, inadequate physical activity (PA), and poor nutritional choices) are often acquired in youth or early adulthood, and they are associated with a fourfold increase in total mortality among men and women in the general adult population [17]. However, despite the obvious consequences of such lifestyles, a high proportion of young people lead unhealthy lives, indulging in habits such as the avoidance of PA, an unsuitable diet, and a high intake of alcohol, tobacco, and illegal drugs [18].

Physical activity is considered ideal in promoting healthy brain functioning, cognition, and mental health throughout one's life. PA has been broadly defined as any bodily movement produced by the contraction of skeletal muscle that increases energy expenditure above a basal level and involves detailed parameters such as intensity, type, and duration [19]. Among youth, PA has been shown to reduce substance abuse and symptoms of depression and anxiety while offering substantial benefits to physical and mental health [20]. These benefits can occur quickly, inducing positive moods and attitudes [21], or they may require weeks of consistent exercise before emerging [22]. Research into youth PA highlights the difficulty of initiating and maintaining this behavior, especially among university students who are often sedentary [23]. Studies have also found that those who initiate an exercise program do so sporadically or stop completely before reaping any of its many potential benefits [24,25]. By contrast, habitual exercise is associated with better emotional regulation strategies [26], greater inhibitory control [27], and greater resilience, strengthening self-regulation through top-down control of bottom-up processing [28]. Studies on young people suggest that high-intensity interval training (HIIT) could have more positive effects on cognitive performance and psychological outcomes [29], promoting higher levels of neurotrophic factors, such as brain-derived neurotrophic factors [30], synaptic plasticity [31], and increased cerebral blood flow [32]. Nonetheless, more studies on the intensity of PA among young people and its relationship with positive emotional and cognitive variables must be carried out.

Few studies have explored the effect of PA intensity on healthy behavior (drug use, sleep quality, leisure activities, etc.) and the psychological and cognitive variables among the young according to gender. These studies are even less common in Spain, where the limited evidence available suggests a high prevalence of alcohol and tobacco use and a low prevalence of PA, especially among women [33,34]. Unfortunately, approximately one third of Spanish university students reported suffering from a common mental disorder in the past year, and one third of those reported severe role impairment [35]. Women reported a higher prevalence of mood and anxiety disorders, while men showed higher levels of substance abuse [36]. Taking this into account, this study aimed to explore how regular PA at different intensities (light, moderate, and vigorous) can variously impact mental well-being and cognition, especially prefrontal-related functions and healthy lifestyle choices, among a sample of Spanish university students. We considered the obtained results to be relevant since, as we mentioned, there are few studies on the impact of exercise on lifestyle, cognition, and emotion, as well as potential gender-related differences, among young people in Spain. Likewise, understanding whether these changes may be greater or not depending on the intensity of physical activity can help promote specific physical activity guidelines for young people based on their physical and mental state. Finally, we hypothesized that certain mental difficulties are more prevalent among more sedentary participants, whereas moderate or vigorous PA will be related to mental well-being and other healthy behaviors, including sleep quality or reduced substance abuse. Moreover, we expected women to be more sedentary, with more frequent anxiety or emotional alterations in line with the findings of the existing literature. Thus, PA may constitute an interesting and non-stigmatizing activity to improve the well-being, habits, and competences of university students.

2. Method

2.1. Participants

This study used cross-sectional data from undergraduate students aged between 18 and 25 years. The recruitment followed the snow-ball sampling technique through verbal disclosure, e-mails, and notice boards at the Autonomous University of Madrid, Francisco de Vitoria, and the Complutense University of Madrid. The inclusion criteria were as follows: (1) aged 18–25 years; (2) college students; and (3) absence of diagnosed psychological disorders (anxiety, depression, substance use disorders, etc.). Volunteers were excluded if they presented severe difficulties in understanding the test instructions, altered consciousness or agitation, if they consumed prescription drugs affecting the central nervous system (mainly anxiolytics and antidepressants), and PA addiction, as revealed by the Spanish version of the Exercise Addiction Inventory (EAI—with a score above 12) [37]. The final sample was 103 Caucasians, of which 30 were male and 73 female, and they were aged 19.85 ± 0.25 and matched for education level. All volunteers included in this study signed an informed consent form accompanied by an informative note, and they created an alphanumeric code based on the first letter of their first name, the last letter of their first surname, followed by their date of birth (e.g., P02712) to guarantee privacy during the data processing and analysis phases. First, to collect information about PA performance, substance use, anxiety traits, emotional regulation, impulsivity, prefrontal symptoms, and personality traits, several online standardized questionnaires were administered (Qualtrics, Silver Lake Partners, 2002): the International Physical Activity Questionnaire-Short form (IPAQ-SF [38]; the Alcohol Use Disorder Identification Test (AUDIT, Spanish adaptation [39]; the Cannabis Abuse Screening Test (CAST) [40]; the State-Trait Anxiety Inventory (STAI-t) [41]; the Difficulties in Emotion Regulation Scale (DERS) Spanish adaptation [42]; the Impulsive Behavior Scale (UPPS-P) Spanish adaptation [43]; the Prefrontal Symptoms Inventory (PSI-20) [44]; and the Mini-IPIP [45]. Regarding physical activity, participants were asked in the IPAQ-SF to report the days, hours, and minutes spent last week on vigorous-intensity PA, moderate-intensity PA, and walking (which reflected light-intensity PA). IPAQ-SF is a widely used and valid 7-day recall measure for assessing various types of PA. The amount of PA was indicated by the metabolic equivalent (MET) of minutes per week, and this was calculated by multiplying the MET value (3.3 METs for walking, 4.0 METs for moderate-intensity PA, and 8.8 METs for vigorous-intensity PA) by the total minutes per week of each type of PA. Higher scores in MET-minutes per week indicated higher levels of PA [46]. Based on the classification criteria of the IPAQ-SF, we divided the sample into 3 groups according to their weekly PA intensity: light PA (mean MET = 436.58 + 48.47, n = 47), moderate PA (MET = 2062.69 + 75.31, n = 29), and vigorous PA (3994.04 + 172.29, n = 27).

This study was approved by the Ethics Committee of the Autonomous University of Madrid (code: CEI-122-2490) and conducted in accordance with the Ethical Principles for Medical Research Involving Human Subjects adopted in the Declaration of Helsinki by the World Medical Association (64th WMA General Assembly, Fortaleza, Brazil, October 2013), Recommendation No. R (97) 5 of the Committee of Ministers to Member States on the Protection of Medical Data (1997), and the Spanish Data Protection Act (Ley Orgánica 15/1999 de Protección de Datos, LOPD). All participants were duly informed about the study prior to their participation and provided their informed consent in writing.

2.2. Procedure

After completing the online questionnaires using the Qualtrics® survey platform (Qualtrics, Silver Lake Partners, 2002), the participants were contacted by email and interviews were arranged to collect more details about sociodemographic variables, lifestyle behaviors (sleep: hours, difficulty in falling asleep, or sleep disorders; drug abuse: type of drug, onset, quantity, etc.; sedentary behavior: hours per day sitting, leisure activities, etc.) [47], and any diagnosed psychological disorders or medication. Participants also performed two prefrontal-dependent tests: the d2 test [48] to measure attentional and speed processing, and the Digit span test [49] to evaluate their working memory. Details of the testing procedures are as follows.

- *d2* test [48]: In this test, participants must cross out any letter "d" with two marks around, above, or below in any order. There are also surrounding distractors that are similar to the target stimulus, e.g., a p with two marks or a d with one or three marks. The time limit per line of the test is 20 s.
- Digit span test [49]: This is used to measure the working memory's number storage capacity. Participants hear a sequence of numbers and are required to recall the sequence correctly, with increasingly longer sequences being tested in each trial. Digit span tasks are given forward or backward, meaning that once the sequence is presented, the participant is asked to recall the sequence in either normal or reverse order.

Finally, the volunteers were instructed to record their daily steps using their watches or mobile devices with pedometers for 7 days, reporting the average number of steps taken at the end of the week. This helped to control the overestimated or biased score of the IPAQ-SF questionnaire, observing a positive Pearson correlation between both results ($r = 0.85$, $p = 0.001$). Table 1 shows the mean ± standard error of the mean (SEM) for each experimental condition (light PA; moderate PA; and vigorous PA).

Table 1. The emotional, cognitive, and behavioral results for each PA group.

	Light PA (n = 47)	Moderate PA (n = 29)	Vigorous PA (n = 27)	*p*
Age	20.19 ± 0.41	19.55 ± 0.33	19.59 ± 0.52	0.47
AUDIT	8.83 ± 1.08	7.07 ± 0.98	4.07 ± 0.89	0.008 **
Age at onset for alcohol use	15.23 ± 0.27	15.41 ± 0.37	16.04 ± 0.30	0.18
CAST	2.17 ± 0.65	2.14 ± 0.83	1.74 ± 0.90	0.92
Cannabis use (YES %)	23.4%	20.7%	11.1%	
Nicotine (YES %)	55.3%	48.3%	25.9%	
Cigarettes/day	7.83 ± 1.29	4.28 ± 1.02	2.04 ± 0.77	<0.001 *
Sleep hours	6.83 ± 0.21	7.52 ± 0.25	8.44 ± 0.22	<0.001 ***#
Sleep difficulties	51.1%	41.4%	11.1%	
IPAQ-SF	436.58 ± 48.47	2062.69 ± 75.31	3994.04 ± 172.29	<0.001 ***###
EAI	6.12 ± 0.45	7.87 ± 0.98	7.02 ± 1.03	0.69
Type of PA (individual %)	100%	100%	74.1%	
Steps/week	4075.06 ± 253.31	5938.72 ± 361.67	9832.81 ± 461.56	<0.001 ***###
Sitting hours/day				
6–8 h	29.8%	62.1%	22.2%	
8–10 h	59.6%	37.9%	70.4%	
>10 h	10.6%	-	7.4%	
CSAs	68.38 ± 2.38	81.21 ± 2.17	88.96 ± 2.88	<0.001 ***###
STAI trait	30.66 ± 1.53	25.93 ± 1.61	20.15 ± 1.81	<0.001 ***#
DERS	75.66 ± 3.27	65.07 ± 3.47	48.70 ± 3.12	<0.001 ***###
Emotional neglect	12.70 ± 0.59	10.69 ± 0.58	9.93 ± 0.62	0.004 ***###
Emotional confusion	7.57 ± 0.49	6.79 ± 0.36	4.67 ± 0.31	<0.001 ***###
Emotional interference	13.81 ± 0.54	12.03 ± 0.65	8.56 ± 0.61	<0.001 ***###
Emotional dysregulation	22.77 ± 1.32	18.79 ± 1.33	12.52 ± 0.90	<0.001 ***###
Emotional rejection	18.81 ± 1.06	16.76 ± 1.57	13.04 ± 1.43	0.007 **
UPPS-P	46.51 ± 1.06	48.24 ± 1.48	42.04 ± 1.59	0.01 *###
Negative urgency	9.64 ± 0.40	9.90 ± 0.42	8.04 ± 0.54	0.03 *
Lack of perseverance	8.49 ± 0.32	8.07 ± 0.51	6.52 ± 0.45	0.003 **
Lack of premeditation	7.72 ± 0.28	7.90 ± 0.40	7.33 ± 0.39	0.56
Sensation seeking	10.62 ± 0.44	11.86 ± 0.50	10.85 ± 0.65	0.21
Positive urgency	10.04 ± 0.45	10.52 ± 0.51	9.30 ± 0.62	0.32

Table 1. *Cont.*

	Light PA (n = 47)	Moderate PA (n = 29)	Vigorous PA (n = 27)	p
PSI-20	30.43 ± 1.37	30.90 ± 2.03	20.48 ± 2.06	<0.001 ***###
Emotional behavior	6.32 ± 0.60	7.31 ± 0.71	4.81 ± 0.61	0.06
Social behavior	3.74 ± 0.47	5.24 ± 0.56	2.89 ± 0.62	0.02 *
Behavioral control	20.36 ± 0.92	18.34 ± 1.38	12.78 ± 1.35	<0.001 ***###
Mini-IPIP	65.43 ± 1.06	65.76 ± 1.01	67.26 ± 1.14	0.49
Openness	10.87 ± 0.23	11.17 ± 0.33	11.63 ± 0.41	0.23
Conscientiousness	13.85 ± 0.36	12.62 ± 0.53	12.37 ± 0.55	0.11
Extraversion	13.34 ± 0.52	14.83 ± 0.55	16.22 ± 0.49	0.08
Agreeableness	15.34 ± 0.38	14.62 ± 0.55	15.52 ± 0.44	0.39
Neuroticism	12.02 ± 0.42	12.52 ± 0.43	11.19 ± 0.41	0.15
		COGNITIVE VARIABLES		
d2–correct	158.62 ± 6.68	158.14 ± 7.65	178.59 ± 6.01	0.09
d2–omissions	21.87 ± 3.07	21.03 ± 4.10	13.41 ± 2.73	0.19
d2–commissions	2.66 ± 0.70	4.17 ± 1.17	1.30 ± 0.58	0.10
d2–TOT	414.13 ± 12.61	407.86 ± 15.14	436.52 ± 11.96	0.36
d2–VAR	12.13 ± 0.61	12.10 ± 1.10	11.41 ± 0.78	0.80
d2–CON	155.98 ± 7.07	153.93 ± 8.37	176.59 ± 6.41	0.09
Forward digits	9.36 ± 0.38	9.69 ± 0.42	10.22 ± 0.36	0.32
Backward digits	7.19 ± 0.39	7.38 ± 0.43	7.56 ± 0.39	0.82
Total digits	16.47 ± 0.74	17.21 ± 0.82	17.78 ± 0.70	0.48

Values are the means ± SEM or percentages. (* vigorous vs. low; # vigorous vs. moderate). All data are the mean + SEM, and statistically significant differences were considered when $p < 0.05$ (*) (#), $p < 0.01$ (**), and $p < 0.005$ (***) (###). AUDIT: Alcohol Use Disorders Identification Test. CAST: Cannabis Abuse Screening Test. IPAQ-SF: International Physical Activity Questionnaire—Short form. EAI: Exercise Addiction Inventory. CSAs: Cognitively Stimulating Activities scale. STAI trait: State-Trait Anxiety Inventory. DERS: Difficulties in Emotion Regulation Scale. UPPS-P: Impulsive Behavior Scale. PSI-20: The Prefrontal Symptoms Inventory—20. Mini-IPIP: Mini-International Personality Item Pool.

2.3. Statistical Analysis

All statistical analyses were performed using SPSS 25 (IBM SPSS Statistics, Corporate headquarters, New Orchard Road, Armonk, New York 10504-1722, USA), and all p values were two-tailed; the level of significance was taken as $p \leq 0.05$. Descriptive analyses (mean ± SEM) were performed on the demographic variables, the information related to drug use, and the online questionnaire and cognitive test results (see Table 1). When the assumption of normality was not met, MANOVA or non-parametric Kruskal–Wallis tests were performed for all measurements taken throughout this study (health behaviors and emotional and cognitive variables). Appropriate post hoc comparisons were conducted when significant differences were found. Additionally, a multiple linear regression analysis was performed in order to determine the relationship of physical exercise with the significant variables.

3. Results

Statistically significant differences were found in the physical activity of the groups in terms of lifestyle variables, substance abuse, leisure activities, psychological traits, and prefrontal-dependent tests. First, and as an objective validation of the self-report questionnaire IPAQ-SF, the number of steps measured by their mobile or smart devices was significantly different in each group ($F_{(2,100)} = 72.21$, $p = 0.0001$; Table 1). Tukey post hoc analysis revealed that these differences were level-dependent, with the vigorous PA group showing the highest levels, followed by the moderate PA group, and then, finally, the light PA group (with the lowest average number of steps) (Figure 1a).

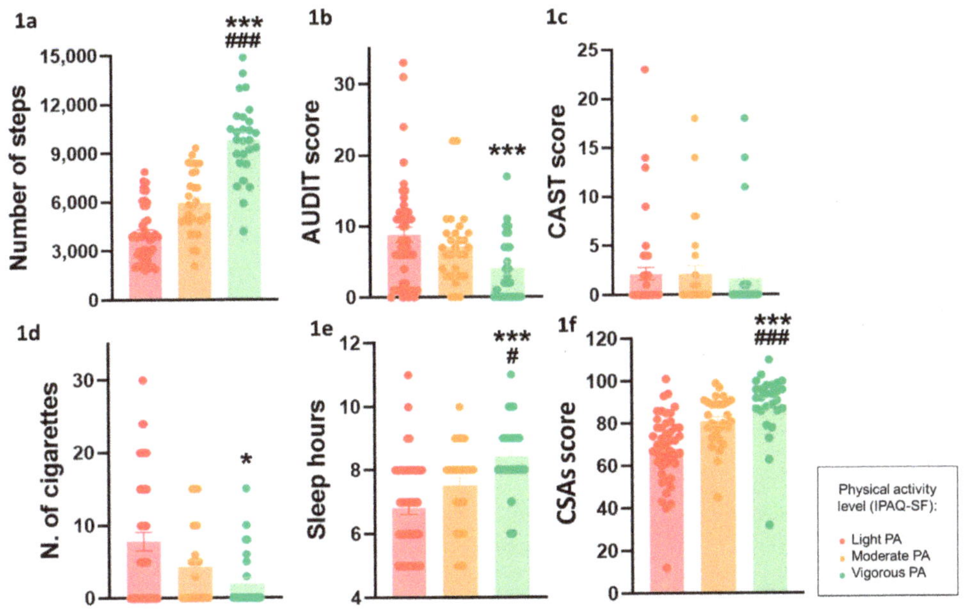

Figure 1. Differences among the light, moderate, and vigorous PA conditions in the average number of steps during a week (**1a**); alcohol (AUDIT) (**1b**), cannabis (CAST) (**1c**), and tobacco abuse (**1d**); sleep hours (**1e**); and CSAs questionnaire results (**1f**) (* vigorous vs. low; # vigorous vs. moderate). All data are the mean ± SEM, and statistically significant differences were considered when $p \leq 0.05$ (*) (#) and $p \leq 0.005$ (***) (###).

3.1. Health- and Lifestyle-Related Variables

The results showed that alcohol use, assessed by AUDIT, was significantly less frequent in the vigorous PA group than in the light PA group ($F(_{2,100}) = 5.04$, $p = 0.008$) (Figure 1b), whereas no differences were observed in cannabis use (CAST score, Figure 1c). Also, the tobacco consumption of the vigorous PA group was also significantly lower than the light PA group ($H(_2) = 9.05$, $p = 0.01$) (Figure 1d). The average number of hours of sleep ($F(_{2,100}) = 12.44$, $p = 0.00001$) was lower in the light PA group than in the moderate and vigorous group (Figure 1e). Regarding leisure activities, the vigorous PA group scored higher than both moderate and light groups ($F(_{2,100}) = 17.92$, $p = 0.00001$) (Figure 1f) (see Table 1).

3.2. Psychological Variables

With regard to emotional regulation, the DERS scores (Figure 2a) were significantly higher in the light PA group ($H_{(2)} = 24.83$, $p = 0.00001$), with levels of difficulty receding as PA increased in the subscales: "Emotional neglect" ($F_{(2,100)} = 5.96$, $p = 0.004$), "Emotional confusion" $H_{(2)} = 18.63$, $p = 0.0001$), "Emotional interference" ($F_{(2,100)} = 19.11$, $p = 0.00001$), "Emotional dysregulation" ($H_{(2)} = 26.69$, $p = 0.00001$), and "Emotional rejection" ($F_{(2,100)} = 4.86$, $p = 0.0097$) (Table 1). The total score of the UPPS-P was also lower in the vigorous PA group ($F_{(2,100)} = 4.82$, $p = 0.01$) (Figure 2b), particularly in the subscales of "Negative urgency" ($F_{(2,100)} = 4.27$, $p = 0.01$) and "Lack of perseverance" ($F_{(2,100)} = 5.90$, $p = 0.004$). The total score of the PSI-20 was also lower in the vigorous PA group (Figure 2c) ($F_{(2,100)} = 9.84$, $p = 0.0013$), where the subscales of "Social behavior" ($F_{(2,100)} = 3.99$, $p = 0.021$) and "Behavioral control" ($F_{(2,100)} = 10.76$, $p = 0.000001$) were found to be significant (Table 1). Finally, we also found that the vigorous PA group displayed significantly less anxiety traits (STAI-t; $F(2,100) = 10.13$, $p = 0.00001$) than the other two groups (Figure 2d) (see Table 1).

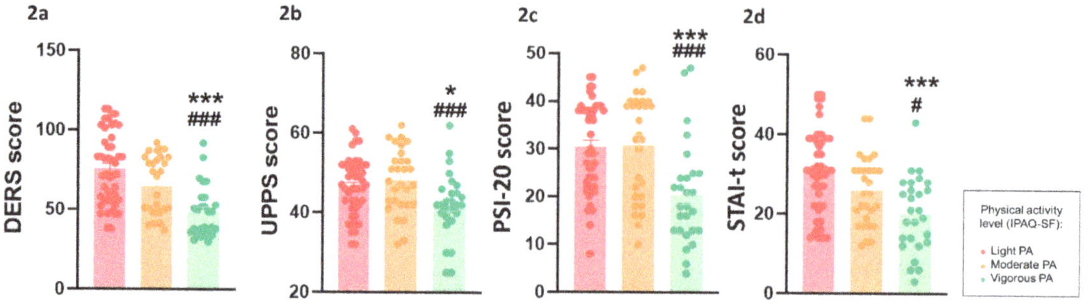

Figure 2. The differences among the light, moderate, and vigorous PA conditions in the total score of the DERS (**2a**), UPPS-P (**2b**), ISP-20 (**2c**), and STAI-t (**2d**) questionnaires, as well as in the sub-scales of the Extraversion and Conscientiousness of Mini-IPIP (* vigorous vs. low; # vigorous vs. moderate). All data are the mean ± SEM, and statistically significant differences were considered when $p \leq 0.05$ (*) (#), $p \leq 0.005$ (***) (###).

3.3. Cognitive Variables

Finally, no statistically significant differences were found in either the attention task (d2) or the working memory test (Digit Span). The only tendency toward significance was in the attentional scores of correct responses ($F_{(2,100)} = 2.39$, $p = 0.09$) and the CON index ($F_{(2,100)} = 2.37$, $p = 0.09$), implying subtle differences in favor of the vigorous PA group with the highest scores (see Table 1).

3.4. Multiple Linear Regression

According to a linear regression analysis of the statistically significant variables above, we found a model with four predictors of the IPAQ score (R^2Adjusted = 0.554, $F(7,95) = 16.879$, $p < 0.0001$=, with two negatives of DERS ($b = -0.31$, $p = 0.016$) and PSI-20 ($b = -0.26$, $p = 0.013$), and two positives of sleep hours ($b = 0.34$, $p < 0.0001$) and leisure activities ($b = 0.42$, $p < 0.0001$)). This result suggests that regular PA is, above all, associated with emotional- and health-related variables.

A supplementary material of this study (Table S1) shows the mean ± SEM by PA and gender. As this study did not focus on gender differences, these data were not included in the main manuscript.

4. Discussion

This study found that individuals engaging in vigorous PA demonstrated superior emotional regulation skills, enhanced impulse control, and fewer prefrontal symptoms in their daily routines compared to those in other groups. Moreover, the vigorous PA group exhibited a lower prevalence of unhealthy behaviors such as alcohol, cannabis, or tobacco use. Members of this group also reported better sleep quality and participated in a more diverse range of leisure activities compared to those with light or moderate PA. However, there were no notable differences among the groups in the evaluated cognitive functions, including attentional processes and working memory. Our linear regression analysis also revealed that self-reported PA intensity by IPAQ-SF was predicted by fewer emotional regulation difficulties, as well as prefrontal symptoms, and higher number of sleep hours and leisure activities. It constitutes a relevant finding highlighting how the higher the intensity of PA, the better emotional regulation and behavioral control, as well as the greater degree of healthier lifestyle habits in young people. This can also lead university campus contexts in which, through access to and promotion of PA, other types of psycho-affective and social aspects can be addressed with young people to improve their wellbeing.

4.1. A Higher Intensity of PA Was Related to Healthy Behaviors

We found that greater PA coincides with less consumption of substances such as alcohol or tobacco among university students. Studies in clinical samples have demonstrated the positive influence of physical activity, in conjunction with standard treatment, in reducing cravings, improving mood, and aiding in abstinence [50]. By contrast, data regarding youth populations with high-risk alcohol consumption are unclear, with contradictory findings in the literature on the relationship between levels of physical activity and alcohol consumption [51]. This effect is particularly pronounced in team and high-competition sports, where it is common to celebrate victories together and the team encourages and sometimes pressures players into alcohol consumption. Additionally, it appears that the association between moderate exercise and alcohol use is often strongest in men [52]. In our study, as shown in Table 1, most of the sample engaged in individual physical activity, primarily at the gym, while a small percentage in the vigorous group participated in team sports but not in a competitive setting. Furthermore, prior studies suggest that certain personality traits, such as extroversion, may serve as moderators in the relationship between exercise and alcohol [53]. To analyze these personality factors, we used the Mini-IPIP questionnaire, but we found no significant differences among the groups in this regard, nor in the rest of the sub-scales assessed. According to our results, highly extroverted individuals or those with pronounced levels of neuroticism were not found to be specifically at risk for increased alcohol abuse when participating in PA [54]. Additionally, it is important to note that some findings indicate a positive relationship between alcohol consumption and PA for men but not women [55], and the sample for this study consisted of 30 men and 73 women.

The average number of hours of sleep was lower in the light PA group than in the moderate and vigorous groups. Several studies have suggested that PA is an effective, non-pharmacological approach for improving sleep. In addition, PA is recommended as an alternative or complementary approach to existing therapies for sleep problems throughout life [56]. Inadequate sleep and irregular sleep–wake patterns observed in younger adolescents raises concerns about similar problems among university students. Poor quality of sleep is associated with reduced neurocognitive and academic performance, which persists from high school into the years in higher education [57]. Interestingly, other studies have also found that vigorous PA has a positive impact on sleep quality and is a predictor of better sleep than moderate PA [58]. Hence, greater effort must be made to promote PA among young people and to understand the impact of different intensities of PA.

Finally, the vigorous PA group not only spent their time performing PA, but also showed high scores in other healthy leisure activities, such as reading, listening to music, going to the cinema or theater, traveling, going out with friends, drawing, playing music, among other activities. Some studies have suggested that participation in leisure activities is a measure of the physical and mental health of an individual [59]. Thus, the evidence suggests that socially active leisure time during adolescence is a protective factor against the appearance of psychiatric disorders such as anxiety or substance abuse disorders in young adulthood [60].

4.2. Higher Intensity of PA Was Associated with Better Emotional and Impulse Control Skills

In line with previous research, the vigorous PA group exhibited better emotional regulation skills, specifically in the sub-scales of "Emotional neglect", "Emotional confusion", "Emotional interference", "Emotional dysregulation", and "Emotional rejection" compared to the other groups. Additionally, the sub-scales of PSI-20 "Social behavior" and "Behavioral control" also showed more positive outcomes with higher intensity PA. Finally, in relation to the UPPS-P questionnaire, the vigorous PA group showed lower scores in "Negative urgency" and "Lack of perseverance", which may have been due to the ability of the vigorous PA group to implement positive re-interpretations and a fewer number of de-emphasizing reappraisals [61]. This positive appraisal style, which can be fostered, at least in part, by PA, was found to predict greater stress resilience [62]. Nonetheless, although numerous studies have found general positive associations between PA and mood, more research is needed to understand the nature of these effects. It has been suggested that PA can generate several physiological changes and mechanisms in the body, which, in turn, may lower stress levels or buffer the stress response protecting against the negative health effects of stress and improving mood and positive affect [63]. It has been also suggested that exercise relieves depressive and anxious symptoms by accumulating recurring mood enhancements. On the physiological level, regular PA is commonly associated with more flexible and adaptive stress responses of the cardiovascular and cortisol system, which may represent biological adaptations in terms of lower reactivity to or faster recovery from stressful events. Thus, it is expected that habitual PA should foster long-term mood elevation [26].

4.3. *Prefrontal-Related Functions Were Not Affected by Different Intensities of PA*

In contrast to previous research, we did not find a positive association between the intensity of PA and attention and working memory, despite there being evidence suggesting that sedentary habits are associated with poorer working memory while moderate and vigorous PA show the opposite [64]. Nonetheless, the exercise–cognition relationship is a complex phenomenon, and it is affected by several factors such as the modality, intensity, and duration of the exercise regime; age; physical fitness; and the cognitive domain being assessed [65]. These discrepant findings in the existing literature and our study may also reflect varying operational definitions of PA. Moreover, we should also consider that most studies have assessed the impact of PA on prefrontal-related functions immediately post-exercise while little is known about its long-term effectiveness or influence [66,67]. It is possible that many cognitive benefits of an intensive PA protocol are due to an increase in lactate and, consequently, the levels of the brain-derived neurotrophic factor (BDNF), which plays a key role in the promotion and maintenance of synaptic connections [68–70].

All in all, our study suggests that young people, given their vulnerability to emotional and impulsivity traits, may be at increased risk for developing future mental health disorders. However, engaging in physical activity, particularly at high intensity, shows promise as an effective approach for managing and reducing these symptoms during this critical developmental period, as well as for supporting improved emotional regulation, impulse control, sleep quality, and overall healthy lifestyle behaviors. Despite these promising results, it is important to note certain limitations in our study. Regarding the sample, although they are not very small, the use of a larger sample would increase the statistical evidence needed to draw stronger conclusions from the findings. Furthermore, the ratio of men to women was not homogenous in each group; thus, the findings of this study may be attributed to differential gender ratios in the different groups. First, our sample primarily consisted of women and Caucasian young adult university students; thus, the findings may not necessarily be generalizable to more diverse groups of young adults. Also, the participants were university students, and their data cannot be generalized to the general youth population. Second, the data were drawn from cross-sectional questionnaires, and a causal relationship between physical activity and the other analyzed variables could not be precisely determined. Additionally, the data from the self-report questionnaires may be overestimated or biased. Thus, for PA, we attempted to resolve these possible inaccuracies by including objective data from pedometers. Nevertheless, accelerometers may better reflect the actual level of the PA of participants. However, despite these limitations, we believe that the findings of this research constitute an advance for the development of prevention and intervention programs within the university context, where the aim is to build emotional competences, impulsivity control, and healthy lifestyles habits, which can help to optimize emotional, affective, academic, and social competences.

Supplementary Materials: The following supporting information can be downloaded at: https://www.mdpi.com/article/10.3390/bs14100935/s1, Table S1. Emotional, cognitive and behavioral results for each group and sex.

Author Contributions: Methodology, A.S.E., R.D.M.-F., A.C.-M. and P.S.-P.; Validation, R.D.M.-F.; Formal analysis, R.D.M.-F. and P.S.-P.; Investigation, A.S.E., R.D.M.-F., A.C.-M. and P.S.-P.; Resources, P.S.-P.; Data curation, P.S.-P.; Writing—original draft, A.S.E., R.D.M.-F. and P.S.-P.; Writing—review and editing, R.D.M.-F. and P.S.-P.; Project administration, P.S.-P.; Funding acquisition, P.S.-P. All authors have read and agreed to the published version of the manuscript.

Funding: This study was funded by the Spanish Ministry of Health (Government Delegation for the National Plan on Drugs, code 2022I004 to P.S.-P.) and the Spanish Ministry of Science and Innovation (MCIN/AEI/10.13039/501100011033/FEDER, UE, code PID2022-137601OA-I00 to P.S.-P.).

Institutional Review Board Statement: The study was conducted in accordance with the Declaration of Helsinki, and approved by the Autonomous University of Madrid (code: CEI-122-2490, 25 April 2022) and the World Medical Association (64th WMA General Assembly, Fortaleza, Brazil, October 2013), Recommendation No. R (97) 5 of the Committee of Ministers to Member States on the Protection of Medical Data (1997), and the Spanish Data Protection Act (Ley Orgánica 15/1999 de Protección de Datos, LOPD).

Informed Consent Statement: Informed consent was obtained from all the subjects involved in this study.

Data Availability Statement: Data are available on request from the corresponding authors.

Acknowledgments: We would like to thank the English editing service of UAM for improving the quality of the manuscript (OAL, FUAM). We wish to also thank our funding institutions for supporting this publication. We gratefully acknowledge the collaboration of our participants.

Conflicts of Interest: The authors declare no conflicts of interest.

References

1. Arnett, J.J. Emerging adulthood. A theory of development from the late teens through the twenties. *Am. Psychol.* **2000**, *55*, 469–480. [CrossRef] [PubMed]
2. Bruffaerts, R.; Mortier, P.; Kiekens, G.; Auerbach, R.P.; Cuijpers, P.; Demyttenaere, K.; Green, J.G.; Nock, M.K.; Kessler, R.C. Mental health problems in college freshmen: Prevalence and academic functioning. *J. Affect. Disord.* **2018**, *225*, 97–103. [CrossRef] [PubMed]
3. Erickson, E.H. *Identity Youth Crisis New York*; W.W. Norton Company: New York, NY, USA, 1968.
4. Limone, P.; Toto, G.A. Factors That Predispose Undergraduates to Mental Issues: A Cumulative Literature Review for Future Research Perspectives. *Front. Public Health* **2022**, *10*, 831349. [CrossRef] [PubMed]
5. Pedrelli, P.; Nyer, M.; Yeung, A.; Zulauf, C.; Wilens, T. College Students: Mental Health Problems and Treatment Considerations. *Acad. Psychiatry* **2015**, *39*, 503–511. [CrossRef]
6. Bewick, B.; Koutsopoulou, G.; Miles, J.; Slaa, E.; Barkham, M. Changes in undergraduate students' psychological well-being as they progress through university. *Stud. High. Educ.* **2010**, *35*, 633–645. [CrossRef]
7. Snedden, T.R.; Scerpella, J.; Kliethermes, S.A.; Norman, R.S.; Blyholder, L.; Sanfilippo, J.; McGuine, T.A.; Heiderscheit, B. Sport and physical activity level impacts health-related quality of life among collegiate students. *Am. J. Health Promot.* **2019**, *33*, 675–682. [CrossRef] [PubMed]
8. Schlack, R.; Peerenboom, N.; Neuperdt, L.; Junker, S.; Beyer, A.K. The effects of mental health problems in childhood and adolescence in young adults: Results of the KiGGS cohort. *J. Health Monit.* **2021**, *6*, 3–19. [CrossRef]
9. Leach, L.S.; Butterworth, P. Depression and anxiety in early adulthood: Consequences for finding a partner, and relationship support and conflict. *Epidemiol. Psychiatr. Sci.* **2020**, *29*, e141. [CrossRef]
10. Daros, A.R.; Daniel, K.E.; Boukhechba, M.; Chow, P.I.; Barnes, L.E.; Teachman, B.A. Relationships between trait emotion dysregulation and emotional experiences in daily life: An experience sampling study. *Cogn. Emot.* **2020**, *34*, 743–755. [CrossRef]
11. Zeman, J.; Cassano, M.; Perry-Parrish, C.; Stegall, S. Emotion regulation in children and adolescents. *J. Dev. Behav. Pediatr.* **2006**, *27*, 155–168. [CrossRef]
12. Berg, J.M.; Latzman, R.D.; Bliwise, N.G.; Lilienfeld, S.O. Parsing the heterogeneity of impulsivity: A meta-analytic review of the behavioral implications of the UPPS for psychopathology. *Psychol. Assess.* **2015**, *27*, 1129–1146. [CrossRef] [PubMed]
13. Bos, J.; Hayden, M.J.; Lum, J.A.G.; Staiger, P.K. UPPS-P impulsive personality traits and adolescent cigarette smoking: A meta-analysis. *Drug Alcohol. Depend.* **2019**, *197*, 335–343. [CrossRef] [PubMed]
14. Stautz, K.; Cooper, A. Impulsivity-related personality traits and adolescent alcohol use: A meta-analytic review. *Clin. Psychol. Rev.* **2013**, *33*, 574–592. [CrossRef]

15. Arias-De la Torre, J.; Fernández-Villa, T.; Molina, A.J.; Amezcua-Prieto, C.; Mateos, R.; Cancela, J.M.; Delgado-Rodríguez, M.; Ortíz-Moncada, R.; Alguacil, J.; Almaraz, A.; et al. Drug use, family support and related factors in university students. A cross-sectional study based on the uniHcos Project data. *Gac. Sanit.* **2019**, *33*, 141–147. [CrossRef]
16. Abrantes, L.C.S.; de Souza de Morais, N.; Gonçalves, V.S.S.; Ribeiro, S.A.V.; de Oliveira Sediyama, C.M.N.; do Carmo Castro Franceschini, S.; dos Santos Amorim, P.R.; Priore, S.E. Physical activity and quality of life among college students without comorbidities for cardiometabolic diseases: Systematic review and meta-analysis. *Qual. Life Res.* **2022**, *31*, 1933–1962. [CrossRef]
17. Steptoe, A.; Wardle, J.; Cui, W.; Bellisle, F.; Zotti, A.M.; Baranyai, R.; Sanderman, R. Trends in smoking, diet, physical exercise, and attitudes toward health in European university students from 13 countries, 1990–2000. *Prev. Med.* **2002**, *35*, 97–104. [CrossRef]
18. Patrick, M.E.; Schulenberg, J.E.; O'Malley, P.M.; Johnston, L.D.; Bachman, J.G. Adolescents' reported reasons for alcohol and marijuana use as predictors of substance use and problems in adulthood. *J. Stud. Alcohol Drugs* **2011**, *72*, 106–116. [CrossRef] [PubMed]
19. Piercy, K.L.; Troiano, R.P.; Ballard, R.M.; Carlson, S.A.; Fulton, J.E.; Galuska, D.A.; George, S.M.; Olson, R.D. The Physical Activity Guidelines for Americans. *JAMA* **2018**, *320*, 2020–2028. [CrossRef]
20. Penedo, F.J.; Dahn, J.R. Exercise and well-being: A review of mental and physical health benefits associated with physical activity. *Curr. Opin. Psychiatry* **2005**, *18*, 189–193. [CrossRef]
21. Li, J.; Huang, Z.; Si, W.; Shao, T. The Effects of Physical Activity on Positive Emotions in Children and Adolescents: A Systematic Review and Meta-Analysis. *Int. J. Environ. Res. Public Health* **2022**, *19*, 14185. [CrossRef]
22. Gmmash, A.; Alonazi, A.; Almaddah, M.; Alkhateeb, A.; Sabir, O.; Alqabbani, S. Influence of an 8-week exercise program on physical, emotional, and mental health in saudi adolescents: A pilot study. *Medicina* **2023**, *59*, 883. [CrossRef] [PubMed]
23. Clemente, F.M.; Nikolaidis, P.T.; Martins, F.M.; Mendes, R.S. Physical activity patterns in university students: Do they follow the public health guidelines? *PLoS ONE* **2016**, *11*, e0152516. [CrossRef] [PubMed]
24. Dishman, R.K.; McIver, K.L.; Dowda, M.; Pate, R.R. Declining physical activity and motivation from middle school to high school. *Med. Sci. Sports Exerc.* **2018**, *50*, 1206–1215. [CrossRef] [PubMed]
25. Martens, M.P.; Buscemi, J.; Smith, A.E.; Murphy, J.G. The short-term efficacy of a brief motivational intervention designed to increase physical activity among college students. *J. Phys. Act. Health* **2012**, *9*, 525–532. [CrossRef]
26. Bernstein, E.E.; McNally, R.J. Acute aerobic exercise helps overcome emotion regulation deficits. *Cogn. Emot.* **2017**, *31*, 834–843. [CrossRef]
27. Giles, G.E.; Cantelon, J.A.; Eddy, M.D.; Brunyé, T.T.; Urry, H.L.; Mahoney, C.R.; Kanarek, R.B. Habitual exercise is associated with cognitive control and cognitive reappraisal success. *Exp. Brain Res.* **2017**, *235*, 3785–3797. [CrossRef]
28. Belcher, B.R.; Zink, J.; Azad, A.; Campbell, C.E.; Chakravartti, S.P.; Herting, M.M. The roles of physical activity, exercise, and fitness in promoting resilience during adolescence: Effects on mental well-being and brain development. *Biol. Psychiatry Cogn. Neurosci. Neuroimaging* **2021**, *6*, 225–237. [CrossRef]
29. Alves, A.R.; Dias, R.; Neiva, H.P.; Marinho, D.A.; Marques, M.C.; Sousa, A.C.; Loureiro, V.; Loureiro, N. High-Intensity Interval Training upon Cognitive and Psychological Outcomes in Youth: A Systematic Review. *Int. J. Environ. Res. Public Health* **2021**, *18*, 5344. [CrossRef]
30. Soler, C.T.; Kanders, S.H.; Olofsdotter, S.; Vadlin, S.; Åslund, C.; Nilsson, K.W. Exploration of the Moderating Effects of Physical Activity and Early Life Stress on the Relation between Brain-Derived Neurotrophic Factor (BDNF) rs6265 Variants and Depressive Symptoms among Adolescents. *Genes* **2022**, *13*, 1236. [CrossRef]
31. Ruotsalainen, I.; Gorbach, T.; Perkola, J.; Renvall, V.; Syväoja, H.J.; Tammelin, T.H.; Karvanen, J.; Parviainen, T. Physical activity, aerobic fitness, and brain white matter: Their role for executive functions in adolescence. *Dev. Cogn. Neurosci.* **2020**, *42*, 100765. [CrossRef]
32. Talbot, J.S.; Perkins, D.R.; Tallon, C.M.; Dawkins, T.G.; Douglas, A.J.M.; Beckerleg, R.; Crofts, A.; Wright, M.E.; Davies, S.; Steventon, J.J.; et al. Cerebral blood flow and cerebrovascular reactivity are modified by maturational stage and exercise training status during youth. *Exp. Physiol.* **2023**, *108*, 1500–1515. [CrossRef] [PubMed]
33. Jiménez-Muro Franco, A.; Beamonte San Agustín, A.; Marqueta, A.; Gargallo Valero, P.; Nerín de la Puerta, I. Addictive substance use among first-year university students. *Adicciones* **2009**, *21*, 21–28. [CrossRef] [PubMed]
34. Molina, A.J.; Varela, V.; Fernández, T.; Martín, V.; Ayán, C.; Cancela, J.M. Unhealthy habits and practice of physical activity in Spanish college students: The role of gender, academic profile and living situation. *Adicciones* **2012**, *24*, 319–327. [CrossRef]
35. Vázquez, F.L.; Torres, Á.; Otero, P.; Díaz, O. Prevalence, comorbidity, and correlates of DSM-IV axis I mental disorders among female university students. *J. Nerv. Ment. Dis.* **2011**, *199*, 379–383. [CrossRef] [PubMed]
36. Ballester, L.; Alayo, I.; Vilagut, G.; Almenara, J.; Cebrià, A.I.; Echeburúa, E.; Gabilondo, A.; Gili, M.; Lagares, C.; Piqueras, J.A.; et al. Mental disorders in Spanish university students: Prevalence, age-of-onset, severe role impairment and mental health treatment. *J. Affect. Disord.* **2020**, *273*, 604–613. [CrossRef]
37. Sicilia, Á.; Alías-García, A.; Ferriz, R.; Moreno-Murcia, J.A. Spanish adaptation and validation of the Exercise Addiction Inventory (EAI). *Psicothema* **2013**, *25*, 377–383. [CrossRef] [PubMed]
38. Craig, C.L.; Marshall, A.L.; Sjöström, M.; Bauman, A.E.; Booth, M.L.; Ainsworth, B.E.; Pratt, M.; Ekelund, U.; Yngve, A.; Sallis, J.F.; et al. International physical activity questionnaire: 12-country reliability and validity. *Med. Sci. Sports Exerc.* **2003**, *35*, 1381–1395. [CrossRef]

39. Contel Guillamon, M.; Gual Solé, A.; Colom Farran, J. Test para la identificación de trastornos por uso de alcohol (AUDIT): Traducción y validación del AUDIT al catalán y castellano. *Adicciones* **1999**, *11*, 337–347. [CrossRef]
40. Legleye, S.; Karila, L.; Beck, F.; Reynaud, M. Validation of the CAST, a general population Cannabis Abuse Screening Test. *J. Subst. Use* **2007**, *12*, 233–242. [CrossRef]
41. Spielberger, C.D.; Gorsuchm, R.L.; Lushene, R.E. *Manual for the State-Trait Anxiety Inventory*; Consulting Psychologist Press: Palo Alto, CA, USA, 1970.
42. Hervas, G.; Jódar, R. Adaptación al castellano de la escala de dificultades en regulación emocional. *Clínica Y Salud* **2008**, *19*, 139–156.
43. Cándido, A.; Orduña, E.; Perales, J.C.; Verdejo-García, A.; Billeux, J. Validation of a short Spanish version of the UPPS-P impulsive behaviour scale. *Trastor. Adict.* **2012**, *14*, 73–78. [CrossRef]
44. Pedrero-Perez, E.J.; Ruiz-Sanchez de Leon, J.M.; Rojo-Mota, G.; Morales-Alonso, S.; Pedrero-Aguilar, J.; Lorenzo, I.; Gonzalez, A. Prefrontal Symptoms Inventory (PSI): Ecological validity and convergence with neuropsychological measures. *Rev. De Neurol.* **2016**, *63*, 241–251.
45. Martínez-Molina, A.; Arias, V.B. Balanced and positively worded personality short-forms: Mini-IPIP validity and cross-cultural invariance. *PeerJ* **2018**, *6*, e5542. [CrossRef] [PubMed]
46. Ainsworth, B.E.; Haskell, W.L.; Herrmann, S.D.; Meckes, N.; Bassett, D.R., Jr.; Tudor-Locke, C.; Greer, J.L.; Vezina, J.; Whitt-Glover, M.C.; Leon, A.S. Compendium of Physical Activities: A second update of codes and MET values. *Med. Sci. Sports Exerc.* **2011**, *43*, 1575–1581. [CrossRef] [PubMed]
47. León-Estrada, I.; García-García, J.; Roldán-Tapia, L. Escala de reserva cognitiva: Ajuste del modelo teórico y baremación. *Rev. De Neurol.* **2017**, *64*, 7–16. [CrossRef]
48. Brickenkamp, R.; Cubero, N.S. *D2: Test de Atención*; TEA Ediciones: Madrid, Spain, 2002.
49. Wechsler, D. *WMS-III Escala de memoria de Wechsler-III*; TEA: Madrid, Spain, 2004.
50. Lardier, D.T.; Coakley, K.E.; Holladay, K.R.; Amorim, F.T.; Zuhl, M.N. Exercise as a useful intervention to reduce alcohol consumption and improve physical fitness in individuals with alcohol use disorder: A systematic review and meta-analysis. *Front. Psychol.* **2021**, *12*, 675285. [CrossRef]
51. Leasure, J.L.; Neighbors, C.; Henderson, C.E.; Young, C.M. Exercise and alcohol consumption: What we know, what we need to know, and why it is important. *Front. Psychiatry* **2015**, *6*, 156. [CrossRef]
52. Buscemi, J.; Martens, M.P.; Murphy, J.G.; Yurasek, A.M.; Smith, A.E. Moderators of the relationship between physical activity and alcohol consumption in college students. *J. Am. Coll. Health* **2011**, *59*, 503–509. [CrossRef]
53. Allen, M.S.; Vella, S.A.; Laborde, S. Health-related behaviour and personality trait development in adulthood. *J. Res. Personal.* **2015**, *59*, 104–110. [CrossRef]
54. Boland, J.K.; Henderson, C.E. The impact of personality on the physical activity and alcohol use relationship. *Clin. Psychol. Spec. Educ.* **2020**, *9*, 62–75. [CrossRef]
55. Sanz-Martín, D.; Zurita-Ortega, F.; Melguizo-Ibáñez, E.; Alonso-Vargas, J.M.; Caracuel-Cáliz, R.; Ubago-Jiménez, J.L. Physical Activity Time, Alcohol Consumption, Mediterranean Diet, and Anxiety in Education Science Students. *Eur. J. Investig. Health Psychol. Educ.* **2024**, *14*, 87–102. [CrossRef] [PubMed]
56. Wang, F.; Boros, S. The effect of physical activity on sleep quality: A systematic review. *Eur. J. Physiother.* **2021**, *23*, 11–18. [CrossRef]
57. Curcio, G.; Ferrara, M.; De Gennaro, L. Sleep loss, learning capacity and academic performance. *Sleep Med. Rev.* **2006**, *10*, 323–337. [CrossRef] [PubMed]
58. Lang, C.; Brand, S.; Feldmeth, A.K.; Holsboer-Trachsler, E.; Pühse, U.; Gerber, M. Increased self-reported and objectively assessed physical activity predict sleep quality among adolescents. *Physiol. Behav.* **2013**, *120*, 46–53. [CrossRef]
59. Eime, R.M.; Young, J.A.; Harvey, J.T.; Charity, M.J.; Payne, W.R. A systematic review of the psychological and social benefits of participation in sport for children and adolescents: Informing development of a conceptual model of health through sport. *Int. J. Behav. Nutr. Phys. Act.* **2013**, *10*, 98. [CrossRef]
60. Timonen, J.; Niemelä, M.; Hakko, H.; Alakokkare, A.; Räsänen, S. Associations between adolescents' social leisure activities and the onset of mental disorders in young adulthood. *J. Youth Adolesc.* **2021**, *50*, 1757–1765. [CrossRef]
61. Perchtold-Stefan, C.M.; Fink, A.; Rominger, C.; Weiss, E.M.; Papousek, I. More habitual physical activity is linked to the use of specific, more adaptive cognitive reappraisal strategies in dealing with stressful events. *Stress Health* **2020**, *36*, 274–286. [CrossRef] [PubMed]
62. Kalisch, R.; Müller, M.B.; Tüscher, O. A conceptual framework for the neurobiological study of resilience. *Behav. Brain Sci.* **2015**, *38*, e92. [CrossRef]
63. Gerber, M.; Pühse, U. Review article: Do exercise and fitness protect against stress-induced health complaints? A review of the literature. *Scand. J. Public Health* **2009**, *37*, 801–819. [CrossRef]
64. Ekelund, U.; Sanchez-Lastra, M.A.; Dalene, K.E.; Tarp, J. Dose-response associations, physical activity intensity and mortality risk: A narrative review. *J. Sport Health Sci.* **2024**, *13*, 24–29. [CrossRef]
65. Williams, R.A.; Hatch, L.; Cooper, S.B. A review of factors affecting the acute exercise-cognition relationship in children and adolescents. *OBM Integr. Complement. Med.* **2019**, *4*, 24. [CrossRef]

66. Browne, R.A.; Costa, E.C.; Sales, M.M.; Fonteles, A.I.; Moraes, J.F.; Barros, J. Acute effect of vigorous aerobic exercise on the inhibitory control in adolescents. *Rev. Paul. De Pediatr.* **2016**, *34*, 154–161. [CrossRef] [PubMed]
67. Soga, K.; Shishido, T.; Nagatomi, R. Executive function during and after acute moderate aerobic exercise in adolescents. *Psychol. Sport Exerc.* **2015**, *16*, 7–17. [CrossRef]
68. Hötting, K.; Röder, B. Beneficial effects of physical exercise on neuroplasticity and cognition. *Neurosci. Biobehav. Rev.* **2013**, *37*, 2243–2257. [CrossRef] [PubMed]
69. Müller, P.; Duderstadt, Y.; Lessmann, V.; Müller, N.G. Lactate and BDNF: Key Mediators of Exercise Induced Neuroplasticity? *J. Clin. Med.* **2020**, *9*, 1136. [CrossRef]
70. Jacob, N.; So, I.; Sharma, B.; Marzolini, S.; Tartaglia, M.C.; Oh, P.; Green, R. Effects of High-Intensity Interval Training Protocols on Blood Lactate Levels and Cognition in Healthy Adults: Systematic Review and Meta-Regression. *Sports Med.* **2023**, *53*, 977–991. [CrossRef]

behavioral sciences

Article

Exploring Constraints and Sport Experiences: A Case Study of Adult Workers in Singapore

Heetae Cho [1,2], Ghazanfar Ali Abbasi [3], Hyoung-Kil Kang [4,*] and Ye Hoon Lee [5,*]

1 Department of Sport Science, Sungkyunkwan University, Suwon 16419, Republic of Korea; htcho@g.skku.edu
2 Department of Physical Education and Sport Science, Nanyang Technological University, Singapore 637616, Singapore
3 Management and Marketing Department, KFUPM Business School, King Fahd University of Petroleum and Minerals, Dharan 31261, Saudi Arabia
4 Department of Physical Education, Kyungnam University, Changwon 51767, Republic of Korea
5 Division of Global Sport Industry, Hankuk University of Foreign Studies, Yongin 17035, Republic of Korea
* Correspondence: hkilkang@kyungnam.ac.kr (H.-K.K.); leeye22@o365.hufs.ac.kr (Y.H.L.)

Abstract: Although rapid economic growth can produce various positive outcomes, the fast-paced society that inevitably accompanies it often results in longer working hours and higher stress levels, leading to reduced participation in sport activities among employees. To better understand this phenomenon, we aimed to explore the constraints and experiences of adult workers. We collected data from adult workers in Singapore who desired to participate in sport activities but were unable to do so due to various constraints. A total of 10 individuals were purposefully selected for interviews. This study identified four key themes: (a) factors causing the reduction of sport participation opportunities, (b) changes in sport activities and satisfaction, (c) nostalgic feelings associated with sport activities, and (d) the role of nostalgia in enhancing sport involvement. The findings of this study suggest the possibility of adapting the conceptual model of nostalgia to sport activities, as well as identifying four factors that hinder employees from engaging in sport activities.

Keywords: constraint; sport experience; nostalgia; satisfaction; sport involvement

1. Introduction

Sport is a significant aspect of life [1,2] that individuals engage in via personal choice due to the inherently exciting nature of these activities (i.e., intrinsic motivation) and their potential for personal development [3]. Researchers have noted that sport participation benefits an individual's health [4,5]. For example, Passmore [6] found that sport activities could improve mental health and social inclusiveness, encourage self-expression, and foster an individual's potential. Additionally, sport activities help prevent stress and aid in coping with it effectively [7–9], making them beneficial for psychological well-being [10,11] and therapeutic for psychological therapy [5].

Active sport participation also has a positive effect on participants' physical health [12,13]. Previous research has shown that exercise can reduce the mortality rate by up to 50% for individuals who shift from a sedentary lifestyle to moderate activity [14]. Thus, sport activities that include physical activity enhance physical fitness and reduce the risk of mortality [15,16]. In summary, active sport participation can result in multiple benefits for individuals, including physical and psychological health, overall well-being, and meaningful activities with cumulative effects [17,18].

In the past, leisure was often viewed negatively, as it was thought to be in conflict with work [19]. This perspective, rooted in an industrialized worldview, has persisted in our society, particularly in Singapore, where work is often given greater priority [20,21]. Although this perception has evolved over time, it remains a prominent feature of Singaporean culture. Comparing Singapore's work culture with that of the United Kingdom, which is often seen as representative of Western culture, can shed light on this issue. According to data from the UK Office for National Statistics, the average working hours per week in 2023 were 36.2 h, while in Singapore the average was 44.2 h [22,23]. Additionally, the GDP per capita ratios of Singapore and the UK were SGD 52,962 and SGD 40,367, respectively [24]. Based on these statistics, it can be inferred that Singapore's higher GDP was the result of a proportionally larger workforce with longer working hours, resulting in less leisure time for individuals working full-time [25]. Sport Singapore reported that 51% of participants lacked sufficient time to engage in sporting activities due to work, while others cited family or work commitments or a lack of interest [26]. This suggests that individuals in Singapore, a highly work-oriented nation, may have limited opportunities to engage in sport activities and may be unable to fully enjoy them. Although sport can offer numerous benefits to individuals [4], many face constraints that prevent them from participating fully, such as cost, time constraints, the availability and quality of sport facilities, social and geographical isolation and personal skills and abilities [27–30].

Researchers have found that long working hours and high stress levels are associated with an increased risk of cardiovascular disease, morbidity, disability [31–33] and common mental disorders [34,35]. The intensive working culture in Singapore has reduced workers' leisure time, leading to constraints that may have negative consequences, such as a decline in physical and mental health [36]. The primary research gap this study addresses is the lack of focused investigation into the specific constraints faced by adult workers in Singapore regarding their sport participation. While existing research has examined constraints in various countries, including the impact of work culture on leisure activities [37–40], there is limited empirical evidence on how the unique work environment in Singapore—a high-pressure, high-hour culture—specifically affects sport participation. Thus, this study aims to fill this gap by providing an in-depth exploration of how working adults in Singapore navigate and experience constraints that lead to reduced physical activity. In addition, Singapore's high-pressure work culture significantly impacts the work-life balance of its residents. This work-life balance refers to the equilibrium between professional commitments and personal time, which enables participation in leisure activities, such as sport [41,42]. The tension between work and leisure is particularly acute in Singapore, where the demands of employment frequently leave little room for personal pursuits [43]. Furthermore, Godbey et al. [44] noted that individuals in different social, cultural, and historical contexts experience different constraints. Therefore, this study identifies the causes of reduced sport activities among participants in Singapore and explore their psychological responses to such constraints, such as satisfaction, nostalgia, and sport involvement. In particular, recent research has highlighted nostalgia as a key emotional factor influencing behavioral outcomes [45]. For adult workers facing various physical and psychological obstacles to sport participation, nostalgia may serve as a unique motivational tool. By evoking memories of previous engagement in sport or leisure activities, nostalgia can rekindle a desire to re-experience joy and satisfaction of physical movement [45].

This study explores how nostalgia can help buffer and overcome such barriers, positioning it as a central motivational factor for re-engagement in sport among adult workers in Singapore. To further deepen the investigation into the phenomenon of reduced sport participation among adult workers in Singapore, the following research questions were developed: (1) What are the specific constraints faced by adult workers in Singapore regarding sport participation? (2) How does nostalgia function as a motivational tool for overcoming barriers to sport participation among Singaporean workers? These research questions allow for a comprehensive exploration of the phenomena and provide important insights into the complex interplay between work-related pressures, cultural influences, and sport participation. The findings illuminate the distinctive challenges encountered by individuals in the Singaporean context, which may diverge from those experienced in other cultural milieus. By elucidating the specific constraints and their psychological ramifications, such as satisfaction and nostalgia, this study offers invaluable perspectives on the relationship between work and leisure in a highly work-centric society. This understanding is crucial for developing targeted interventions to foster enhanced sport participation and overall well-being among workers facing similar high-pressure environments.

2. Literature Review

2.1. Constraints

Constraint refers to the factor that limits an individual's ability to participate in sport activities [46,47]. This concept has been of interest to scholars for several decades. Crawford et al. [48] proposed the earliest theory of constraints, suggesting that constraints could be categorized into three types: intrapersonal, interpersonal and structural. Intrapersonal constraints relate to factors within an individual, such as lack of skills, interests or motivation [47,49]. Interpersonal constraints relate to factors in a person's social environment, such as lack of social support or conflicts with others [46,50]. Structural constraints refer to factors outside of an individual's control, such as lack of time, money or access to sport facilities [48]. Time and money are commonly cited structural constraints to sport participation [51,52]. Scott [47] proposed a fourth category of constraint, cultural constraints, which refer to the influence of cultural norms and values on sport participation. Cultural constraints are also found to shape sport participation with demographic factors such as gender, race and ethnicity [53,54].

Recent studies have further examined the role of sport constraints in different contexts. For example, Lee et al. [55] found that technology-related constraints were a significant barrier to sport participation and argued that lack of technology skills and access to technology were important factors that limited individuals' ability to engage in sport activities. Chen and Petrick [56] found that intrapersonal constraints were the most significant barriers to travel, followed by interpersonal and structural constraints. Similarly, Darcy et al. [57] noted that women and older adults were more likely to experience time- and family-related constraints, while men and younger adults were more likely to experience financial and work-related constraints. Although several scholars have attempted to emphasize the importance of understanding constraints in promoting sport participation, more research is needed to examine the intersection of multiple constraints and how they interact to limit sport participation [58]. In addition, it is necessary to examine how constraints vary across different domains and how they impact participation [59].

2.2. Satisfaction

Satisfaction in the context of sport refers to the contentment and positive feelings individuals derive from engaging in sport and leisure [60]. Previous research suggests that satisfaction with sport and leisure is a significant construct that is influenced by a wide range of individual, social, and contextual factors. For instance, it was found that leisure time spent with family, friends and other social networks is an important factor in increasing leisure satisfaction [61–64]. In addition, the levels of satisfaction can vary depending on demographic factors, such as age, gender, income and education level, which can all impact satisfaction [65,66]. Contextual elements, such as the accessibility of sport facilities and opportunities, as well as the specific sport activities individuals engage in, can also shape their level of satisfaction [67].

Another important finding from the literature is that satisfaction has significant implications for mental health and overall well-being. Previous studies have found that individuals experiencing high levels of leisure satisfaction show high mental wellness and low levels of stress and depression [68]. Similarly, Cho [69] explored the relationship between leisure satisfaction and well-being and highlighted that leisure satisfaction played a significant role in enhancing well-being.

Despite these findings, however, there are research gaps and limitations that should be noted. Previous studies have used self-reported measures of satisfaction, which may be subject to biases and other limitations [65]. Additionally, there is still much to learn about the mechanisms underlying satisfaction, and more research is needed to explore the potential role of cultural factors in shaping satisfaction. Thus, further studies are of high importance to enrich this research field. In this study, we explore the sport satisfaction experiences of adult employees in Singapore. Comprehending them is vital, as greater satisfaction can foster enhanced motivation and sustained engagement in sport. Conversely, dissatisfaction, frequently stemming from constraints such as time limitations, resource deficiencies, or insufficient support, may contribute to diminished participation.

2.3. Nostalgia

Nostalgia can be defined as a longing or sentimental yearning for past experiences or activities [45,70]. Nostalgia has garnered attention as researchers seek to understand why people often look back on experiences with such fondness [71]. Holbrook and Schindler [72] noted that nostalgia was more likely to occur when people perceived a discontinuity between their current and past experiences, such as moving to a new location or entering a new life stage. Similarly, Cho et al. [70] found that people were more likely to experience nostalgia when they felt a sense of loss or absence in their current sport activities.

Researchers have noted that nostalgia can generate positive psychological and behavioral outcomes [45,73,74]. For instance, Kim et al. [75] found that individuals experience nostalgia for past experiences, such as going on school trips and participating in extracurricular activities. In a recent study, Cho [1] found that individuals with nostalgia showed a high level of life satisfaction and tended to engage in sport activities, suggesting that nostalgia may motivate individuals to seek out sport experiences that are meaningful and enjoyable. Additionally, inducing feelings of nostalgia has been found to increase feelings of social connectedness and reduce feelings of loneliness [76]. Likewise, Huddart and Stott (2018) noted that nostalgia could help people cope with negative life events by providing a source of comfort and familiarity. However, some researchers have cautioned that nostalgia may also have negative effects, particularly if it leads to excessive dwelling on the past or a reluctance to engage with current sport activities [77]. In sum, nostalgia is a complex and multifaceted psychological construct; there may be individual differences in how people experience nostalgia for sport activities. While many studies have found that nostalgia can have positive effects on behavioral and psychological responses, there is a need for more research to examine the underlying mechanisms of its linkage with sport experiences.

2.4. Sport Involvement

Sport involvement refers to the extent to which individuals engage in sport activities and the psychological significance that these activities hold for them [78,79]. In previous studies, researchers have explored various factors that contribute to sport involvement and have examined how it varies across different demographic groups. For instance, one of the earliest studies on involvement was conducted by Iso-Ahola and Mannell [80], who proposed a model of leisure involvement. They noted that people with high motivation to engage in leisure activities participate in a wide range of activities and have positive personal attributes, such as self-esteem and a sense of control over their lives [80]. Additionally, previous research has found that the availability of sport facilities and programs, as well as accessibility to transportation and information, are important factors in promoting sport participation [81,82]. Researchers have also highlighted factors that contribute to differences in sport involvement across different demographic groups [8,83] and further identified a relationship between sport involvement and diverse psychological factors, particularly its benefits for individual well-being and quality of life [84–87]. Although involvement is a complex construct that has been studied extensively in the literature, most studies have focused on the psychological and behavioral outcomes of involvement. Therefore, this study focuses on the process that leads to sport involvement to gain a broader understanding of it.

3. Materials and Methods

This study utilizes a qualitative research approach, which is grounded in constructivist and interpretivist paradigms. These paradigms highlight the subjective nature of reality and the significance of understanding individuals' experiences from their own perspectives. By employing a qualitative methodology, we aimed to explore and interpret the complex, nuanced experiences and constraints of individuals in Singapore regarding their sport activities. This approach enables an in-depth examination of the participants' personal narratives, yielding rich, detailed insights that may not be captured through quantitative methods.

3.1. Data Collection and Participants

To recruit research participants, this study employed a combination of snowball and purposeful sampling. Initially, we utilized social media platforms and sport community groups to identify individuals who expressed a high intention to participate in sport activities but were experiencing constraints. Additionally, participants were required to work more than 45 h per week for inclusion in this study. Before collecting data, this study obtained Institutional Review Board (IRB) approval from a university in Singapore. Purposeful sampling allowed us to select participants who met specific criteria relevant to our study, ensuring a focused and relevant sample. Participants were chosen based on their self-reported decrease in sport participation due to various constraints. Once initial participants were identified, snowball sampling was employed to expand the sample. For example, Darren (male, 44) introduced Fiona (female, 44) and Tom (male, 49) introduced Perry (male, 36) and Jane (female, 36). This method helped us reach additional participants who fit our criteria through referrals from the initial participants.

We conducted semi-structured interviews, crafting questions along the topics of constraints and sport experiences to gather their past and current experiences in sport. The interview questions were structured to explore the main research question while allowing for unanticipated themes to emerge [88]. The interview protocol was developed through a collaborative process to ensure its theoretical and practical robustness. The initial draft was created by the first author based on a thorough review of the relevant literature and research objectives. This draft was reviewed by a panel of four experts in the fields of sport psychology, sport management and leisure. They provided feedback on relevance and clarity of the questions. It consisted of semi-structured questions designed to explore various facets of the participants' experiences, including introductory (e.g., what is the most frequent or enjoyable leisure activity that you participated in?); constraint-related (e.g., what factors have affected your ability to participate in sport activities recently?); attitude and negotiation (e.g., how has your participation in sport activities changed over time?); nostalgia (do you feel nostalgic about any past sport experiences? If so, how does this nostalgia affect your current participation?); and future involvement (e.g., what are your future plans or goals related to sport activities?) themes. The interview guide was customized to elicit in-depth responses on these key areas, while also allowing flexibility to investigate emerging topics as necessary.

All interviews were recorded using an audio recording device to facilitate efficient transcription. Each interview lasted between 20 to 40 min and was conducted at the convenience of the interviewee, either at their residence or a nearby café. The average duration of the interviews was 32.67 min, with a standard deviation of 6.25 min. Although one interview lasted only 20 min, we ensured that sufficient information was collected through a combination of well-structured questions and a flexible interview approach that allowed participants to elaborate on their experiences. Each interview was designed to cover all the essential topics related to constraints and sport experiences while allowing for deeper exploration based on participants' responses.

The final selection of participants was based on achieving data saturation. Specifically, we determined that data collection and analysis had reached saturation through an iterative process. We continuously compared new data to existing themes using the constant comparison method, until no additional themes emerged [89]. In other words, data saturation was considered to have been achieved when further interviews did not uncover new information or themes, existing themes were consistently supported by new data, and peer debriefing sessions confirmed that saturation had been reached. In total, 10 participants residing in Singapore were interviewed. These participants consisted of seven males and two females, aged between 33 to 49 years (Table 1). Among them, nine were married with children and one was single. The majority of participants held a college degree and had an average working hour per week of 53.3 h.

Table 1. Characteristics of participant.

Name	Age	Gender	Marital Status	Presence of Children	Occupation	Working Hours per Week	Education
Perry	36	Male	Married	Yes	Financial Service Manager	50	Bachelor's degree
Jane	36	Female	Married	Yes	Account Executive	45	Diploma
Tom	49	Male	Married	Yes	Remisier	40	Bachelor's degree
Darren	44	Male	Married	Yes	Deputy Chief Executive Officer (CEO)	50	Bachelor's degree
Fiona	44	Female	Married	Yes	Manager	50	Bachelor's degree
Mark	40	Male	Married	Yes	Chief Operating Officer	50	Master's degree
Jet	42	Male	Married	Yes	Sport Manager	40	Bachelor's degree
Ali	44	Male	Married	Yes	Taxi Driver	45	Secondary School
Peter	33	Male	Single	No	Claims Executive	40	Bachelor's degree
George	63	Male	Married	Yes	Taxi Driver	70	Secondary School

After the interview, the recordings were transcribed, and participants were provided with the details of the study, including the purpose, confidentiality, time frame, waiver and contact information. We also explained the study to the participants to ensure a better understanding of the research. Contact information, including the participant's contact number and email address, was collected for future communication if needed.

3.2. Data Analysis

To provide an archive of a more specific targeted group for future research with similar topics [90], the interviews and analysis of the transcripts from the collected data were conducted simultaneously using the constant comparison method [91]. This methodological approach was chosen because it systematically compares data elements, helping to develop and refine concepts and categories through an iterative process. This aligns well with our constructivist and interpretivist research paradigms, which emphasize understanding participants' subjective experiences and constructing theory grounded in their perspectives. During the analysis, the transcripts were examined in detail to gain a deeper understanding of the participants' responses. The data analysis involved three coders to ensure a rigorous thematic analysis. Coding was placed along the margins of the document in alignment with the transcript text. This process was repeated for the other transcripts, with the audio files being played several times to ensure accuracy. The location and time of the interview were labelled in each transcript. The main themes drawn from the responses were compiled and compared to the original transcripts of the participants to ensure validity. Further, to ensure trustworthiness, we conducted member checking, wherein preliminary findings were shared with participants for validation. We returned the findings to the participants to confirm the accuracy of the data and interpretations. Additionally, peer debriefing sessions were conducted to validate the data analysis. Specifically, we shared our findings with five professors in the field of sport psychology to receive their feedback on the interpretations. Data triangulation was used by selecting participants from diverse sectors and age groups to provide a broader range of experiences. Additionally, theory triangulation was applied by integrating perspectives from emotion-related and leisure constraint theories to offer a comprehensive understanding of the role of nostalgia in sport participation. Finally, the themes were categorized with the research topic to evaluate the data. In particular, the main topic of this study is related to constraints. Therefore, this study adopted a deductive approach, utilizing Crawford and Godbey's [92] constraints model to classify the qualitative data. This model categorizes leisure constraints into intrapersonal, interpersonal and structural constructs. We used this framework to organize and interpret our findings, providing a structured lens through which to analyze the constraints experienced by participants.

4. Results

The aim of this study was to investigate constraints and sport experiences among individuals in Singapore. We identified four main themes from the interviews: *factors causing the reduction of sport opportunities, changes in sport activities and satisfaction, nostalgic feelings associated with sport activities and the role of nostalgia in enhancing sport involvement*. Each theme highlights different aspects of participants' sport experiences and constraints.

4.1. Factors Causing the Reduction of Sport Opportunities

Participants reported various constraints that contributed to a reduction in their sport participation. A common factor was physical limitations due to injury or aging. For example, Peter (33, male) described how an ACL injury reduced his soccer participation from once a week to once a month, due to limitations in his ability to play and the need to manage his injury. Additionally, another participant, Jet (42, male), had started playing badminton when he was six years old and had enjoyed the activity with his family and relatives in his younger days. However, as Jet grew older, he found that his recovery period after badminton games had significantly slowed down, preventing him from maintaining the high intensity of the games he used to enjoy. Even though Jet still played badminton once a week, he was not able to enjoy it as much as before due to his physical constraints and the natural aging process. The psychological fear of getting injured and the long recovery period associated with aging were the barriers that Jet did not want to go through. That is, aging affects his ability to play badminton at high intensity, leading to reduced enjoyment and participation:

> *Around 3–4 years ago, I suffered an ACL injury, and it doesn't mean that I can't play. I still can, but there were limitations to it. So that is the reason why I have to reduce the playing time.* (Peter)

> *As you grow older, injuries and recovery are much slower than before, so you don't expect to play at very high intensity when you haven't been doing it frequently. One of my biggest worries is also injuries and age.* (Jet)

Environmental constraints such as family and work commitments also played a significant role. Darren (44, male) emphasized the difficulty of balancing family responsibilities with sport participation, particularly when considering the risk of injury:

> *We still have a family to take care of. I can't afford to play a football game, and then tomorrow, tell my boss that I will be on medical leave for a week because of a sprained ankle, even though it is very hard to justify that.* (Darren)

Apart from age, other factors, such as the availability of facilities, family commitments and work commitments, have also limited the sport participation of participants like Darren and Jet. Previous studies on constraints have also identified similar factors, including a lack of time, money, and information [40]. While this study's findings showed similarities in terms of time constraints, other constraints, such as insufficient information and economic affordability from Scott et al.'s [40] study, were not applicable in the context of Singapore.

Another participant, Perry (male, 36), who had been actively trekking for the past 7–8 years, saw a significant decrease in his engagement in this sport activity due to social factors, such as the personalities of other participants and interactions between them during his sport activity. Perry found it challenging to deal with multiple inputs from different people, and friction within the group of friends that was inevitable due to the nature of the activity itself.

> *Different people have different personalities, so when you explore and you go trekking with a different group of people, different inputs will come in, so that's the part that so-called the organizer has to handle.* (Perry)

In addition, another psychological factor that led to a reduction in sport participation was pressure. Tom (49, male), an avid golf player who has been playing golf for around 25 years, mentioned that stress sometimes made him reconsider his participation in the sport activity as he could not enjoy the game if he was under too much pressure. Overall, constraints such as physical limitations, psychological constraints, environmental factors and social dynamics were key reasons for reduced sport participation.

4.2. Changes in Sport Activities and Satisfaction

Participants also reported changes in their sport activities and associated levels of satisfaction. For instance, Darren (44, male) transitioned from playing football to watching soccer due to physical constraints, resulting in dissatisfaction with his current level of engagement:

> *Although my passion for football remains, I have shifted to watching soccer due to physical constraints. The alternative of watching the sport isn't as fulfilling as participating.* (Darren)

Jet (42, male) similarly experienced dissatisfaction due to limitations on court availability, which prevented him from playing badminton as often as he would like. Despite these changes, some participants found new forms of enjoyment. Jane (36, female) and Mark (40, male) expressed positive outcomes from their sport activities, such as social bonding and stress relief:

> *I enjoy the competitive element in badminton and the social interactions with friends during leisure time.* (Jet)

> *Bowling provides a break from work and family, allowing me to enjoy the sport without worrying about standards.* (Mark)

For these participants, the outcomes of their sport activities were the main motivators for maintaining their lives. During follow-up interviews, positive feelings were expressed, with some participants recalling specific details of their sport experiences vividly from memory.

4.3. Nostalgic Feelings Associated with Sport Activities

The theme of nostalgia emerged strongly, highlighting how past sport experiences evoke significant emotional responses among participants. This theme not only reflects their personal experiences but also how their current circumstances, including family dynamics, influence their nostalgic feelings. Several participants expressed vivid nostalgic memories related to their past sport activities. Perry (36, male), an avid trekker, shared detailed recollections of a memorable trek, describing the landscape and environmental conditions that evoked a deep sense of nostalgia:

> *We went during autumn, so we shouldn't see any snow, but when we reached the base camp which is around 4900 m above sea level, we managed to see snow and the whole scenery really resembles the north pole, basically those houses painted blue on the rooftop. You see the whole place in white, it was nice, really nice.* (Perry)

This sense of nostalgia was further amplified when Perry reflected on past experiences and how they shaped his current motivations for trekking. His nostalgia was not only about the physical experiences but also the emotional connections formed during these treks.

Darren (44, male) provided an additional dimension to the theme of nostalgia by relating his past sport experiences to his present life through his children. He mentioned watching his son play soccer, which evoked nostalgic feelings as he recalled his own days of playing soccer:

> *Seeing my son play soccer reminds me of my own days on the field. It is a mixed feeling of joy and longing for those times when I was actively playing.* (Darren)

This reflection illustrates how observing his son's participation in soccer rekindled Darren's own memories of the sport, blending his past with his current experiences.

Similarly, Tom (49, male) experienced nostalgia as he used to play golf once a week when he was younger, but the time he spent on golf gradually decreased as he aged due to other commitments. Although his time for golf diminished, he found joy in seeing his children partake in sport, which provided him with a sense of connection to his own past:

> *Even though I don't play golf as often, watching my children take part in sport brings back memories of when I was actively involved. It's a way of reliving those experiences through them.* (Tom)

Another form of nostalgia expressed by participants was related to their social interactions during their sport activities. Jane (36, female) expressed her longing for past badminton training sessions, where she and her classmates would gather on weekends and enjoy each other's company.

> *As I said, I spent a lot of time training, so I missed the time I spent with my own classmates. When my classmate gathers together on the weekend, I am unable to because I have the training to attend to.* (Jane)

Cho et al. [93] noted that nostalgia can develop from objects and interpersonal relationships, while Korte [94] stated that socialization can increase an individual's sense of identity, leading to the development of nostalgia for group identity. Tajfel's [95] view on social identity suggests that an individual's emotional attachment to a specific group establishes a sense of belonging, and Jane's expression during the interview evoked those feelings. Specifically, nostalgia for group identity surfaced during Jane's representation of her school team's badminton tournament, highlighting her motivation and continued participation in badminton. This study also found that a participant's sport experience is associated with nostalgia for personal identity. For example, Perry took pride in being an avid trekker and had nostalgic feelings toward his personal identity. He also felt nostalgia for the time, effort and resources he had invested in the activity.

4.4. The Role of Nostalgia in Enhancing Sport Involvement

This section specifically explores how nostalgic feelings impact participants' current involvement in sport activities. While previous sections discussed constraints and general changes in sport participation, this section focuses on how nostalgia not only triggers past memories, but also motivates continued or renewed engagement in sport.

Nostalgia played a significant role in motivating participants to remain involved in or return to sport. For example, Perry (36, male) experienced a strong connection between his nostalgic memories of trekking and his motivation to continue the activity. Perry missed those sport experiences and the valuable feedback he received, which he regarded as lifelong tips. Although he cannot turn back time, the feedback he gained had a lasting impact on his current trekking skills. This indicates how past sport involvement can affect current sport involvement. In addition, Perry experienced nostalgia due to the unique experiences of each trek, which helped motivate him to continue his passion for trekking. It suggests that nostalgia can enhance current sport involvement by providing positive memories and motivation to continue participating in sport activities.

> *I would say I have the feelings because every trek is different. I think that is the key part of trekking. So, when I look back at this mountain or that mountain, I feel nostalgic. It is related to how that particular trip is heavy or how eventful.* (Perry)

However, Perry also noted the need for lifestyle changes to fully enjoy his sport activities, suggesting that nostalgia alone may not be sufficient to sustain involvement.

Nostalgia also influenced participants' choices of sport activities. Darren (44, male), although physically constrained from playing soccer, expressed a renewed connection to the sport through watching his son play. This experience underscored how nostalgia for his own soccer days fueled his ongoing interest. Similarly, Tom (49, male) found that nostalgic feelings associated with his past golf activities helped him stay engaged with the sport, even if his participation had decreased:

> *Watching my son play soccer reminds me of my own playing days. It's a joy to see him and relive those memories through him.* (Darren)
>
> *I don't play golf as often, but the memories and seeing my children in sport remind me of my love for it. It's a way of holding onto those past experiences.* (Tom)

Nostalgia sometimes helped participants overcome the constraints that limited their sport activities. For instance, Jane (36, female) used her nostalgic memories of past badminton training sessions to sustain her interest in the sport, despite current barriers:

> *I miss the social interactions and training sessions. These memories keep my interest in badminton alive, even though I can't participate as much.* (Jane)

Overall, the findings suggest that nostalgic feelings have a significant impact on one's sport involvement in the present, influenced by specific sport experiences and past involvement levels. Some participants expressed their willingness to change their current lifestyles to enhance their sport experiences. The constraints that trigger nostalgia and motivate participants to make changes can ultimately lead to an increase in current sport activity participation and a more positive mindset toward participating in sport activities. Therefore, constraints may trigger nostalgia, encourage motivation, diminish the perception of constraints and facilitate negotiation efforts, ultimately leading to positive actions toward sport participation.

5. Discussion

This study aimed to identify the types of constraints and their relationship with satisfaction, benefits of sport, nostalgia and sport involvement among Singaporean adults, as there are limited studies on constraints among this population. In this study, we identified four main themes related to sport experiences and constraints among individuals in Singapore. These themes provide insight into the various factors affecting sport participation and the role of nostalgia. The first theme, *factors causing the reduction of sport opportunities*, indicates that participants experienced certain constraints, which resulted in negative emotions and dissatisfaction with their limited engagement in sport activities. The second theme, *changes in sport activities and satisfaction*, highlights the fact that participants highlighted multiple advantages that they could gain from sport. The third theme, *nostalgic feelings associated with sport activities*, refers to nostalgia related to these sport activities. Finally, the last theme, the role of nostalgia in enhancing sport involvement, focus on how nostalgic feelings influence participants' current sport involvement and how they can change individuals' current lifestyle to continue their sport activities. We discuss these themes in detail, exploring how each contributes to our understanding of sport participation and the influence of nostalgia.

The constraints identified in this study were classified into four main groups: physical, environmental, psychological and social factors. To contextualize these constraints within existing theoretical frameworks, we used Crawford and Godbey's [92] constraints model, which classifies leisure constraints into three constructs: intrapersonal, interpersonal and structural. Physical and psychological constraints belong to the intrapersonal construct. These constraints include personal health issues and psychological barriers, which directly impact an individual's ability to engage in sport. Social factors, such as family commitments and social interactions, align with the interpersonal construct. These constraints relate to how interactions with others affect one's participation in sport. Environmental factors, including facility availability and work commitments, correspond with the structural construct. Structural constraints involve external barriers that could be addressed through policy changes, such as adjustments to working hours or improved access to sport facilities. Our findings indicate that addressing structural constraints, particularly those related to working hours, could help Singaporean adults engage in more sport activities, leading to improved satisfaction, reduced stress and better health outcomes. For instance, participants highlighted work commitments and family responsibilities as significant barriers to sport participation. Singaporeans work more hours per week compared to individuals in some other countries, resulting in less time for sport and increased stress. Hence, revising working hour policies or encouraging companies to implement flexible working arrangements could enhance quality of life and reduce health issues among Singaporean workers.

However, this may present a compromise for workers who have to choose between income and leisure time. Participants often expressed a sense of being torn between earning a livelihood and having time for leisure activities, including sport. This tension is not unique to Singapore but is also seen in other countries, such as Australia, where work-time reduction is a topic of debate [96]. According to Gerold and Nocker [96], workers' working-time preferences are shaped by social norms (i.e., full-time working norm) and personal priorities, such as the need for financial security versus the desire for leisure time. Furthermore, participants in this study expressed dissatisfaction with their current situation, where they could not maintain their sport participation as they used to. This dissatisfaction is consistent with Hughes and Bozionelos' [97] findings that work–life imbalance is a significant source of dissatisfaction among workers, leading to labor turnover and other work withdrawal behaviors.

Work–life balance refers to the balance of work, whether done on the job or at home, and leisure time for working individuals to enjoy life to its fullest [41]. In contrast, individuals who feel in control of their work are more likely to perceive a balanced life. Mitigating structural impediments, particularly those pertaining to working time arrangements, could substantially improve the quality of life for Singaporean adults. Introducing policies that foster a better equilibrium between professional and personal domains, such as flexible or reduced work schedules, may stimulate increased engagement in sport activities. This shift could yield enhanced job satisfaction, diminished stress and improved health outcomes. Incentivizing organizations to implement these policies and disseminate the corresponding findings may represent a strategic approach to elevating the overall well-being of the workforce.

Another significant finding of this study is the relationship between constraints and nostalgia among Singaporean adults. Individuals encountering physical and psychological barriers to sport participation may experience an increased sense of nostalgia, as they look back on past sport activities in the context of their present limitations. This feeling of nostalgia can act as a motivational factor, alleviating some of the constraints and potentially fostering renewed interest in sport. By exploring this dynamic, we offer a deeper insight into how nostalgic emotions can affect sport engagement, despite the constraints outlined in our study.

Participants' nostalgic feelings toward their sport activities were associated with their past experiences, social interactions and personal identity. The conceptual model of nostalgia by Cho et al. [93] can be incorporated into the findings of this study. The model was designed to explain the feelings of nostalgia through a scope of memories, and Cho et al. [1,70] further provided five different aspects of nostalgia (i.e., experience, environment, socialization, personal identity and group identity) and discussed how those nostalgic feelings affect one's sport activity. Individuals' nostalgia regarding past sport participation is not simply a yearning for past activities, but rather encompasses a multifaceted interplay of experiences and emotions that influence their current behaviors.

Participants frequently reflected on their younger years, during which they engaged in sport alongside friends, enjoyed communal spaces and experienced a profound sense of belonging. For example, one participant reminisced about playing soccer in the past, emphasizing how these memories evoke nostalgic feelings. This nostalgia motivates them to seek analogous experiences in their present-day lives, though these may be modified by their current circumstances. In addition, the role of nostalgia in sport participation may vary across cultural contexts. For example, the nostalgia associated with outdoor ice rinks in Canada appears to be a significant attraction for sport tourists, evoking a sense of place identity and an idealized past [98]. In the American context, research suggests that sport halls of fame and museums also serve as sites of collective and private nostalgia, allowing visitors to engage with cherished memories and a romanticized vision of sporting history [99]. These nostalgic memories can inspire continued engagement in physical activities and sport, as individuals seek to reconnect with their personal or cultural past.

Moreover, the level of an individual's participation in sport activities in the past can be used to predict their current frequency of sport activity. Specifically, sport activities can be classified based on the level of commitment by applying the six different features of serious leisure pursuits from the past [100]. These include perseverance, significant personal efforts, unique ethos, strong identification with the activity, durable individual benefits and involvement in a career. Stebbins' [100] model enables a better understanding of the relationship between past leisure activities and their impact on current involvement, contrasting casual and serious leisure. As serious leisure is considered significantly more rewarding and fulfilling compared to casual leisure, participants with such a level of commitment are more likely to overcome the adversity posed by the various costs of that leisure, suggesting a higher level of participation in leisure in the future.

This study has contributed to the understanding of constraints and sport experience among individuals in Singapore and the level of commitment to their sport activities in the past, predicting their sport activities in the present or future. Moreover, understanding the role of nostalgia in sport participation can provide practical insights for policymakers and sport organizations. For example, organizations could incorporate nostalgia into wellness programs by creating opportunities for employees to engage in activities that evoke positive past experiences. Additionally, developing community programs that revive traditional or culturally meaningful sport activities could leverage nostalgic feelings to enhance participation. Similarly, in the Singaporean context, programs that incorporate traditional games or sport familiar to older adults could potentially foster greater engagement among this demographic. Finally, we recommend that policymakers develop targeted strategies to overcome barriers that hinder employee engagement in sport and physical activities. Suggested interventions might involve introducing flexible work hours or establishing on-site fitness centers, which could alleviate the adverse effects of high-pressure work settings and contribute to improved employees' well-being.

Limitations and Future Research

This study has some limitations that should be considered. The qualitative approach used in this study provides insights into the subjective experiences of Singaporean workers. However, it also faces certain methodological limitations. Relying on self-reported data may introduce biases, as participants may not fully or accurately recollect their experiences. Moreover, qualitative findings from a single cultural context can be challenging to generalize. Additionally, the heterogeneity in participant age, occupation and other characteristics may have contributed to variability in the study's findings, while this diversity could limit the generalizability of the results to broader populations. Future research should explore a more homogeneous sample or utilize additional methods to account for these demographic factors. In addition, increasing the sample size and conducting diversified studies across countries can facilitate higher generalizability for this research. Second, the findings of this study suggest that nostalgia can be a powerful motivator for sport participation, but its manifestations and impacts can differ significantly across cultures. Thus, future research should explore these cultural intricacies to develop a more comprehensive understanding of how nostalgia influences sport participation globally. In addition, by being more specific and looking into each constraint meticulously, researchers might be able to locate new findings, and it will benefit the understanding for future studies on sport-specific nostalgia.

6. Conclusions

According to Sport Singapore [26], 51% of participants do not participate in sport activities due to their long working hours, indicating that working adults in Singapore seldom engage in sport activities because of their long working hours. However, it should be noted that life satisfaction, physical and mental health have positive relationships with outdoor, physical and social activities. If constraints continue to dominate an individual's life, it will lead to negative health and wellness consequences, and the number of inactive individuals in sport activities would gradually increase. Since nostalgia is generated by sport activities that cannot be enjoyed currently, it motivates and increases individuals' willingness to participate in their preferred sport activities. That is, the findings highlight the significant role of nostalgia as a motivational force for adult workers facing barriers to sport participation. By reconnecting individuals with positive memories of their past sport involvement, nostalgia acts as an emotional catalyst, encouraging them to renew their interest and commitment to physical activity. This suggests a valuable application for sport promotion strategies, where nostalgia is intentionally employed to motivate adults to overcome present challenges and re-engage in active lifestyles. Future research could explore the nostalgic feelings within each of the four constraints discussed in this study, including physical, environmental, social, and psychological constraints. The findings of this study provide a foundation that shows the current constraints faced by Singaporean working adults and how these constraints affect their nostalgia and involvement. By extending the research on each constraint, researchers may be able to identify new findings or emerging themes within each factor itself, which would contribute to a better understanding for future studies on sport-specific nostalgia. Additionally, this study encourages the government, private and public organizations to take further action to develop policies that facilitate participation in sport activities for workers in the long term.

Author Contributions: Conceptualization, H.C.; methodology, H.C.; validation, H.-K.K. and Y.H.L.; writing—original draft preparation, H.C. and G.A.A.; writing—review and editing, H.-K.K. and Y.H.L. All authors have read and agreed to the published version of the manuscript.

Funding: This research received no external funding.

Institutional Review Board Statement: The study was conducted in accordance with the Declaration of Helsinki, and approved by the Institutional Review Board of Nanyang Technological University (IRB-2017-06-029, 28 July 2017).

Informed Consent Statement: Informed consent was obtained from all subjects involved in the study.

Data Availability Statement: The data presented in this study are available on request from the first author. The data are not publicly available due to privacy.

Acknowledgments: We appreciate Ngo Yi Chye for his help with data collection and all research participants for their invaluable contributions to this study.

Conflicts of Interest: The authors declare no conflicts of interest.

References

1. Cho, H. Importance of leisure nostalgia on life satisfaction and leisure participation. *Serv. Ind. J.* **2020**, *40*, 90–109. [CrossRef]
2. Sato, M.; Jordan, J.S.; Funk, D.C. The role of physically active leisure for enhancing quality of life. *Leis. Sci.* **2014**, *36*, 293–313. [CrossRef]
3. Sivan, A.; Tam, V.; Siu, G.; Stebbins, R. Adolescents' choice and pursuit of their most important and interesting leisure activities. *Leis. Stud.* **2019**, *38*, 98–113. [CrossRef]
4. Arai, S.M.; Mock, S.E.; Gallant, K.A. Childhood traumas, mental health and physical health in adulthood: Testing physically active leisure as a buffer. *Leisure/Loisir* **2011**, *35*, 407–422. [CrossRef]
5. García-Villamisar, D.A.; Dattilo, J. Effects of a leisure programme on quality of life and stress of individuals with ASD. *J. Intellect. Disabil. Res.* **2010**, *54*, 611–619. [CrossRef]
6. Passmore, A. The occupation of leisure: Three typologies and their influence on mental health in adolescence. *OTJR Occup. Particip. Health* **2003**, *23*, 76–83. [CrossRef]
7. Bandura, A. *Self-Efficacy*; W. H. Freeman and Company: New York, NY, USA, 1997.
8. Chang, H.H. Gender differences in leisure involvement and flow experience in professional extreme sport activities. *World Leis. J.* **2017**, *59*, 124–139. [CrossRef]
9. Iwasaki, Y. Examining rival models of leisure coping mechanisms. *Leis. Sci.* **2003**, *25*, 183–206. [CrossRef]
10. Fancourt, D.; Aughterson, H.; Finn, S.; Walker, E.; Steptoe, A. How leisure activities affect health: A narrative review and multi-level theoretical framework of mechanisms of action. *Lancet Psychiatry* **2021**, *8*, 329–339. [CrossRef]

11. Molina-García, J.; Castillo, I.; Queralt, A. Leisure-Time Physical Activity and Psychological Well-Being in University Students. *Psychol. Rep.* **2011**, *109*, 453–460. [CrossRef]
12. Hills, A.P.; Street, S.J.; Byrne, N.M. Physical activity and health: "what is old is new again". *Adv. Food Nutr. Res.* **2015**, *75*, 77–95. [PubMed]
13. Iso-Aloha, S.; Mannell, R.C. *Work and Leisure*; Routledge: London, UK, 2004.
14. Blair, S.; Connelly, J. How much physical activity should we do? The case for moderate amounts and intensities of physical activity. *Res. Q. Exerc. Sport* **1996**, *67*, 193–205. [CrossRef]
15. Arem, H.; Moore, S.C.; Patel, A.; Hartge, P.; De Gonzalez, A.B.; Visvanathan, K.; Campbell, P.T.; Freedman, M.; Weiderpass, E.; Adami, H.O.; et al. Leisure time physical activity and mortality: A detailed pooled analysis of the dose-response relationship. *JAMA Intern. Med.* **2015**, *175*, 959–967. [CrossRef] [PubMed]
16. Glass, T.; DeLeon, C.; Marottoli, R.; Berkman, L. Population based study of social and productive activities as predictors of survival among elderly Americans. *Br. Med. J.* **1999**, *319*, 478–483. [CrossRef] [PubMed]
17. Hooker, S.A.; Masters, K.S.; Vagnini, K.M.; Rush, C.L. Engaging in personally meaningful activities is associated with meaning salience and psychological well-being. *J. Posit. Psychol.* **2020**, *15*, 821–831. [CrossRef]
18. O'Connor, D.; Smith, J. Relationship Between Meaningful Activity Engagement and Well-Being Moderated by Race. *Innov. Aging* **2021**, *5*, 867–868. [CrossRef]
19. Beatty, J.E.; Torbert, W.R. The false duality of work and leisure. *J. Manag. Enq.* **2003**, *12*, 239–252. [CrossRef]
20. Hilbrecht, M. Changing perspectives on the work–leisure relationship. *Annals of Leisure Research* **2007**, *10*, 368–390. [CrossRef]
21. Robinson, J.; Godbey, G. *Time for Life: The Surprising Ways Americans Use Their Time*; Pennsylvania State University Press: University Park, PA, USA, 1997.
22. Clark, D. Average Weekly Hours of Work for Full-Time Workers in the United Kingdom from May 1992 to December 2022. Available online: https://www.statista.com/statistics/280763/average-working-hours-uk/ (accessed on 14 February 2023).
23. Dayani, D. What Is the Average Working Hours in Singapore for Full-Tie and Part-Time Employees. Available online: https://dollarsandsense.sg/business/what-is-the-average-working-hours-in-singapore/ (accessed on 11 September 2022).
24. The Global Economy. Compare Countries Using Data from Official Sources. Available online: https://www.theglobaleconomy.com/compare-countries/ (accessed on 16 September 2024).
25. Payne, C.S. Leisure Time in the UK: 2015. Available online: https://www.ons.gov.uk/economy/nationalaccounts/satelliteaccounts/articles/leisuretimeintheuk/2015 (accessed on 24 October 2017).
26. Sport Singapore. Sports Index Participation Trends. 2015. Available online: https://www.sportsingapore.gov.sg/files/About%20Us/Sports%20Participation/Sports%20Index%202015.pdf (accessed on 16 September 2024).
27. Aslan, N. The impact of leisure constraints on leisure participation. *Ege Eğitim Derg.* **2002**, *2*, 11–24.
28. Chick, G.; Hsu, Y.C.; Yeh, C.K.; Hsieh, C.M. Leisure constraints, leisure satisfaction, life satisfaction, and self-rated health in six cities in Taiwan. *Leis. Sci.* **2015**, *37*, 232–251. [CrossRef]
29. Jackson, E.L. Will research on leisure constraints still be relevant in the twenty-first century? *J. Leis. Res.* **2000**, *32*, 62–68. [CrossRef]
30. Tan, W.K. Repeat visitation: A study from the perspective of leisure constraint, tourist experience, destination images, and experiential familiarity. *J. Destin. Mark. Manag.* **2017**, *6*, 233–242. [CrossRef]
31. Kivimäki, M.; Virtanen, M.; Elovainio, M.; Kouvonen, A.; Väänänen, A.; Vahtera, J. Work stress in the etiology of coronary heart disease—A meta-analysis. *Scand. J. Work. Environ. Health* **2006**, *32*, 431–442. [CrossRef] [PubMed]
32. Härmä, M. Workhours in relation to work stress, recovery and health. *Scand. J. Work. Environ. Health* **2006**, *32*, 502–514. [CrossRef] [PubMed]
33. Steptoe, A.; Kivimäki, M. Stress and cardiovascular disease: An update on current knowledge. *Annu. Rev. Public Health* **2013**, *34*, 337–354. [CrossRef]
34. Stansfeld, S.; Candy, B. Psychosocial work environment and mental health—A meta-analytic review. *Scand. J. Work. Environ. Health* **2006**, *32*, 443–462. [CrossRef]
35. Szeto, A.C.; Dobson, K.S. Mental disorders and their association with perceived work stress: An investigation of the 2010 Canadian Community Health Survey. *J. Occup. Health Psychol.* **2013**, *18*, 191–197. [CrossRef]
36. Caldwell, L.L. Leisure and health: Why is leisure therapeutic? *Br. J. Guid. Couns.* **2005**, *33*, 7–26. [CrossRef]
37. Dong, E.; Chick, G. Leisure constraints in six Chinese cities. *Leis. Sci.* **2012**, *34*, 417–435. [CrossRef]
38. Ito, E.; Kono, S.; Walker, G.J. Development of cross-culturally informed leisure-time physical activity constraint and constraint negotiation typologies: The case of Japanese and Euro-Canadian adults. *Leis. Sci.* **2020**, *42*, 411–429. [CrossRef]
39. Lewis, S.T.; Puymhroeck, M.V. Obesity-stigma as a multifaceted constraint to leisure. *J. Leis. Res.* **2008**, *40*, 574–588. [CrossRef]
40. Scott, D.; Lee, S.; Lee, J.J.; Kim, C. Leisure constraints and acculturation among Korean immigrants. *J. Park Recreat. Adm.* **2006**, *24*, 63–86.
41. Simmons, S. Striving for work-life balance. *Nursing* **2012**, *42*, 25–26. [CrossRef] [PubMed]
42. Clark, S.C. Work/family border theory: A new theory of work/family balance. *Hum. Relat.* **2000**, *53*, 747–770. [CrossRef]
43. Alavanza, M. Singapore's Working Hours: Longer Days, More Productivity or Just More Stress? The Independent Singapore. Available online: https://theindependent.sg/sg-working-hours-do-we-really-have-more-to-do/ (accessed on 20 September 2023).

44. Godbey, G.; Crawford, D.W.; Shen, X.S. Assessing hierarchical constraints theory after two decades. *J. Leis. Res.* **2010**, *42*, 111–134. [CrossRef]
45. Cho, H. Nostalgia in sport and leisure. *Curr. Opin. Psychol.* **2023**, *49*, 101551. [CrossRef]
46. Lee, K.J.; Scott, D. Interracial contact experience during recreational basketball and soccer: Korean American males' perspectives. *J. Leis. Res.* **2013**, *45*, 267–294. [CrossRef]
47. Jackson, E.L.; Scott, D. Constraints to Leisure. In *Leisure Studies: Prospects for the Twenty-First Century*; Jackson, E.L., Burton, T.L., Eds.; Venture Publishing: State College, PA, USA, 1999; pp. 299–321.
48. Crawford, D.W.; Jackson, E.L.; Godbey, G. A hierarchical model of leisure constraints. *Leis. Sci.* **1991**, *13*, 309–320. [CrossRef]
49. Skowron, M.A.; Stodolska, M.; Shinew, K.J. Determinants of leisure time physical activity participation among Latina women. *Leis. Sci.* **2008**, *30*, 429–447. [CrossRef]
50. Klenosky, D.B.; Gitelson, R.E. Travel agents' destination recommendations. *Ann. Tour. Res.* **1998**, *25*, 661–674. [CrossRef]
51. Floyd, M.F. Social justice as an integrating force for leisure research. *Leis. Sci.* **2014**, *36*, 379–387. [CrossRef]
52. Roberts, K. Sociology of Leisure and the Wars of the Lifestyle Gurus. In *Idleness, Indolence and Leisure in English Literature*; Palgrave Macmillan: London, UK, 2014; pp. 273–292.
53. Stodolska, M.; Shinew, K.J.; Camarillo, L.N. Constraints on recreation among people of color: Toward a new constraints model. *Leis. Sci.* **2020**, *42*, 533–551. [CrossRef]
54. Jeanes, R.; Magee, J.; Spaaij, R. Understanding leisure in a complex world: Promoting a critical leisure studies. *Ann. Leis. Res.* **2014**, *17*, 351–353. [CrossRef]
55. Lee, O.E.; Kim, D.H.; Lee, H.; Beum, K.A. Information Communication Technology Use to Improve eHealth Literacy, Technophobia, and Social Connection among Community Dwelling Older Adults. *Educ. Gerontol.* **2022**, *48*, 445–457. [CrossRef]
56. Chen, C.C.; Petrick, J.F. The roles of perceived travel benefits, importance, and constraints in predicting travel behavior. *J. Travel Res.* **2016**, *55*, 509–522. [CrossRef]
57. Darcy, S.; Lock, D.; Taylor, T. Enabling inclusive sport participation: Effects of disability and support needs on constraints to sport participation. *Leis. Sci.* **2017**, *39*, 20–41. [CrossRef]
58. Lee, N.; Kim, J.J.; Shin, Y.B.; Eom, H.; Kim, M.K.; Kyeong, S.; Jung, Y.H.; Min, S.; Kwon, J.H.; Kim, E. Choice of leisure activities by adolescents and adults with internet gaming disorder: Development and feasibility study of a virtual reality program. *JMIR Serious Games* **2020**, *8*, e18473. [CrossRef]
59. Kim, Y.J.; Cho, J.H.; Park, Y.J. Leisure sports participants' engagement in preventive health behaviors and their experience of constraints on performing leisure activities during the COVID-19 pandemic. *Front. Psychol.* **2020**, *11*, 589708. [CrossRef]
60. Chick, G.; Hsu, Y.C.; Yeh, C.K.; Hsieh, C.M.; Bae, S.Y.; Iarmolenko, S. Cultural consonance in leisure, leisure satisfaction, life satisfaction, and self-rated health in urban Taiwan. *Leis. Sci.* **2016**, *38*, 402–423. [CrossRef]
61. Coleman, D.; Iso-Ahola, S.E. Leisure and health: The role of social support and self-determination. *J. Leis. Res.* **1993**, *25*, 111–128. [CrossRef]
62. Kawachi, I.; Berkman, L.F. Social ties and mental health. *J. Urban Health* **2001**, *78*, 458–467. [CrossRef] [PubMed]
63. Kim, J.; Tussyadiah, I.P. Social networking and social support in tourism experience: The moderating role of online self-presentation strategies. *J. Travel Tour. Mark.* **2013**, *30*, 78–92. [CrossRef]
64. Wu, H.Y.; Chiou, A.F. Social media usage, social support, intergenerational relationships, and depressive symptoms among older adults. *Geriatr. Nurs.* **2020**, *41*, 615–621. [CrossRef] [PubMed]
65. Akyüz, H.; Aydin, I. Investigation of the relationship between leisure satisfaction and life satisfaction levels of individuals participating in physical activity education programs in civil society organizations. *Afr. Educ. Res. J.* **2020**, *8*, 11–19.
66. Khalaf, M.A.R.; Elias, W.; Wafik, G.M. Evaluating the Optional Tours Service Quality and its Effect on Tourist's Satisfaction in Marsa Alam City. *Minia J. Tour. Hosp. Res. MJTHR* **2020**, *10*, 51–80.
67. Tian, H.B.; Qiu, Y.J.; Lin, Y.Q.; Zhou, W.T.; Fan, C.Y. The role of leisure satisfaction in serious leisure and subjective well-being: Evidence from Chinese marathon runners. *Front. Psychol.* **2020**, *11*, 581908. [CrossRef]
68. Yoon, H.; Lee, W.S.; Kim, K.B.; Moon, J. Effects of leisure participation on life satisfaction in older Korean adults: A panel analysis. *Int. J. Environ. Res. Public Health* **2020**, *17*, 4402. [CrossRef]
69. Cho, H. The impacts of leisure nostalgia on well-being and turnover intention: The mediating roles of leisure satisfaction and work commitment. *Leis. Sci.* **2024**, *46*, 618–638. [CrossRef]
70. Cho, H.; Pyun, D.Y.; Wang, C.K.J. Leisure nostalgia: Scale development and validation. *J. Leis. Res.* **2019**, *50*, 330–349. [CrossRef]
71. Wang, J.; Xia, L. Revenge travel: Nostalgia and desire for leisure travel post COVID-19. *J. Travel Tour. Mark.* **2021**, *38*, 935–955. [CrossRef]
72. Holbrook, M.B.; Schindler, R.M. Echoes of the dear departed past: Some work in progress on nostalgia. *Adv. Consum. Res.* **1991**, *18*, 330.
73. Faul, L.; De Brigard, F. The moderating effects of nostalgia on mood and optimism during the COVID-19 pandemic. *Memory* **2022**, *30*, 1103–1117. [CrossRef] [PubMed]
74. Wildschut, T.; Sedikides, C.; Arndt, J.; Routledge, C. Nostalgia: Content, triggers, functions. *J. Personal. Soc. Psychol.* **2006**, *91*, 975–993. [CrossRef] [PubMed]
75. Kim, J.; Kim, M.; Han, A. Exploring the relationship between types of leisure activities and life satisfaction, health perception, and social support among Korean individuals with physical disabilities. *Am. J. Health Behav.* **2018**, *42*, 34–44. [CrossRef] [PubMed]

76. Sedikides, C.; Wildschut, T.; Cheung, W.Y.; Routledge, C.; Hepper, E.G.; Arndt, J.; Vail, K.; Zhou, X.; Brackstone, K.; Vingerhoets, A.J. Nostalgia fosters self-continuity: Uncovering the mechanism (social connectedness) and consequence (eudaimonic well-being). *Emotion* **2016**, *16*, 524. [CrossRef] [PubMed]
77. Cho, H. Work-leisure conflict and well-being: The role of leisure nostalgia. *Leis. Sci.* **2023**, *45*, 309–330. [CrossRef]
78. Alexandris, K.; Douka, S.; Balaska, P. Involvement with active leisure participation: Does service quality have a role? *Manag. Leis.* **2012**, *17*, 54–66. [CrossRef]
79. Li, J.; Zeng, B.; Li, P. The Influence of Leisure Activity Types and Involvement Levels on Leisure Benefits in Older Adults. *Front. Public Health* **2021**, *9*, 659263. [CrossRef]
80. Iso-Ahola, S.E.; Mannell, R.C. *Social and Psychological Constraints on Leisure*; Charles C. Thomas: Springfield, IL, USA, 1985; pp. 111–151.
81. Chua, S. The Sociology of Leisure: An Examination of the Relationship between Perceived Experience and Leisure Participation. Ph.D. Thesis, University of Surrey, Guildford, UK, 2001.
82. Chun, S.; Lee, Y.; Kim, B.; Heo, J. The contribution of leisure participation and leisure satisfaction to stress-related growth. *Leis. Sci.* **2012**, *34*, 436–449. [CrossRef]
83. Wiley, C.G.; Shaw, S.M.; Havitz, M.E. Men's and women's involvement in sports: An examination of the gendered aspects of leisure involvement. *Leis. Sci.* **2000**, *22*, 19–31.
84. Chin-Tsai, K. Leisure involvement, leisure benefits, quality of life, and job satisfaction. A case study on 2011 creating sports island plan in ChiaYi City, Taiwan held by sports affairs council, executive yuan. *Int. Rev. Manag. Bus. Res.* **2013**, *2*, 421–428.
85. Ho, T.S. An exploration of relationship among leisure involvement, leisure benefits, quality of life, and training effects of collegiate athletes. *Int. J. Organ. Innov.* **2018**, *10*, 327–344.
86. Kara, F.M.; Sarol, H. Level up the Life!! Leisure Involvement, Basic Psychological Need Satisfaction and Life Satisfaction among University Students. *High. Educ. Stud.* **2021**, *11*, 91–101. [CrossRef]
87. Wu, J.; Li, X.; Gao, B.; Su, X. The effects of serious leisure involvement on subjective well-being and successful aging: A case study of young-old participants in Chinese seniors' universities. *Sage Open* **2020**, *10*, 2158244020914559. [CrossRef]
88. Kvale, S.; Brinkmann, S. *InterViews: Learning the Craft of Qualitative Research Interviewing*; Sage Publications: New York, NY, USA, 2009.
89. Saunders, B.; Sim, J.; Kingstone, T.; Baker, S.; Waterfield, J.; Bartlam, B.; Burroughs, H.; Jinks, C. Saturation in qualitative research: Exploring its conceptualization and operationalization. *Qual. Quant.* **2018**, *52*, 1893–1907. [CrossRef]
90. Milliken, P. Grounded theory. In *Encyclopedia of Research Design*; Salkind, N., Ed.; SAGE Publications, Inc.: New York, NY, USA, 2010; pp. 549–554.
91. Merriam, S.B. *Qualitative Research and Case Study Application in Education*; Jossey-Bass: Hoboken, NJ, USA, 1998.
92. Crawford, D.W.; Godbey, G. Reconceptualizing barriers to family leisure. *Leis. Sci.* **1987**, *9*, 119–127. [CrossRef]
93. Cho, H.; Ramshaw, G.; Norman, W.C. A conceptual model for nostalgia in the context of sport tourism: Re-classifying the sporting past. *J. Sport Tour.* **2014**, *19*, 145–167. [CrossRef]
94. Korte, R.F. A review of social identity theory with implications for training and development. *J. Eur. Ind. Train.* **2007**, *31*, 166–180. [CrossRef]
95. Tajfel, H. *Human Groups and Social Categories: Studies in Social Psychology*; Cambridge University Press: Cambridge, UK, 1981.
96. Gerold, S.; Nocker, M. More leisure or higher pay? A mixed-methods study on reducing working time in Austria. *Ecol. Econ.* **2018**, *143*, 27–36. [CrossRef]
97. Hughes, J.; Bozionelos, N. Work-life balance as source of job dissatisfaction and withdrawal attitudes. *Pers. Rev.* **2007**, *36*, 145–154. [CrossRef]
98. Ramshaw, G.; Hinch, T. Place identity and sport tourism: The case of the heritage classic ice hockey event. *Curr. Issues Tour.* **2006**, *9*, 399–418. [CrossRef]
99. Snyder, E. Sociology of nostalgia: Sport halls of fame and museums in America. *Sociol. Sport J.* **1991**, *8*, 228–238. [CrossRef]
100. Stebbins, R.A. *Amateur, Professional, and Serious Leisure*; McGill-Queen's University Press: Montreal, QC, Canada, 1992.

behavioral sciences

MDPI

Article

Analysis of Bullying in Physical Education: Descriptive Study of Spanish Adolescents

Juan de Dios Benítez-Sillero [1,2], Diego Corredor-Corredor [3], Álvaro Morente-Montero [1,2], Javier Murillo-Moraño [2,4,*] and José Manuel Armada-Crespo [1,2]

[1] Department of Specific Didactics, Universidad de Córdoba, 14071 Córdoba, Spain; eo1besij@uco.es (J.d.D.B.-S.); eo1momoa@uco.es (Á.M.-M.); m62arcrj@uco.es (J.M.A.-C.)
[2] Research Group in Sport and Physical Education for Personal and Social Development, 14071 Córdoba, Spain
[3] Counselling of Education, Junta de Andalucía, 14071 Córdoba, Spain; dcorcor015@g.educaand.es
[4] Teacher Training College "Sagrado Corazón", University of Córdoba, 14006 Córdoba, Spain
* Correspondence: z02mumoj@uco.es

Abstract: Physical education classes can be a place where both bullying and harassment take place, and a powerful strategy is needed to prevent it. The present study analyses bullying and students' behaviour as active or passive observers in a general educational context and physical education lessons. A sample of 958 adolescents aged 12 to 18 was studied. A questionnaire was used to analyse the victimisation and the bullying and behaviour observed. The results showed a lower incidence rate than that observed in other studies in physical education classes with a higher level of perpetration by boys than by girls and a more active rejection of aggression by victims and girls. On the other hand, passive attitudes were greater among perpetrators and boys. The observers' attitudes were similar in both contexts. The scenario in which this subject takes place could reduce the risk of these phenomena occurring. Therefore, physical education teachers should analyse these behaviours and intervene, especially when creating awareness in boys.

Keywords: bullying; observation; physical education; victimisation; perpetration; adolescents

1. Introduction

Bullying is a phenomenon in which interpersonal aggression among students occurs repeatedly and is sustained over time with an imbalance of power between the aggressor(s) or perpetrators and the victim [1]. It is not a fight or a conflict although this can be a trigger; it is a behaviour or attitude of social exclusion which may involve psychological or verbal abuse in addition to intentional and repeated physical attacks by a schoolchild. The prevalence of bullying is between 10 and 35% [2]. Various factors can influence this variability, such as the behaviours studied and the contexts in which descriptive studies are carried out [3,4]. Bullying is considered one of the most damaging phenomena to students' well-being at school. Since the first such research was conducted in the 1970s, it has been known that the incidence rates are the highest in the last years of primary school and the first years of compulsory secondary school [5]. The most recent systematic reviews and meta-analyses have indicated that the highest incidence takes place between 11 and 14 years of age [4]. It is also known that there is a gender difference in the profiles of the participants in the phenomenon, with males being more involved in any of the roles, particularly in the role of the aggressor [4,6], but they are equally involved as the victims of their peers.

Bullying has terrible consequences, especially for the victims, such as lower academic performance [4], sleep disorders [4], and even suicidal ideation [7]. However, not only does it affect the victims: it also creates an atmosphere of detachment, coldness, and lack of respect that contaminates school life [8]. This creates a serious problem within the educational community [9]. All scenarios and all activities and communications are affected when, in a school, negative interpersonal relationships and socio-moral issues, which are implicit in the phenomenon of school bullying, are allowed to continue [10,11], but some scenarios and some activities, due to important factors such as communication and interactive relationships, seem to be more exposed to the processes of bullying and harassment.

However, when a physical education (PE) class is carried out in a cordial environment and aspects of interpersonal relationships are considered relevant educational factors [12] in an appropriate way, the activities and the social interactions that they imply seem to contribute to a better coexistence climate and a lower incidence of bullying [13,14]. On another note, there is some evidence that students excluded from PE classes due to health problems suffer more bullying at school and are even bullied more than those who participate normally in their school PE classes [15]. Some studies have indicated that the prevalence of bullying in PE classrooms may be high if the class is not properly managed; specific scenarios (playgrounds, gymnasiums, and external exits) seem to have less teacher vigilance toward students, who often interact in large or closed spaces (locker rooms) where teachers do not enter [16–18].

Some research has focused on the study of bullying and PE, physical activity, and sports in adolescents [17,19] with controversial results. Studies such as [20–22], among others, have used disparate methodologies and procedures, producing equally mixed results. For example, questions can be asked about the occurrence of bullying over an entire school year or a limited situation of two months; the victims or perpetrators are considered if the occurrence is only on a one-off occasion (which is excluded from the definition of bullying itself) or if it is something that occurs with a certain frequency and involves the same protagonists (aggressor(s) and victim(s)). In just one study [21], the occurrence of bullying was analysed both at a general level and in PE classes for the same sample, and it obtained results where, compared to the 23% perpetrators and 39% victims at the general level in the whole-school context, in the PE classes, 15% were perpetrators and 28% were victims among the same students.

Bullying is considered a group phenomenon which, in addition to bullies and victims, involves many participants who are, to some extent, informed or directly witness the events and are more or less inhibited or involved [23]. In this regard, it has been described that observers can adopt the following four roles: (1) assistants, who join the side of the bully; (2) reinforcers, who encourage the bully and reinforce the bullying behaviour with their support; (3) passive observers, who simply watch what is happening; and (4) advocates or proactive observers that are against what is happening and stand up on behalf of the victims to try to prevent a repetition of the events, explicitly supporting the victim [23]. When peers intervene in situations of bullying (i.e., exclusion or unjustified aggression) by reproaching the bully, expressing such behaviour is not permissible, or alerting teachers to intervene, these bullying behaviours decrease significantly, although this proactive attitude of an observer is not common in this complex phenomenon [24]. Moreover, the profiles and attitudes of observers are less studied than anything related to the profiles and attitudes of the protagonists. More is known about victimisation and perpetration than about what affects the observers of the phenomenon in general [25]. Similarly, there is more knowledge about passive bystanders or observers and proactive defenders as categories within bullying, differentiating them from the other roles, but few studies have analysed the observational attitudes of all those involved [26,27]. We also must consider that victims or perpetrators may be victims or perpetrators in specific situations at school, but they may also act as protagonists or in another role in the social fabric of their school groups. Being an observer of bullying situations can even have negative personal and social consequences for the individual due to the vicarious impacts [28–30].

This study aimed to analyse the occurrence of bullying in PE classes compared to general bullying in schools, focusing on analysing the behaviours and roles of observers in both educational contexts. It is hypothesised that PE is an educational setting that, being not free from the risks of bullying, is less likely to present a lower incidence than bullying in general at school, with perpetration being higher among boys. It is also presumed that observers' profiles and behaviours are more active among victims and girls.

2. Materials and Methods

2.1. Design and Participants

A descriptive, cross-sectional study design with non-probability sampling was carried out. A total of 958 students aged between 12 and 18 (50% girls M = 14.65, SD = 1.36) participated in the study. Participants were selected from four public schools in Huelva and Córdoba (Spain) due to accessibility for the researchers. The participants ranged from the first to the fourth year of compulsory secondary education (12–16 years old) and the first year of upper secondary education (17–18 years old). No exclusion criteria were applied, accepting all collected questionnaires. The study was carried out in the academic year 2020–2021, during March to May 2021. In this year, the restrictions due to the COVID-19 pandemic consisted of the use of masks, the predominance of the use of outdoor spaces, the limitation of the use of changing rooms in shifts, and increased hygienic measures.

The study was conducted as a part of an educational research project funded and authorised by the Regional Ministry of Education and Sport of the Andalusian Regional Government. All the national and international ethical standards such as the Declaration of Helsinki and personal data protection laws were followed. Permissions to conduct the research project were granted by the school boards, and informed consents were provided by the families of the participants. The objective of the study was explained to the participants, and the anonymous, confidential, and voluntary nature of their participation was stressed. The project was approved by the Ethics Committee of the University of Córdoba.

2.2. Instruments

2.2.1. Bullying

The Spanish version of the European Bullying Intervention Project Questionnaire (EBIPQ) [1] was used to measure bullying victimisation and perpetration at a general level. It includes 14 items of which seven are focused on victimisation and seven are focused on perpetration. Questions were answered on a Likert-type response scale that ranges from 0 to 4, (0 = never, 1 = once or twice, 2 = once or twice a month, 3 = about once a week and 4 = more than once a week). This questionnaire obtained good Cronbach's alphas for victimisation ($\alpha = 0.84$) and perpetration ($\alpha = 0.82$). Students were considered to be perpetrators or victims if they claimed to have answered once or twice a month or more frequently for any of the behaviours presented for victimisation or perpetration. Students who were involved in both victimisation and perpetration at that frequency were considered perpetrator–victimised. This data collection methodology was used because it was validated with good psychometric properties and highly cited in peer-reviewed journals [2,4,8,13].

The same questionnaire was used, but with the nuance "in PE classes", to investigate the same phenomena (victimisation/perpetration) occurring in PE lessons. To date, this study represents the first attempt to analyse bullying in physical education using this questionnaire; thus, there is no known evidence regarding its utilisation in this context. Therefore, it was necessary to conduct a confirmatory factor analysis of the current data, which showed they adjusted properly: $\chi^2_{91} = 10{,}938.15$, $p = 0.022$; $\chi^2/gl = 120.20$; NNFI = 0.997; CFI = 0.998; TLI = 0.997; RMSEA = 0.019, 90% CI [Li = 0.008, Ls = 0.028], $p = 1.000$ y SRMR = 0.074. The Cronbach's alpha tests for victimisation ($\alpha = 0.85$) and perpetration ($\alpha = 0.76$) showed good internal consistency. To ensure that students did not confuse harassment experiences in PE with those in general school environments, the questionnaire assessing bullying in PE was administered after the questionnaire assessing harassment in general environments. This sequence allowed students to notice that it was the same question but with a different purpose. Additionally, it was indicated in bold and large font that the questions specifically referred to PE. The researcher administering the questionnaires also verbally emphasised that, after responding in the general educational context, they should exclusively respond about bullying behaviours in the PE classes.

2.2.2. Observation Bullying

To analyse the role of observers in bullying situations, the two dimensions proposed by Caballo et al. [26] in the following instrument "Multimodal School Interaction Questionnaire" (CMIE-IV) were used. This questionnaire consists of five factors, although only two of them were considered. The first of the dimensions considered was the active observation in defence of the bullied factor, in which 6 items were taken into account. The second factor was the passive observation in which 4 items were considered. In this questionnaire, the subjects were asked "How many times have you experienced these situations in the last two months?" The response options were (1 = never, 2 = few, 3 = quite a few and 4 = many). As with the bullying questionnaire, subjects were first asked about the occurrence of these behaviours at a general level. A confirmatory factor analysis of the current data showed they adjusted properly: $\chi^2_{45} = 24{,}846.97$, $p < 0.001$; $\chi^2/gl = 512.15$; NNFI = 0.997; CFI = 0.997; TLI = 0.997; RMSEA = 0.045, 90% CI [Li = 0.035, Ls = 0.055]; $p = 0.782$; and SRMR = 0.047. The Cronbach´s alpha tests for active observation in defence of the harassed ($\alpha = 0.88$) and passive observation ($\alpha = 0.79$) showed good internal consistency. Subsequently, the same questionnaire was carried out at the level of the PE class. A confirmatory factor analysis of the current data showed they adjusted properly: $\chi^2_{45} = 67{,}717.87$, $p < 0.001$; $\chi^2/gl = 1504.84$; NNFI = 0.999; CFI = 0.999; TLI = 0.999; RMSEA = 0.037, 90% CI [Li = 0.026, Ls = 0.048], $p = 0.782$ y SRMR = 0.040. The Cronbach´s alphas tests for active observation in defence of the harassed ($\alpha = 0.93$) and passive observation ($\alpha = 0.86$) showed good internal consistency.

2.3. *Statistical Analysis*

First, after checking the non-normality of the sample data, Spearman's bivariate correlations of the quantitative variables were analysed. Student's t-test to contrast the existence of differences by gender, and Cohen's d was considered to control the effect size. To determine the relationship between observation as a function of the roles of involvement in bullying, an ANOVA analysis with Tukey's post hoc test was carried out. Subsequently, a linear regression analysis was performed with the dependent variable being observation and the independent variables being sex, victimisation and bullying perpetration as quantitative variables. The analyses were carried out using the IBM SPSS Statistics 25 statistical package.

3. Results

Table 1 shows the bivariate correlations among the different study variables. The negative relationships between age or year with victimisation, both in general and in PE, and the decrease in the active role observers stand out.

Table 1. Spearman's correlations between all studied variables.

Variable	1	2	3	4	5	6	7	8	9
1. Age	-	-	-	-	-	-	-	-	-
2. Grade	0.915 **	-	-	-	-	-	-	-	-
3. Victimisation GE	−0.084 **	−0.132 **	-	-	-	-	-	-	-
4. Perpetration GE	0.008	−0.034	0.531 **	-	-	-	-	-	-
5. Victimisation PE	−0.070 *	−0.103 **	0.559 **	0.399 **	-	-	-	-	-
6. Perpetration PE	−0.029	−0.044	0.321 **	0.567 **	0.436 **	-	-	-	-
7. Acti. Observ. GE	−0.115 **	−0.144 **	0.214 **	0.066 *	0.106 **	0.020	-	-	-
8. Pasi. Obersv. GE	0.006	−0.010	0.127 **	0.219 **	0.104 **	0.166 **	0.195 **	-	-
9. Acti. Observ. PE	−0.142 **	−0.164 **	0.169 **	0.057	0.108 **	0.036	0.764 **	0.210 **	-
10. Pasi. Obersv. PE	−0.013	−0.052	0.172 **	0.251 **	0.154 **	0.184 **	0.179 **	0.717 **	0.373 **

Notes. GE = general; PE = physical education; Acti. = active; Pasi. = passive; Observ. = observation. * Established level of significance: $p < 0.05$; ** Established level of significance; $p < 0.01$.

Table 2 shows the variables of victimisation and perpetration of bullying as a function of gender. Both in the general exploration and in the exploration in the PE classes, perpetration was higher in boys. There were no significant differences in the sample in victimisation.

Table 2. Descriptive statistics and differences by gender for all variables of bullying.

Variable/Condition	Total (n = 958)		Boys (n = 479)		Girls (n = 479)				
	M	SD	M	SD	M	SD	*t*	*p*	*d*
Victimisation general	0.40	0.59	0.38	0.61	0.41	0.58	−0.55	0.581	−0.05
Perpetration general	0.16	0.35	0.19	0.40	0.13	0.30	20.83	0.005 **	0.17
Victimisation PE	0.12	0.35	0.13	0.38	0.12	0.82	0.28	0.780	0.02
Perpetration PE	0.05	0.18	0.07	0.22	0.04	0.13	20.08	0.038 *	0.39

Notes. M = mean; SD = standard deviation; t = Student's t; d = Cohen's d. * Established level of significance: $p < 0.05$; ** Established level of significance; $p < 0.01$.

Table 3 shows the differences in the role of observers according to gender. Overall, girls showed higher levels of active observation and lower levels of passive observation. In PE, only passive observation was significant, being lower in girls.

Table 3. Descriptive statistics and differences by gender for all variables of observation.

Variable/Condition	Total (n = 958)		Boys (n = 479)		Girls (n = 479)				
	M	SD	M	SD	M	SD	*t*	*p*	*d*
Active observation general	2.63	0.83	2.58	0.81	2.69	0.85	−2.05	0.041 *	−0.13
Passive observation general	1.83	0.59	1.93	0.62	1.74	0.55	4.99	≤0.001 ***	0.32
Active observation PE	2.50	0.95	2.47	0.92	2.53	0.98	−0.93	0.353	0.06
Passive observation PE	1.78	0.65	1.88	0.69	1.67	0.58	5.08	≤0.001 ***	0.33

Notes. M = mean; SD = standard deviation; t = Student's t; d = Cohen's d; PE = physical education. * Established level of significance: $p < 0.05$; *** Established level of significance: $p \leq 0.001$.

Table 4 shows the occurrence of bullying at a general level in the whole educational context with the victims being 18% plus 6% of the perpetrators–victimised, totalling 24%, and the perpetrators 2% plus 6% of the perpetrators–victimised, i.e., 8%. The percentage of students not involved was 74%. Subjects are also categorised according to the roles they adopt in bullying at a general level and then compared according to their attitude as observers. In relation to active observation, when comparing according to the roles adopted in bullying, this was significant (F = 12.79; $p \leq 0.001$), and average differences were found among some groups with higher values for victims compared to those not involved. The passive attitude was also significant (F = 5.37; $p \leq 0.001$); at the group level, the perpetrators–victimised presented higher values than those not involved at the mean level.

Table 4. Comparisons of their observational attitude in terms of their role in general bullying.

Condition		Active Observation General		Passive Observation General	
	N (%)	M (SD)	Post-Hoc	M (SD)	Post-Hoc
0. Not involved	709 (74)	2.55 (0.85)	1 **	1.80 (0.59)	3 *
1. Victims	172 (18)	2.97 (0.68)	0 **	1.91 (0.55)	
2. Perpetrators	20 (2)	2.44 (0.99)		1.97 (0.72)	
3. Perpetrators-Victims	57 (6)	2.77 (0.74)		2.07 (0.62)	0 *

Notes. M = mean; SD = standard deviation. * Established level of significance: $p < 0.05$; ** Established level of significance; $p < 0.01$.

Table 5 shows the occurrence of bullying in PE and compares the different groups according to their attitude as observers in PE classes according to the roles adopted in bullying. Differences were found in the active observation attitude (F = 7.04; $p \leq 0.001$) with higher levels in the victims than in those not involved. In the passive attitude, there were also significant differences (F = 8.09; $p \leq 0.001$) with the non-involved showing lower values than the victims and perpetrators.

Table 5. Comparisons of their observational attitude according to their role in bullying in PE.

Variable/Condition		Active Observation PE		Passive Observation PE	
	N (%)	M (SD)	Post-Hoc	M (SD)	Post-Hoc
0. Not involved	880 (92)	2.45 (0.96)	1 ***	1.74 (0.64)	1 ** 0.2 *
1. Victims	53 (6)	3.02 (0.62)	0 ***	2.06 (0.63)	0 **
2. Perpetrators	13 (1)	2.88 (0.79)		2.30 (0.77)	0 *
3. Perpetrators-Victims	12 (1)	2.71 (0.70)		2.12 (0.71)	

Notes. M = mean; SD = standard deviation. * Established level of significance: $p < 0.05$; ** Established level of significance: $p < 0.01$; *** Established level of significance: $p \leq 0.001$.

Table 6 represents the attitude of active and passive observation at the general level as a dependent variable in a linear regression analysis with the independent variables of grade, gender, victimisation, and perpetration. Relationships are found for active observation with the student's grade, being lower as one moves up to higher grades, and a positive relationship with general victimisation. In relation to passive observation, it was lower in boys and was related to perpetration behaviour. The year of study variable was used instead of age, as it showed higher levels of significance.

Table 6. Linear regression with grade, gender, victimisation, and perpetration as predictors of behaviour when observing bullying situations in general.

Variable/Condition	Active Observation General		Passive Observation General	
	β	t	β	t
Grade	−0.077 ***	−3.656	0.02	0.108
Gender (female)	0.093	1.772	−0.174 ***	−4.610
Victimisation general	0.292 ***	5.516	0.021	0.562
Perpetration general	−0.136	−1.545	0.235 ***	3.716
	F = 14.51 $p < 0.001$ $R^2 = 0.06$		F = 12.16 $p < 0.001$ $R^2 = 0.05$	

Notes. *** Established level of significance: $p \leq 0.001$.

Finally, Table 7 presents active and passive observation in PE as the dependent variable in a linear regression analysis with the independent variables grade, gender, victimisation and perpetration in PE. The active observation was negatively related to the grade studied and positively related to victimisation. In passive observation, lower levels were found in girls, and higher levels were found in those who presented greater perpetration behaviour.

Table 7. Linear regression with grade, gender, victimisation and perpetration as predictors of behaviour when observing bullying situations in PE.

Variable/Condition	Active Observation PE		Passive Observation General	
	β	t	β	t
Grade	−0.117 ***	−4.824	−0.015	−0.917
Gender (female)	0.056	0.927	−0.200 ***	−4.881
Victimisation PE	0.285 *	2.934	0.144 *	−2.166
Perpetration PE	−0.007	−0.069	0.421 **	−3.252
	F = 9.36 $p < 0.001$ $R^2 = 0.04$		F = 13.93 $p < 0.001$ $R^2 = 0.06$	

Notes. PE = physical education. * Established level of significance: $p < 0.05$; ** Established level of significance: $p < 0.01$; *** Established level of significance: $p \leq 0.001$.

4. Discussion

In this study, we have focused on the PE class as a particularly relevant setting and the prevention of bullying. Although it is presumed that PE lessons are not free from this phenomenon of mistreatment among students, its incidence is differential both for the protagonists of the problem and for the observers of it. Based on the results obtained, we can argue, with reference to the levels of occurrence that other studies [3] have shown, that the general trend indicating that more than three quarters of the school population is unaffected by the phenomenon of bullying, i.e., they state that they are neither involved in nor affected by these problems, is fulfilled. Nevertheless, this prevalence is lower in the PE classes in this sample: less than one schoolchild out of ten is involved in bullying in any of its protagonist roles (victim/bully). This confirms our initial hypothesis, as in the only previous study [21] that analysed this difference. The trends previously reported by other studies [6,8,20] that indicate that boys are more involved (both in general and PE classes) than girls are also maintained. Indeed, boys showed higher values in perpetration behaviour both at the general and PE level with no significant differences in victimisation according to gender. That is to say, the role of victims is evenly distributed between girls and boys in PE classrooms.

Concerning the occurrence of school bullying at a general level, the data from our study indicate that 26% of adolescents of these ages have been framed within the leading roles involved in it. These data are very similar to studies that place the prevalence at around 25–30% [31]. It is noteworthy that the incidence of bullying seemed to remain constant in recent years [2,32]. In our study, boys were more involved in aggressive behaviour than girls, as in other studies [6,8,33], although there were no significant differences with respect to victimisation as in recent studies in adolescents [8,13]. In relation to the age and school year of the participants, less victimisation was observed as age and school year increased. However, there was no significant relationship between age and school year with perpetration behaviour. These results align with other studies regarding victimisation [8,26], but not with perpetration, where it seems that perpetration behaviour increases with age [26,33].

Regarding the occurrence of bullying in PE classrooms, the overall prevalence was 8% (including 1% of perpetrators and 1% of victimised perpetrators). These results are lower than the few previous studies where bullying in PE classrooms has been analysed. But as we have seen, only one previous study analysed the occurrence of bullying in the same population at the general level and in PE [21]. In this study, 15% of 10–15-year-olds were perpetrators in PE classes compared to 23% overall, a difference of 8 percentage points, while in our study, the difference was 6 points but with lower results both in PE (2%) and overall (8%). In relation to victimisation, the Gano-Overway study [21] reported a prevalence of 28% in PE versus 39% overall, while in our study, the prevalence of both was lower (7% PE and 24% overall). However, it has already been noted that the methodology was different in terms of the time being investigated. The Gano-Overway [21] study asked about the occurrence in the last 30 days and considered that bullying was prevalent when they answered that such behaviour had occurred at least once, while our study considered the perpetrator or victim to be those who indicated that the events had occurred two or more times a month during the last two months. Therefore, the probability of prevalence in our study is clearly lower and more in line with the concept itself that defines bullying [34,35], which requires repetition over a clearly defined period of time. The use of such a cut-off point to consider the involvement in each bullying role in our study is argued by the definition of bullying itself, which requires the occurrence to be repeated and sustained over time, as well as by the greater psychometric value of the scale used [1].

With respect to other studies that have also focused on bullying in PE classes [22], studying Portuguese students aged between ten and eighteen, considering the period of the entire academic year, and recording the event as bullying when there is at least one event, they found that 30% of students reported victimising behaviours and 29% reported having carried out perpetrating behaviours. Therefore, the results were higher in incidence in our study, although this could be explained by the fact that it was asked for the occurrence in a full academic year and in our study in only two months. It was also considered involved if the behaviour is experienced or carried out only once, while in our study, it takes place once or twice a month.

The most recent study analysing bullying in PE is that of Borowiec et al. [20] in Poland with adolescents aged 14–16. In this one, as in ours, they asked about bullying in the last two months, considering the person involved if they answered "rarely" or "often", categories 2 and 3 of a three-dimensional scale. In this study, in contrast to those previously reviewed, the percentage of perpetrators was 23% higher than that of victims 19%.

The explanations for the lower levels of occurrence of both victimisation and perpetration in physical education in our study, compared to previously published studies [20–22], could be due in part to methodological issues and the very concept of the phenomenon of bullying itself, since the other studies asked about a different time period and the repetition of bullying was excluded, which is a defining characteristic of bullying. The instrument used here, the EBIPQ, defines a specific, standardised, and validated period for the measurement of the prevalence of bullying in any setting, and it includes repetition of aggression as a constituent element of the construct, as mentioned above. Other possible explanations could be that this study was carried out when some measures of social distance in PE were still in place due to the COVID-19 pandemic. For example, students did not use the locker rooms to a large extent, and they did so without crowding. Some studies claim that many bullying situations occur in the locker rooms in PE because they are outside the supervision of teachers [16–18].

In relation to gender and grade, our study found that there are no significant differences in the victimisation of students in PE classes. However, other studies found, both in this specific scenario and at a general level, that boys recognised themselves as more victimised than girls, coinciding with what occurs in other studies on bullying at a general level [8,36]. In reference to the perpetration in our study, boys were more perpetrators than girls, which is consistent with other studies [20,37].

As far as grade is concerned, our results found greater victimisation as the grade increased, both in physical education classes [20] and at a general level [8]. Differences in perpetration were not significant with grade, contrasting with other studies in PE that claim that violence and perpetration tendencies increase with grade [20,38].

When we moved on to the analysis of active or passive observation behaviour in bullying situations, girls showed higher levels of proactive observation in general bullying, which were differences that were not found in PE classes. On the other hand, in passive observation, boys showed higher values both in general level and in PE. This coincides with the results of other studies that analyse it at a general level in the whole educational context [26,27,39] with no analysis in physical education.

With grade, proactive observation decreases both in general and in PE classrooms, which is consistent with what has been stated in other studies [26,27]. In relation to passive observation, we found no significant differences as published in the study by Parris et al. [27], in contrast to Caballo et al. [26], in which passive observation increased with grade. When studying the relationships among the attitude as observers depending on the roles in bullying, higher levels of proactive observation were found in victims, which agree with the results of Wu et al. [30]. We interpret these results, which reinforce previous studies, in a double sense. On the one hand, perhaps victims have, due to their experience, more pronounced peer-supportive behaviours compared to non-involved and perpetrators [30]. On the other hand, perhaps some of these victims belong to that group that has been given different names (paradoxical victims, victimised aggressors) that participate in traits of both roles. A complementary explanation would suggest that perhaps some victims have a higher level of empathy and anti-bullying sentiment [40,41]. In any case, victims' experiences make them more familiar with the signs of bullying, and they may be better able to detect it in order to act, than perpetrators or those not involved [42].

In relation to passive observation, it was higher in boys and among students with more aggressive behaviour, which was also replicated for PE victimisation. This passive attitude of perpetrators when observing other bullying situations in which they are not involved could again be associated with the perpetrators' lack of empathy [40], which is consolidated, uncontroversial knowledge among previous research. In our study, the highest levels of passive at a general level were found in victimised perpetrators. Nonetheless, in physical education, differences were significant also between victims and non-victims and were related to victimisation. In the absence of previous studies in this area, it is risky to seek an explanation, and more knowledge and research are needed. Stein and Jimerson [11] found that perpetrators had the highest levels of moral disengagement in bullying situations, which could also be related to this passive attitude [40]. Another aspect that could explain these relationships could be the lower social competences and skills of bystanders who display these passive attitudes. Likewise, this attitude that leads them to ignore bullying situations could be due to a lower knowledge or ability to intervene in defence of the victim [39]. For this reason, teachers should not assume that young people who do not intervene in defence of others do so not because they are unwilling to do so but perhaps because they are unable to find the mechanisms to intervene. It is therefore important to know whether young people know how to intervene in a bullying situation when they are bystanders and how they feel about it [39]. It is also desirable that in-service teachers and future teachers receive training on bullying in physical education [43].

5. Conclusions

From the results, and in relation to the objectives that were set out, this paper can point to several conclusions: bullying in PE classes in our study was lower than the prevalence levels that have been published by the few that exist in the scientific literature that have focused on the specific scenario of this area of the school curriculum. There are methodological and construct differences that may be at the basis of this difference in prevalence, as we have mentioned. Yet, we also believe that the scenario itself, which is more open to physical activity, and perhaps for many students is more fun and relaxing (although obviously not for all), reduces the risk of the emergence of these phenomena. Therefore, we will have to continue studying this incidence in the future to find the keys to this decrease in risk and learn to transfer these keys to other educational scenarios.

Boys, as all studies admit, also showed higher levels of perpetration than girls in PE, but this was not replicated among girls in terms of victimisation. Active observation behaviour was higher among victims of bullying and among girls. Passive observing behaviour was higher among perpetrators and boys. The dynamics of observers' attitudes were similar in the general educational context and in PE classes. Therefore, PE teachers should analyse and intervene especially in raising the awareness of boys.

With this study, we have tried to provide a more in-depth understanding of what bullying in PE classes is like in comparison with that which occurs at a general level and the attitude of observation of all those involved. But more studies are needed to know the specificity of this phenomenon, since the subject of PE, due to its specific characteristics, can become both a space where bullying can occur and a powerful tool to promote strategies and values in students that help against this problem.

This study is limited by the specificity of the sample, which has not been randomised. Questionnaire-based measurement of the occurrence of bullying may not be as accurate, so conclusions should be taken with caution. Nevertheless, the study presented here shows evidence of the importance of the settings in which educational activities take place in the school context. In this sense, there is no doubt that the setting of PE is particularly interesting as a framework in which, even with a certain level of risk, bullying can be reduced. This will increase if, as Jiménez-Barbero et al. [17] state, PE programmes continue to include social competence and moral values among their objectives and intentions. Furthermore, other practical measures to reduce bullying in the physical education classroom could involve implementing supervision strategies in the locker rooms through designated student monitors, as well as adopting a teaching style that is less controlling [41] and more open to activities with adaptable difficulty levels, allowing students to feel comfortable in class.

Finally, it is important to consider the possible political implications derived from the findings. As noted, the subject of physical education provides an opportunity to implement school-based anti-bullying programs, which could be crucial in preventing and reducing bullying in physical education as well as in other educational settings. Therefore, it would be necessary to direct new modifications in educational laws where sufficient importance is given to this subject to achieve not only the physical benefits it provides but also social well-being. Additionally, the adoption of specific measures in school policies that reflect the commitment of schools as safe environments where tolerance and respect are promoted is essential. This underscores the need to train current and future teachers not only in physical education but in all areas so they can design joint intervention programs with the aim of preventing and reducing school bullying. It is therefore crucial that these measures are not limited to reactive action in bullying situations but also focused on active prevention.

Author Contributions: Conceptualisation, J.d.D.B.-S. and D.C.-C.; methodology, J.d.D.B.-S. and D.C.-C.; software, J.d.D.B.-S. and D.C.-C.; validation, J.d.D.B.-S., D.C.-C., Á.M.-M., J.M.-M. and J.M.A.-C.; formal analysis, J.d.D.B.-S. and D.C.-C.; investigation, J.d.D.B.-S., J.M.-M. and Á.M.-M.; resources, J.d.D.B.-S., J.M.-M. and J.M.A.-C.; data curation, J.d.D.B.-S., J.M.-M. and D.C.-C.; writing—original draft preparation, J.d.D.B.-S., D.C.-C. and J.M.A.-C.; writing—review and editing, J.d.D.B.-S., D.C.-C., J.M.-M. and J.M.A.-C.; visualisation, J.d.D.B.-S., D.C.-C., Á.M.-M., J.M.-M. and J.M.A.-C.; supervision, J.d.D.B.-S., D.C.-C., Á.M.-M., J.M.-M. and J.M.A.-C.; project administration, J.d.D.B.-S.; funding acquisition, J.d.D.B.-S. All authors have read and agreed to the published version of the manuscript.

Funding: This research was funded by the Regional Ministry of Education and Sport of the Andalusian Regional Government, as educational research grant number (PIV-021/20).

Institutional Review Board Statement: This study was conducted in accordance with the Declaration of Helsinki and approved by the Ethics Committee of the University of Córdoba (17 June 2020).

Informed Consent Statement: Written consent was obtained from the parents of all participants involved in the study.

Data Availability Statement: The data presented in this study are available on request from the corresponding author. The data are not publicly available due to ethical and privacy considerations to protect the confidentiality of participants.

Acknowledgments: The authors would like to thank the schools that participated in the study.

Conflicts of Interest: The authors declare no conflicts of interest.

References

1. Ortega-Ruiz, R.; Del Rey, R.; Casas, J.A. Evaluar El Bullying y El Cyberbullying Validación Española Del EBIP-Q y Del ECIP-Q. *Psicol. Educ.* **2016**, *22*, 71–79. [CrossRef]
2. Carmona-Rojas, M.; Ortega-Ruiz, R.; Romera Félix, E.M. Bullying and Cyberbullying, What Do They Have in Common and What Not? A Latent Class Analysis. *An. De Psicol.* **2023**, *39*, 435–445. [CrossRef]
3. Biswas, T.; Scott, J.G.; Munir, K.; Thomas, H.J.; Huda, M.M.; Hasan, M.M.; David de Vries, T.; Baxter, J.; Mamun, A.A. Global Variation in the Prevalence of Bullying Victimisation amongst Adolescents: Role of Peer and Parental Supports. *EClinicalMedicine* **2020**, *20*, 100276. [CrossRef]
4. Zych, I.; Ortega-Ruiz, R.; Del Rey, R. Systematic Review of Theoretical Studies on Bullying and Cyberbullying: Facts, Knowledge, Prevention, and Intervention. *Aggress. Violent. Behav.* **2015**, *23*, 1–21. [CrossRef]
5. Olweus, D. School Bullying: Development and Some Important Challenges. *Annu. Rev. Clin. Psychol.* **2013**, *9*, 751–780. [CrossRef]
6. Martínez, J.; Rodríguez-Hidalgo, A.J.; Zych, I. Bullying and Cyberbullying in Adolescents from Disadvantaged Areas: Validation of Questionnaires; Prevalence Rates; and Relationship to Self-Esteem, Empathy and Social Skills. *Int. J. Environ. Res. Public Health* **2020**, *17*, 6199. [CrossRef]
7. Suárez-Soto, E.; Guilera, G.; Pereda, N. Victimization and Suicidality among Adolescents in Child and Youth-Serving Systems in Spain. *Child Youth Serv. Rev.* **2018**, *91*, 383–389. [CrossRef]
8. Romera, E.M.; Luque-González, R.; García-Fernández, C.M.; Ortega-Ruiz, R. Competencia Social y Bullying: El Papel de La Edad y El Sexo. *Educ. XX1* **2022**, *25*, 309–333. [CrossRef]
9. Timmons-Mitchell, J.; Levesque, D.A.; Harris, L.A.; Flannery, D.J.; Falcone, T. Pilot Test of StandUp, an Online School-Based Bullying Prevention Program. *Child. Sch.* **2016**, *38*, 71–79. [CrossRef]
10. Romera, E.M.; Ortega-Ruiz, R.; Runions, K.; Falla, D. Moral Disengagement Strategies in Online and Offline Bullying. *Psychosoc. Interv.* **2021**, *30*, 85–93. [CrossRef]
11. Stein, R.; Jimerson, S. An Examination of Bullying Roles and Moral Disengagement Using Latent Analysis. *J. Sch. Violence* **2020**, *19*, 485–498. [CrossRef]
12. Wei, M.; Graber, K.C. Bullying and Physical Education: A Scoping Review. *Kinesiol. Rev.* **2023**, *12*, 217–234. [CrossRef]
13. Benítez-Sillero, J.D.; Corredor-Corredor, D.; Córdoba-Alcaide, F.; Calmaestra, J. Intervention Programme to Prevent Bullying in Adolescents in Physical Education Classes (PREBULLPE): A Quasi-Experimental Study. *Phys. Educ. Sport Pedagog.* **2021**, *26*, 36–50. [CrossRef]
14. Benítez-Sillero, J.D.; Córdoba-Alcaide, F.; Moyano, M.; Rodríguez-Hidalgo, A.J.; Calmaestra, J. Prevention and Educational Intervention on Bullying: Physical Education as an Opportunity. *Mov. (ESEFID/UFRGS)* **2020**, *26*, e26091. [CrossRef]
15. Jesina, O.; Baloun, L.; Kudlacek, M.; Dolezalova, A.; Badura, P. Relationship of Exclusion From Physical Education and Bullying in Students With Specific Developmental Disorder of Scholastic Skills. *Int. J. Public Health* **2022**, *67*, 1604161. [CrossRef] [PubMed]
16. Atkinson, M.; Kehler, M. Boys, Bullying and Biopedagogies in Physical Education. *Thymos J. Boyhood Stud.* **2012**, *6*, 166–185. [CrossRef]
17. Jiménez-Barbero, J.A.; Jiménez-Loaisa, A.; González-Cutre, D.; Beltrán-Carrillo, V.J.; Llor-Zaragoza, L.; Ruiz-Hernández, J.A. Physical Education and School Bullying: A Systematic Review. *Phys. Educ. Sport Pedagog.* **2020**, *25*, 79–100. [CrossRef]
18. Vaillancourt, T.; Brittain, H.; Bennett, L.; Arnocky, S.; McDougall, P.; Hymel, S.; Short, K.; Sunderani, S.; Scott, C.; Mackenzie, M.; et al. Places to Avoid: Population-Based Study of Student Reports of Unsafe and High Bullying Areas at School. *Can. J. Sch. Psychol.* **2010**, *25*, 40–54. [CrossRef]
19. Castañeda-Vázquez, C.; Moreno-Arrebola, R.; González-Valero, G.; Viciana-Garófano, V.; Zurita-Ortega, F. Posibles Relaciones Entre El Bullying y La Actividad Física: Una Revisión Sistemática. *J. Sport Health Res.* **2020**, *12*, 94–111.
20. Borowiec, J.; Król-Zielińska, M.; Osiński, W.; Kantanista, A. Victims and Perpetrators of Bullying in Physical Education Lessons: The Role of Peer Support, Weight Status, Gender, and Age in Polish Adolescents. *J. Interpers. Violence* **2022**, *37*, NP15726–NP15749. [CrossRef]
21. Gano-Overway, L.A. Exploring the Connections Between Caring and Social Behaviors in Physical Education. *Res. Q. Exerc. Sport* **2013**, *84*, 104–114. [CrossRef]
22. Ornelas Melim, F.M.; Ferreira Leite de Oliveira Pereira, M.B. A Influência Da Educação Física No Bullying Escolar: A Solução Ou Parte Do Problema? *Rev. Iberoam. De Educ.* **2015**, *67*, 65–84. [CrossRef]
23. Salmivalli, C.; Lagerspetz, K.; Björkqvist, K.; Österman, K.; Kaukiainen, A. Bullying as a Group Process: Participant Roles and Their Relations to Social Status within the Group. *Aggress. Behav.* **1998**, *22*, 1–15. [CrossRef]
24. Lynn Hawkins, D.; Pepler, D.J.; Craig, W.M. Naturalistic Observations of Peer Interventions in Bullying. *Soc. Dev.* **2001**, *10*, 512–527. [CrossRef]
25. Callaghan, M.; Kelly, C.; Molcho, M. Bullying and Bystander Behaviour and Health Outcomes among Adolescents in Ireland. *J. Epidemiol. Community Health* **2019**, *73*, 416–421. [CrossRef]
26. Caballo, V.; Calderero, M.; Arias, B.; Salazar, I.; Irurtia, M.J. Development and Validation of a New Self-Report Assessment Measure of Bullying. *Behav. Psychol.* **2012**, *3*, 625–647.
27. Parris, L.; Jungert, T.; Thornberg, R.; Varjas, K.; Meyers, J.; Grunewald, S.; Shriberg, D. Bullying Bystander Behaviors: The Role of Coping Effectiveness and the Moderating Effect of Gender. *Scand J. Psychol.* **2020**, *61*, 38–46. [CrossRef]

28. Jenkins, L.N.; Fredrick, S.S. Social Capital and Bystander Behavior in Bullying: Internalizing Problems as a Barrier to Prosocial Intervention. *J. Youth Adolesc.* **2017**, *46*, 757–771. [CrossRef]
29. Lambe, L.J.; Hudson, C.C.; Craig, W.M.; Pepler, D.J. Does Defending Come with a Cost? Examining the Psychosocial Correlates of Defending Behaviour among Bystanders of Bullying in a Canadian Sample. *Child Abus. Negl.* **2017**, *65*, 112–123. [CrossRef]
30. Wu, W.-C.; Luu, S.; Luh, D.-L. Defending Behaviors, Bullying Roles, and Their Associations with Mental Health in Junior High School Students: A Population-Based Study. *BMC Public Health* **2016**, *16*, 1066. [CrossRef]
31. Modecki, K.L.; Minchin, J.; Harbaugh, A.G.; Guerra, N.G.; Runions, K.C. Bullying Prevalence Across Contexts: A Meta-Analysis Measuring Cyber and Traditional Bullying. *J. Adolesc. Health* **2014**, *55*, 602–611. [CrossRef] [PubMed]
32. Zych, I.; Ttofi, M.M.; Llorent, V.J.; Farrington, D.P.; Ribeaud, D.; Eisner, M.P. A Longitudinal Study on Stability and Transitions Among Bullying Roles. *Child Dev.* **2020**, *91*, 527–545. [CrossRef] [PubMed]
33. Romera, E.M.; Ortega-Ruiz, R.; Runions, K.; Camacho, A. Bullying Perpetration, Moral Disengagement and Need for Popularity: Examining Reciprocal Associations in Adolescence. *J. Youth Adolesc.* **2021**, *50*, 2021–2035. [CrossRef] [PubMed]
34. Olweus, D. *Bullying at School: What We Know and What We Can Do*; Blackwell: Berkeley, CA, USA, 1993.
35. Ortega, R. *Agresividad Injustificada Bullying y Violencia Escolar*; Alianza Editorial: Madrid, Spain, 2010.
36. Benítez-Sillero, J.D.; Ortega-Ruiz, R.; Romera, E.M. Victimization in Bullying and Cyberbullying and Organized Physical Activity: The Mediating Effect of Physical Self-Concept in Adolescents. *Eur. J. Dev. Psychol.* **2022**, *19*, 810–827. [CrossRef]
37. Vianna, J.A.; De Souza, S.M.; Dos Reis, K.P. Bullying Nas Aulas de Educação Física: A Percepção Dos Alunos No Ensino Médio. *Rev. Ens. Avaliação E Políticas Públicas Em Educ.* **2015**, *23*, 73–93. [CrossRef]
38. Koc, Y. Relationships between the Physical Education Course Sportsmanship Behaviors with Tendency to Violence and Empathetic Ability (Note 1). *J. Educ. Learn.* **2017**, *6*, 169. [CrossRef]
39. Jenkins, L.N.; Tennant, J. Social-Emotional Skill-Based Differences Between Active and Passive Bystanders of Bullying. *Contemp. Sch. Psychol.* **2023**, *27*, 469–478. [CrossRef]
40. Thornberg, R.; Pozzoli, T.; Gini, G. Defending or Remaining Passive as a Bystander of School Bullying in Sweden: The Role of Moral Disengagement and Antibullying Class Norms. *J. Interpers. Violence* **2022**, *37*, NP18666–NP18689. [CrossRef]
41. Montero-Carretero, C.; Pastor, D.; Santos-Rosa, F.J.; Cervelló, E. School Climate, Moral Disengagement and, Empathy as Predictors of Bullying in Adolescents. *Front. Psychol.* **2021**, *12*, 656775. [CrossRef]
42. Latané, B.; Rodin, J. A Lady in Distress: Inhibiting Effects of Friends and Strangers on Bystander Intervention. *J. Exp. Soc. Psychol.* **1969**, *5*, 189–202. [CrossRef]
43. Ríos, X.; Ventura, C.; Prat, M. "We've Never Studied Bullying at University:" Bullying-Related Beliefs, Training, and Strategies Among Physical Education Preservice Teachers. *J. Teach. Phys. Educ.* **2022**, *42*, 556–562. [CrossRef]

behavioral sciences

MDPI

Article

Physical Exercise and Life Satisfaction of Urban Residents in China

Buerzhasala Ha [1] and Jie Zhang [2,3,*]

1 School of Ethnology and Sociology, Minzu University of China, Beijing 100081, China; harper00@sina.com
2 School of Public Health, Shandong University, Jinan 250012, China
3 Department of Sociology, State University of New York Buffalo State University, Buffalo, NY 14222, USA
* Correspondence: zhangj@buffalostate.edu

Abstract: Currently, an increasing number of Chinese urban citizens are participating in daily physical exercise. Existing research has shown that physical exercise can increase life satisfaction. However, some studies also suggest that the relationship between the two is unstable. The purposes of this study are to examine physical exercise and to test its correlation with life satisfaction of urban residents in China. Data are obtained from the 2018 China Family Panel Studies, and we focus on urban residents. Our overall sample size is 7423 people, including 3641 females (49.05%) and 3782 males (50.95%), with an average age of 49.55 years old. Because the dependent variables are continuous variables, the multiple linear regression model is used for data analysis. We find that the life satisfaction of Chinese urban residents is on the high side. Our core discovery is that there is a significant positive relationship between the frequency and duration of physical exercise and life satisfaction. Our further discovery is that the frequency of physical exercise affects life satisfaction by influencing popularity and positive emotions. Similarly, the duration of physical exercise affects life satisfaction by influencing popularity and positive emotions. Whether it is the frequency or the duration of physical exercise, it can reflect the residents' attention to physical exercise. Physical exercise habits not only promote physical health by strengthening physical fitness but also promote mental health by alleviating depression and promote social communication by increasing social activities in the Chinese context. All of these can improve people's life satisfaction. Our research suggests that the improvement in life satisfaction not only needs the abundance of external material conditions but also needs the individual to improve their physical and mental health through physical exercise.

Keywords: life satisfaction; physical exercise; physical health; mental health; social communication

1. Introduction

Aristotle believed that happiness is the ultimate goal pursued by people, transcending any boundaries of material wealth and rights, and is the greatest value and meaning of life [1]. Life satisfaction refers to an individual's cognitive assessment of his or her quality of life, which is a key indicator to measure his or her subjective well-being [2]. With the emergence of the Easterlin paradox [3], people's understanding of life satisfaction has become more diverse. The Easterlin paradox shows that although the rich are usually happier than the poor within a country, when compared across borders, the happiness levels of poor and rich countries are similar, such as the United States and Cuba. The Easterlin paradox draws attention to the limitations of equating life satisfaction solely with material wealth. It emphasizes the importance of non-material factors such as health [4,5], psychological capital [6], and social relationships [7,8], encouraging people to have a broader understanding of life satisfaction beyond economic indicators.

Existing studies have shown that physical exercise is not only beneficial for physical health [9,10], such as preventing and treating chronic diseases [11], delaying aging [12], improving functional capacity, improving body composition [13,14], reducing risks of cardiovascular disease, obesity, stroke, and cancer [15], but it is also beneficial for mental health [16]. There is already a lot of research on the impact on physical health, so there is no need to elaborate further. The evidence regarding mental health comes from both neuroscience and psychology (The research content of this article is physical exercise rather than physical activity. According to Caspersen et al. [17], physical activity is defined as any bodily movement produced by skeletal muscles that results in energy expenditure. The energy expenditure can be measured in kilocalories. Physical activity in daily life can be categorized into occupational, sports, conditioning, household, or other activities. Exercise is a subset of physical activity that is planned, structured, and repetitive and has as a final or an intermediate objective the improvement or maintenance of physical fitness. However, the distinction between physical activity and physical exercise is not very clear in the existing literature, and the concept of physical activity is often used to measure the content of physical exercise. If the references are limited to the literature with the keyword physical exercise, a large number of valuable literature publications will be missed. Therefore, based on the specific content of the literature, the references in this article will also include the literature with physical activity as the keyword. This article is collectively referred to as physical exercise).

Studies from neuroscience have shown that physical exercise can induce changes in brain structure and function [10], such as increasing gray matter volume in the frontal lobe and hippocampus, reducing gray matter damage, and expanding cortical and basal ganglia volume [10,18–20].

Studies from psychology have shown that physical exercise can reduce psychological disorders such as depression and anxiety [21–23], alcoholism [24], and even the probability of self-injurious behaviors [25]; improve emotional state [26]; and enhance self-esteem [27,28] and self-efficacy [29,30]. It should be noted that some studies have found that although overall exercise is better than not exercising, more exercise was not always associated with better mental health. If the duration exceeds 45 min per session or the frequency exceeds 5 times a week, the mental health burden of participants will increase [31]. There are also studies that have found gender differences in the impact of physical exercise on mental health. Boys and girls have different responses to physical exercise in terms of a reduced risk of depression, anxiety, ADHD, and ODD. For example, for boys, a high frequency of MVPA (Moderate-to-Vigorous Physical Activity) is significantly associated with a lower risk of depression. For girls, both moderate- and high-frequency MVPA are associated with a lower risk of depression, indicating a generally positive impact of physical exercise on the risk of depression in girls [32].

Physical exercise is a social behavior [33]. It can improve self-image and social skills [24]. Teenagers who exercise regularly become more sociable, which makes them happier [34]. When physical exercise is digitized and embedded into social media, it strengthens the existing social network. Research by Gui Xinyu et al. indicates that sharing fitness data with pre-existing social networks motivates users to enhance their existing social relationships [35].

Returning to the research topic of this article, physical exercise and life satisfaction, existing research has shown that physical exercise can improve participant life satisfaction [9,16,36–43]. People who regularly participate in physical exercise have higher life satisfaction than those who do not exercise [44]. Middle-aged adult males who engaged in regular physical exercise reported greater levels of overall life satisfaction [45]. There is a significant positive correlation between the time and frequency of physical exercise and college students' life satisfaction [46]. In the short term, exercise induces positive mood states, and in the long term, regular exercise leads to greater happiness [47]. However, some studies have also pointed out that the correlation between the two is unstable. Sidney and Shephard concluded that although physical exercise improved the physical condition of the elderly, it failed to improve their life satisfaction [48]. The research by Dai Q. and Yao J.-X. shows that there is no direct correlation between physical exercise and the life satisfaction of the elderly. Physical exercise affects the life satisfaction of elderly people through two mediating variables: friend support and self-efficacy [49]. There are also studies indicating that excessive exercise reduces the life satisfaction of elderly people [50]. Maher et al.'s research found that there is no correlation between physical exercise and life satisfaction in young adulthood [51]. Research has also found that moderate-intensity physical exercise can increase happiness, but high-intensity exercise can reduce happiness [52]. Low-intensity and moderate-intensity physical exercise bring happiness, while the effects of high-intensity exercise cannot be verified [53]. First, there is still no final conclusion regarding the relationship between physical exercise and life satisfaction in existing research. Second, most of the existing research has focused narrowly on the relationship between physical exercise and life satisfaction in specific age groups (elderly, young people, etc.), specific gender groups (such as males), and specific identity groups (such as students), lacking a more comprehensive macro perspective that examines this relationship across all age groups, genders, and identities. Third, among the studies that believe there is a correlation between the two, there is no consensus on how the frequency and duration of physical exercise affect life satisfaction. Finally, there is insufficient discussion on the mechanism of the correlation between the two.

The fitness culture [33] is spreading among the urban population in China, with an increasing number of Chinese people participating in daily physical exercise. According to the National Fitness Survey Bulletin of the General Administration of Sports of China in 2014, the percentage of people who regularly took part in physical exercise in 2014 was 33.9% (including children and adolescents), an increase of 5.7 percentage points compared with 2007, and included 14.7% of people aged 20 and over, of which 19.5% were urban residents, an increase of 48.0% compared with 2007. It can be seen that urban citizens' physical exercise activities are increasing day by day.

Based on the previous discussion, we propose the following research hypotheses:

Hypothesis 1. *The more frequent the frequency of physical exercise, the higher the satisfaction of urban residents with their lives.*

Hypothesis 2. *The longer the duration of physical exercise, the higher the satisfaction of urban residents with their lives.*

Hypothesis 3. *The frequency of physical exercise is positively associated with life satisfaction among urban residents, mediated through an increase in personal popularity.*

Hypothesis 4. *The frequency of physical exercise is positively related to life satisfaction among urban residents, mediated through an increase in positive emotions.*

Hypothesis 5. *The duration of physical exercise is positively associated with life satisfaction among urban residents, mediated by an increase in personal popularity.*

Hypothesis 6. *The duration of physical exercise is positively correlated with life satisfaction among urban residents, mediated through an enhancement of positive emotions.*

2. Methods

2.1. Data Source and Analysis Methods

The data used in this study come from the 2018 China Family Panel Studies (CFPS), a panel data collection project managed by Peking University in China. CFPS focuses on the economic and non-economic welfare of Chinese residents, as well as many research topics including economic activities, educational achievements, family relations and family dynamics, population migration, health, etc. It is a national, large-scale, multi-disciplinary social tracking survey project. CFPS samples cover 25 provinces/cities/autonomous regions, and the target sample size is 16,000 households. The respondents include all family members in the sample households. A total of 32,669 valid cases were collected in CFPS 2018, including 7872 urban cases, 22,259 rural cases, and 2538 other cases.

Considering that people in rural areas of China rarely participate in physical exercise, this article only retains urban samples. (Physical exercise is defined as an active and regular physical activity undertaken for the purpose of exercising, excluding passive activities like agricultural labor. While it is often assumed that rural Chinese individuals may not actively engage in physical exercises, we understand this may be a generalization. However, for the sake of clarity and standardization, we have chosen to limit the scope of this article to urban samples, considering the presumed lower participation rate of physical exercise in rural areas.) After handling missing values, the final sample of urban residents was 7423 people. It is worth mentioning that from 2018 to now, CFPS has released the latest data for 2020. Considering that most people affected by the COVID-19 epidemic were isolated at home that year, which seriously affected the results we want to test, the data for 2020 are not used.

We use a multiple linear regression model and StataMP 17 statistical software for data analysis. The set p-values are 0.001, 0.01, and 0.05.

2.2. *Measurements*

2.2.1. Dependent Variable

Following the CFPS 2018 survey questionnaire, we used the question, "How satisfied are you with your life?" to measure the life satisfaction of urban residents. Respondents had five options: 1 = not at all satisfied, 2 = not satisfied, 3 = average, 4 = satisfied, 5 = very satisfied.

2.2.2. Independent Variables

To measure the condition of exercise of urban residents, we selected two questions from the 2018 CFPS questionnaire. One question was, "How many times have you exercised in the past week?" and the other was, "How long have you exercised in the past week?"; the former can be answered from 0 to 50 times, while the latter can be answered from 0.1 to 105.0 h, the higher the value, the higher the frequency and intensity of exercise. The exercises here include walking, long-distance running, jogging, and mountaineering; practicing martial arts such as Tai Chi and qigong; indoor and outdoor dance; fitness exercises; aerobics; yoga; various ball games such as small and large balls; water sports such as swimming, diving, rowing, and sailing; winter ice and snow sports; as well as physical contact sports such as wrestling, judo, and boxing.

2.2.3. Mediating Variables

To reveal the mechanism of the impact of physical exercise on life satisfaction, we used popularity and positive emotions as mediating variables, corresponding to "How good the social relationship is" and "The frequency of various feelings or behaviors occurring in the past week" with 8 statements (the 8 statements are the following: "I feel emotionally low", "I feel that doing anything is difficult", "My sleep is not good", "I feel happy", "I feel lonely", "I live happily", "I feel sad", "I feel that life cannot continue"), respectively. The former has a minimum score of 0 and a maximum score of 10, while the latter has a minimum score of 4 and a maximum score of 32 (each question scores 1–4 points, the more positive the emotion, the higher the score).

2.2.4. Control Variables

To eliminate error caused by the omission of variables from the model estimation to the best extent possible, we introduced other related control variables based on existing research results. The control variables in this article included the following: individual's gender (female = 0; male = 1), marital status (unmarried = 0; married = 1), age, years of education, self-rated income level in local terms (1–5), and self-rated health (1–5).

Regarding years of education, the options provided in the questionnaire include "illiterate/semi-illiterate", "elementary school", "junior high school", "high school/technical school/vocational high school", "associate degree", "undergraduate degree", "master's degree", and "doctoral degree". In China, in most cases, they correspond to education years of 0, 6, 9, 12, 15, 16, 19, and 23 years, respectively. Currently, most studies have shown that relative deprivation of income has a greater impact on happiness compared to absolute income [4,54]. Therefore, we select self-rated income level in local terms as the control variable to control for economic level.

3. Results

3.1. Descriptive Statistical Analysis

Table 1 shows the basic situation of the variables in this study. There are 3641 (49.05%) women and 3782 (50.95%) men in the sample, and 1371 (18.47%) samples are unmarried and 6052 (81.53%) samples are married. The average age is 49.55 years old and the average number of years of education is 10.45 years. Respondents rated their income level in local terms and their health status as medium, giving 2.87 points and 2.94 points, respectively, from the full score of 5 points. The average number of physical exercise sessions per week is 3.41 times, and the average length of physical exercise is 4.74 h per week. The average of life satisfaction with a full score of 5 points is 4.01 points. This illustrates that the life satisfaction of Chinese urban residents is on the high side.

Table 1. Variable descriptive statistical analysis (N = 7423).

Variable	Variable Definition	Freq./Mean	Percent (%)/SD
DV			
Life satisfaction (1–5)	Assign values of 1–5 from "very dissatisfied" to "very satisfied".	4.01	0.89
IV			
Exercise frequency (times/week)	The lowest value is 0, the highest value is 35, among which 2682 are selected as 0, accounting for 36%.	3.41	3.30
Duration of exercise (hour/week)	The lowest value is 0, the highest value is 90, among which 2682 are selected as 0, accounting for 36%.	4.74	6.92
MV			
Popularity (0–10)	Assign values of 0–10 from "very unpopular" to "very popular".	7.17	1.80
Positive emotions (8–32)	It involves 8 CESD variables, with a minimum value of 1 and a maximum value of 4 for each variable. After adding up, the minimum value is 8 and the maximum value is 32. The higher the score, the higher the level of positive emotions.	27.08	3.76
CV			
Gender			
Female (0)		3641	49.05
Male (1)		3782	50.95
Marital status			
Unmarried (0)		1371	18.47
Married (1)		6052	81.53
Age	The minimum age is 16, and the maximum age is 96.	49.55	16.23
Years of education	The minimum education period is 0 years, and the maximum education period is 23 years. Among them, 722 are illiterate, accounting for 9.73%.	10.45	4.70
Self-rated income level in local terms (1–5)	Assign values of 1–5 from "very low" to "very high".	2.87	0.99
Self-rated health (1–5)	Assign values of 1–5 from "unhealthy" to "very healthy".	2.92	1.09

DV: dependent variable, IV: independent variable, MV: mediator variable, CV: control variable.

3.2. Regression Analysis

Table 2 shows the correlation between frequency and duration of exercise and life satisfaction of Chinese urban residents without any control variables. Among them, the p value between exercise frequency and life satisfaction is statistically significant, and the p value between the duration of exercise and life satisfaction is also statistically significant, which indicates that exercise condition affects the life satisfaction of Chinese urban residents.

Table 2. Bi-variate analyses of exercise and life satisfaction.

	Exercise Frequency	Duration of Exercise
Life satisfaction	$r = 9.53, p < 0.001$	$r = 8.79, p < 0.001$

r: Spearman's rank correlation coefficient.

We used multiple regressions in Table 3 to reveal whether the relationship between physical exercise and life satisfaction is still significant when the control variables are added. Model 1 introduced control variables into the model, and we drew the following conclusions by analyzing the model fit results: gender, marital status, age, years of education, income level in local terms, and health condition all had a significant relationship with the life satisfaction of urban residents. Specifically, women have higher life satisfaction than men. Being married has a higher level of life satisfaction than not being married. The higher the age, income level in local terms, and health condition, the higher the life satisfaction. It is worth noting that our study found that the higher the number of years of education, the lower the life satisfaction. One possible reason is that longer years of education in China means greater academic burden and more intense competition among peers, so their life satisfaction is not very high. Studies on education level and depression have also confirmed that after reaching a certain level of education, the higher the level of education, the more likely it is to experience depression [55–57].

Table 3. Multiple regressions with life satisfaction as their dependent variables (N = 7423).

Variables	Model 1	Model 2	Model 3
Gender (male)	−0.0540 **	−0.0572 **	−0.0573 **
	(−2.79)	(−2.96)	(−2.96)
Married	0.179 ***	0.182 ***	0.182 ***
	(7.14)	(7.28)	(7.25)
Age	0.00656 ***	0.00564 ***	0.00613 ***
	(8.85)	(7.28)	(8.11)
Years of education	−0.0114 ***	−0.0122 ***	−0.0117 ***
	(−4.67)	(−5.00)	(−4.77)
Self-rated income level in local terms	0.256 ***	0.255 ***	0.255 ***
	(25.84)	(25.79)	(25.81)
Self-rated health	0.123 ***	0.120 ***	0.121 ***
	(13.19)	(12.90)	(13.01)
Exercise frequency		0.0123 ***	
		(4.05)	
Duration of exercise			0.00423 **
			(2.98)
F	205.94	179.23	177.98
p	<0.001	<0.001	<0.001
R^2	0.1428	0.1447	0.1438

** $p < 0.01$, *** $p < 0.001$.

On this basis, we added the first independent variable exercise frequency in Model 2, and we found that there is still a significant correlation between the frequency of physical exercises and life satisfaction ($p < 0.001$); each time the number of physical exercise sessions increases 1 time, the life satisfaction of urban residents will increase 0.0123 points. On the basis of Model 1, we added the second independent variable duration of exercise in Model 3, and the result is still significant; for every 1 h increase in the length of physical exercise, the life satisfaction of urban residents will be increased by 0.00423 points. Hypotheses 1 and 2 are verified.

To verify hypotheses 3, 4, 5, and 6, namely the mediating role of popularity and positive emotions in the impact of physical exercise frequency and duration on life satisfaction, we conducted regression analysis of the mediating variable on the dependent variable and regression analysis of the independent variable on the mediating variable, respectively. The results are presented in Tables 4 and 5.

Table 4. Regression estimation results of mediating variables on life satisfaction (N = 7423).

Variables	Model 4	Model 5	Model 6	Model 7
Gender (male)	−0.0481 *	−0.0769 ***	−0.0482 *	−0.0772 ***
	(−2.53)	(−4.14)	(−2.53)	(−4.16)
Married	0.182 ***	0.128 ***	0.182 ***	0.128 ***
	(7.40)	(5.31)	(7.38)	(5.30)
Age	0.00453 ***	0.00305 ***	0.00493 ***	0.00324 ***
	(5.91)	(4.08)	(6.60)	(4.43)
Years of education	−0.0141 ***	−0.0179 ***	−0.0136 ***	−0.0177 ***
	(−5.85)	(−7.62)	(−5.66)	(−7.53)
Self-rated income level in local terms	0.233 ***	0.217 ***	0.233 ***	0.217 ***
	(23.67)	(22.66)	(23.68)	(22.66)
Self-rated health	0.101 ***	0.0484 ***	0.102 ***	0.0485 ***
	(10.93)	(5.18)	(11.01)	(5.19)
Exercise frequency	0.0106 ***	0.00591 *		
	(3.53)	(2.02)		
Popularity	0.0842 ***	0.0694 ***	0.0845 ***	0.0696 ***
	(15.67)	(13.18)	(15.73)	(13.20)
Positive Emotions		0.0549 ***		0.0551 ***
		(20.76)		(20.87)
Duration of exercise			0.00368 **	0.00235
			(2.64)	(1.73)
F	192.67	229.06	191.84	228.91
p	<0.001	<0.001	<0.001	<0.001
R^2	0.1721	0.2176	0.1715	0.2175

* $p < 0.05$, ** $p < 0.01$, *** $p < 0.001$.

Table 5. Regression estimation results of the relationship between exercise and mediating variables (N = 7423).

Variables	Popularity	Positive Emotions	Popularity	Positive Emotions
Gender (male)	−0.108 **	0.495 ***	−0.107 **	0.498 ***
	(−2.62)	(6.03)	(−2.61)	(6.06)
Married	−0.00107	0.988 ***	−0.00234	0.980 ***
	(−0.02)	(9.30)	(−0.04)	(9.21)
Age	0.0133 ***	0.0305 ***	0.0141 ***	0.0346 ***
	(8.05)	(9.27)	(8.80)	(10.77)
Years of education	0.0223 ***	0.0752 ***	0.0233 ***	0.0799 ***
	(4.29)	(7.24)	(4.49)	(7.69)
Self-rated income level in local terms	0.265 ***	0.352 ***	0.265 ***	0.355 ***
	(12.60)	(8.40)	(12.62)	(8.45)
Self-rated health	0.228 ***	1.022 ***	0.229 ***	1.031 ***
	(11.47)	(25.84)	(11.57)	(26.03)
Exercise frequency	0.0206 **	0.0911 ***		
	(3.17)	(7.05)		
Duration of exercise			0.00644 *	0.0260 ***
			(2.13)	(4.31)
F	61.45	170.73	60.61	165.61
p	<0.001	<0.001	<0.001	<0.001
R^2	0.0548	0.1388	0.0541	0.1352

* $p < 0.05$, ** $p < 0.01$, *** $p < 0.001$.

Exercise frequency → Popularity and Positive emotions → Life satisfaction. As shown in Model 4, we add the first mediator variable on top of Model 2: popularity. We found a significant correlation between popularity and life satisfaction ($p < 0.001$). For every 1-point increase in popularity, life satisfaction increases by 0.0842 points. As shown in Model 5, based on Model 4, we add a second mediator variable: positive emotions. We found a significant correlation between positive emotions and life satisfaction ($p < 0.001$). For every 1-point increase in positive emotions, life satisfaction increases by 0.0549 points. From Model 2 to Model 4 and then to Model 5, the estimated coefficient of exercise frequency on life satisfaction gradually decreases, from 0.0123 points to 0.0106 points and then to 0.00591 points. Therefore, the two mediating variables of popularity and positive emotions can explain the partial impact of exercise frequency on life satisfaction.

Duration of exercise → Popularity and Positive emotions → Life satisfaction. As shown in Model 6, we add the first mediating variable on top of Model 3: popularity. We conclude that in this model, there is a significant correlation between popularity and life satisfaction ($p < 0.001$). For every 1-point increase in popularity, life satisfaction increases by 0.0845 points. As shown in Model 7, based on Model 6, we add a second mediator variable: positive emotions. We found a significant correlation between positive emotions and life satisfaction ($p < 0.001$). For every 1-point increase in positive emotions, life satisfaction increases by 0.0551 points. From Model 3 to Model 6 and then to Model 7, the estimated coefficient of duration of exercise on life satisfaction gradually decreases, from 0.00423 points to 0.00368 points and then to 0.00235 points. Therefore, the two mediating variables of popularity and positive emotions can explain the partial impact of duration of exercise on life satisfaction.

In order to ultimately confirm whether the two mediating variables of popularity and positive emotions are the mediating mechanisms of the impact of physical exercise on life satisfaction, we further tested the relationship between physical exercise and the two mediating variables, and the results are shown in Table 5.

There is a significant correlation between exercise frequency and popularity ($p < 0.01$). Each time the number of physical exercises increases 1 time, the popularity will increase 0.0206 points. There is a significant correlation between exercise frequency and positive emotions ($p < 0.001$). For every increase in exercise frequency, positive emotions increase by 0.0911 points.

There is a significant correlation between exercise duration and popularity ($p < 0.1$). For every increase in exercise frequency, the popularity is 0.00644 points. There is a significant correlation between exercise frequency and positive emotions ($p < 0.001$). For every increase in exercise frequency, positive emotions increase by 0.0260 points.

It can be seen that physical exercise increases urban residents' popularity and positive emotional level, thereby enhancing life satisfaction. This proves that popularity and positive emotional level are two important mediating mechanisms for the impact of physical exercise on life satisfaction.

4. Conclusions

This study analyzed data from the 2018 China Family Panel Studies to examine the relationship between physical exercise and the life satisfaction of urban residents in China. We found that both the frequency and duration of physical exercise have positive correlations with residents' life satisfaction. The findings verify the previous research results about the positive relationship between physical exercise and life satisfaction [58]. To further reveal the impact mechanism between physical exercise and life satisfaction, we introduce two mediating variables: popularity and positive emotions. The results show that the frequency of physical exercise affects life satisfaction by influencing popularity and positive emotions. Similarly, the duration of physical exercise affects life satisfaction by influencing popularity and positive emotions. Namely, the higher the frequency and duration of physical exercise, the higher the popularity and positive emotion levels among Chinese urban citizens, resulting in an increased life satisfaction.

Residents' life satisfaction is not only affected by objective conditions, but also by individual cognitive characteristics. The improvement in people's life satisfaction not only depends on a good policy, social, and cultural environment but also requires a good habit of physical exercise to improve their physical and mental quality.

To explain the positive relationship towards physical exercise and life satisfaction, one possibility is that physical exercise can strengthen physical quality. Good health can improve people's life satisfaction, especially the elderly [59]. Another possibility is that physical exercise can improve people's psychological well-being or reduce the level of anxiety and depression [60,61], and then produce emotional benefits. Obviously, good emotions can improve people's life satisfaction. The third possibility is that in the context of China, in the middle-aged and elderly groups, the group activities represented by square dance are their main physical exercise methods. In addition to the above two benefits, this kind of physical exercise also has strong social characteristics, and these frequent social activities can increase people's life satisfaction [62].

Although we can infer through the literature references that participating in physical exercise is the reason for increased life satisfaction, the causal relationship between the two cannot be inferred from the data used in this study, which are cross sectional survey data. One possibility is that people with higher life satisfaction are more willing to participate in physical exercise. This is a limitation of our research. In the future, we look forward to research to supplement the limitation at the data level and determine the causal relationship between the two through data analysis.

Author Contributions: Conceptualization, J.Z. and B.H.; methodology, J.Z. and B.H.; software, B.H.; validation, J.Z.; formal analysis, B.H.; data curation, B.H.; writing—original draft preparation, B.H.; writing—review and editing, B.H.; visualization, B.H.; supervision, J.Z.; project administration, J.Z. All authors have read and agreed to the published version of the manuscript.

Funding: This research received no external funding.

Institutional Review Board Statement: Not applicable.

Informed Consent Statement: Not applicable.

Data Availability Statement: The data that support the findings of this study are available from Institute of Social Science Survey, Peking University. Data are available from Peking University Research Data Platform https://opendata.pku.edu.cn/dataset.xhtml?persistentId=doi:10.18170/DVN/45LCSO (accessed on 13 May 2023) with the permission of Institute of Social Science Survey, Peking University.

Conflicts of Interest: The authors declare no conflicts of interest.

References

1. Shin, D.C.; Johnson, D.M. Avowed happiness as an overall assessment of the quality of life. *Soc. Indic. Res.* **1978**, *5*, 475–492. [CrossRef]
2. Diener, E. Subjective well-being. The science of happiness and a proposal for a national index. *Am. Psychol.* **2000**, *55*, 34–43. [CrossRef] [PubMed]
3. Easterlin, R.A. Does Economic Growth Improve the Human Lot? Some Empirical Evidence. In *Nations and Households in Economic Growth*; David, P.A., Reder, M.W., Eds.; Academic Press: New York, NY, USA, 1974; pp. 89–125.
4. Koivumaa-Honkanen, H.; Honkanen, R.; Viinamäki, H.; Heikkilä, K.; Kaprio, J.; Koskenvuo, M. Self-reported Life Satisfaction and 20-Year Mortality in Healthy Finnish Adults. *Am. J. Epidemiol.* **2000**, *152*, 983–991. [CrossRef] [PubMed]
5. Strine, T.W.; Chapman, D.P.; Balluz, L.S.; Moriarty, D.G.; Mokdad, A.H. The Associations Between Life Satisfaction and Health-related Quality of Life, Chronic Illness, and Health Behaviors among U.S. Community-dwelling Adults. *J. Community Health* **2008**, *33*, 40–50. [CrossRef] [PubMed]
6. Youssef-Morgan, C.M.; Luthans, F. Psychological Capital and Well-being. *Stress Health J. Int. Soc. Investig. Stress* **2015**, *31*, 180–188. [CrossRef] [PubMed]
7. House, J.S.; Landis, K.R.; Umberson, D. Social Relationships and Health. *Science* **1988**, *241*, 540–545. [CrossRef] [PubMed]
8. Muhammad, T.; Pai, M.; Afsal, K.; Saravanakumar, P.; Irshad, C.V. The association between loneliness and life satisfaction: Examining spirituality, religiosity, and religious participation as moderators. *BMC Geriatr.* **2023**, *23*, 301. [CrossRef]
9. An, H.-Y.; Chen, W.; Wang, C.-W.; Yang, H.-F.; Huang, W.-T.; Fan, S.-Y. The Relationships between Physical Activity and Life Satisfaction and Happiness among Young, Middle-Aged, and Older Adults. *Int. J. Environ. Res. Public Health* **2020**, *17*, 4817. [CrossRef] [PubMed]

10. Qiao, Y.-C.; Fan, Y.-Z. Interrogation and Response: Eight Basic Problems in the Study of the Relationship Between Physical Activity and Happiness. *J. Shanghai Univ. Sport* **2020**, *44*, 1–15.
11. Grazioli, E.; Dimauro, I.; Mercatelli, N.; Wang, G.; Pitsiladis, Y.; Luigi, L.D.; Caporossi, D. Physical activity in the prevention of human diseases: Role of epigenetic modifications. *BMC Genom.* **2017**, *18*, 802. [CrossRef]
12. Popov, D.; Zinovkin, R.; Karger, E.; Tarasova, O.; Vinogradova, O. Effects of continuous and intermittent aerobic exercise upon mRNA expression of metabolic genes in human skeletal muscle. *J. Sports Med. Phys. Fit.* **2014**, *54*, 362–369.
13. Penedo, F.J.; Dahn, J.R. Exercise and well-being: A review of mental and physical health benefits associated with physical activity. *Curr. Opin. Psychiatry* **2005**, *18*, 189–193. [CrossRef] [PubMed]
14. Vogel, T.; Brechat, P.-H.; Leprêtre, P.-M.; Kaltenbach, G.; Berthel, M.; Lonsdorfer, J. Health benefits of physical activity in older patients: A review. *Int. J. Clin. Pract.* **2009**, *63*, 303–320. [CrossRef] [PubMed]
15. Lee, I.M.; Shiroma, E.J.; Lobelo, F.; Puska, P.; Blair, S.N.; Katzmarzyk, P.T. Effect of physical inactivity on major non-communicable diseases worldwide: An analysis of burden of disease and life expectancy. *Lancet* **2012**, *380*, 219–229. [CrossRef] [PubMed]
16. Fox, K.R. The influence of physical activity on mental well-being. *Public Health Nutr.* **1999**, *2*, 411–418. [CrossRef] [PubMed]
17. Caspersen, C.J.; Powell, K.E.; Christenson, G.M. Physical activity, exercise, and physical fitness: Definitions and distinctions for health-related research. *Public Health Rep.* **1985**, *100*, 126–131. [PubMed]
18. Chaddock, L.; Erickson, K.I.; Prakash, R.S.; Kim, J.S.; Voss, M.W.; VanPatter, M.; Pontifex, M.B.; Raine, L.B.; Konkel, A.; Hillman, C.H.; et al. A neuroimaging investigation of the association between aerobic fitness, hippocampal volume, and memory performance in preadolescent children. *Brain Res.* **2010**, *1358*, 172–183. [CrossRef] [PubMed]
19. Chaddock-Heyman, L.; Erickson, K.I.; Holtrop, J.L.; Voss, M.W.; Pontifex, M.B.; Raine, L.B.; Hillman, C.H.; Kramer, A.F. Aerobic fitness is associated with greater white matter integrity in children. *Front. Hum. Neurosci.* **2014**, *8*, 584. [CrossRef] [PubMed]
20. Erickson, K.I.; Miller, D.L.; Weinstein, A.M.; Akl, S.L.; Banducci, S. Physical activity and brain plasticity in late adulthood: A conceptual and comprehensive review. *Ageing Res.* **2012**, *3*, e6. [CrossRef]
21. Carek, P.J.; Laibstain, S.E.; Carek, S.M. Exercise for the Treatment of Depression and Anxiety. *Int. J. Psychiatry Med.* **2011**, *41*, 15–28. [CrossRef]
22. Salmon, P. Effects of physical exercise on anxiety, depression, and sensitivity to stress: A unifying theory. *Clin. Psychol. Rev.* **2001**, *21*, 33–61. [CrossRef]
23. Ströhle, A. Physical activity, exercise, depression and anxiety disorders. *J. Neural Transm.* **2009**, *116*, 777–784. [CrossRef]
24. Taylor, C.; Sallis, J.; Needle, R. The relation of physical activity and exercise to mental health. *Public Health Rep.* **1985**, *100*, 195–202.
25. Liu, M.-L.; Zhang, J.; Hu, E.; Yang, H.-L.; Cheng, C.; Yao, S.-Q. Combined patterns of physical activity and screen-related sedentary behavior among Chinese adolescents and their correlations with depression, anxiety and self-injurious behaviors. *Psychol. Res. Behav. Manag.* **2019**, *12*, 1041–1050. [CrossRef]
26. Jiang, Y.; Zhang, L.-W.; Mao, Z.-X. Behavior Physical exercise and mental health: The effect of emotion regulation self-efficacy and emotion regulation strategy. *Stud. Psychol. Behav.* **2018**, *16*, 570.
27. Ekeland, E.; Heian, F.; Hagen, K.B.; Abbott, J.; Nordheim, L. Exercise to Improve Self-Esteem in Children and Young People. *Campbell Syst. Rev.* **2005**, *1*, 1–52. [CrossRef]
28. Sonstroem, R.J. Exercise and Self-Esteem. *Exerc. Sport Sci. Rev.* **1984**, *12*, 123–156. [CrossRef]
29. Medrano-Ureña, M.D.; Ortega-Ruiz, R.; Benítez-Sillero, J.D. Physical Fitness, Exercise Self-Efficacy, and Quality of Life in Adulthood: A Systematic Review. *Int. J. Environ. Res. Public Health* **2020**, *17*, 6343. [CrossRef]
30. Pauline, J.S. Physical activity behaviors, motivation, and self-efficacy among college students. *Coll. Stud. J.* **2013**, *47*, 64–74.
31. Chekroud, S.R.; Gueorguieva, R.; Zheutlin, A.B.; Paulus, M.; Krumholz, H.M.; Krystal, J.H.; Chekroud, A.M. Association between physical exercise and mental health in 1·2 million individuals in the USA between 2011 and 2015: A cross-sectional study. *Lancet Psychiatry* **2018**, *5*, 739–746. [CrossRef]
32. Liu, M.-L.; Zhang, J.; Kamper-DeMarco, K.E.; Hu, E.; Yao, S. Associations of moderate-to-vigorous physical activity with psychological problems and suicidality in Chinese high school students: A cross-sectional study. *PeerJ* **2020**, *8*, e8775. [CrossRef] [PubMed]
33. McKenzie, S. *Getting Physical: The Rise of Fitness Culture in America*; University Press of Kansas: Lawrence, KS, USA, 2013.
34. Cheon, H. The Structural Relationship between Exercise Frequency, Social Health, and Happiness in Adolescents. *Sustainability* **2021**, *13*, 1050. [CrossRef]
35. Gui, X.-N.; Chen, Y.; Caldeira, C.; Xiao, D.; Chen, Y. When fitness meets social networks: Investigating fitness tracking and social practices on werun. In Proceedings of the 2017 CHI Conference on Human Factors in Computing Systems, Denver, CO, USA, 6–11 May 2017; pp. 1647–1659. [CrossRef]
36. Hayes, D.; Ross, C.E. Body and Mind: The Effect of Exercise, Overweight, and Physical Health on Psychological Well-Being. *J. Health Soc. Behav.* **1986**, *27*, 387–400. [CrossRef] [PubMed]
37. Kan, B.; Xie, Y. Impact of sports participation on life satisfaction among internal migrants in China: The chain mediating effect of social interaction and self-efficacy. *Acta Psychol.* **2024**, *243*, 104139. [CrossRef] [PubMed]
38. Louise, M.; Tess, K.; Catherine, M.; Lily, G.-D.; Jack, L.; Alistair, J.; Norma, D.; Paul, D.; Stefano, T.; Guy, J.; et al. Sport and dance interventions for healthy young people (15–24 years) to promote subjective well-being: A systematic review. *BMJ Open* **2018**, *8*, e020959. [CrossRef] [PubMed]

39. Riddick, C.C.; Daniel, S.N. The relative contribution of leisure activities and other factors to the mental health of older women. *J. Leis. Res.* **1984**, *16*, 136–148. [CrossRef]
40. Russell, R.V. The Importance of Recreation Satisfaction and Activity Participation to the Life Satisfaction of Age-segregated Retirees. *J. Leis. Res.* **1987**, *19*, 273–283. [CrossRef]
41. Schnohr, P.; Kristensen, T.S.; Prescott, E.; Scharling, H. Stress and life dissatisfaction are inversely associated with jogging and other types of physical activity in leisure time—The Copenhagen City Heart Study. *Scand. J. Med. Sci. Sports* **2005**, *15*, 107–112. [CrossRef] [PubMed]
42. Stubbe, J.H.; de Moor, M.H.M.; Boomsma, D.I.; de Geus, E.J.C. The association between exercise participation and well-being: A co-twin study. *Prev. Med.* **2007**, *44*, 148–152. [CrossRef]
43. Teixeira Vaz, C.; de Souza Andrade, A.C.; Proietti, F.A.; Xavier, C.C.; de Lima Friche, A.A.; Caiaffa, W.T. A multilevel model of life satisfaction among old people: Individual characteristics and neighborhood physical disorder. *BMC Public Health* **2019**, *19*, 861. [CrossRef]
44. Iwon, K.; Skibinska, J.; Jasielska, D.; Kalwarczyk, S. Elevating Subjective Well-Being Through Physical Exercises: An Intervention Study. *Front. Psychol.* **2021**, *12*, 702678. [CrossRef] [PubMed]
45. Gous, G.; Ali, A.; Hadayat, T. Association Between Physical Activity and Life Satisfaction Among Middle-Aged Adult Men. *J. Dev. Soc. Sci.* **2023**, *4*, 131–139. [CrossRef]
46. Liu, L. The Related Research of University Students' Physical Exerciseand Life Satisfaction, a Sense of the Meaning of Life. Master's Thesis, Zhengzhou University, Zhengzhou, China, 10 May 2012.
47. Sran, S.K.; Vats, P.; Wadhawan, P. Effect of Exercise on Life Satisfaction and Happiness. *Indian J. Health Wellbeing* **2021**, *12*, 79–82.
48. Sidney, K.H.; Shephard, R.J. Attitudes towards health and physical activity in the elderly. Effects of a physical training program. *Med. Sci. Sports* **1976**, *8*, 253–257. [CrossRef]
49. Dai, Q.; Yao, J.-X. Relationship between Physical Exercise and Life Satisfaction: The Mediation Effects of Self-efficacy, Social Support and Self-esteem. *J. Beijing Sport Univ.* **2012**, *35*, 67–72.
50. Ma, J.-F.; Wang, H.-T.; Wang, J.-J.; Shi, D.-L. Inverted U-shaped relationship between physical activity and life satisfaction among Chinese older adults: Mediating role of depression. *China J. Health Psychol.* **2024**, *32*, 7–13.
51. Maher, J.P.; Pincus, A.L.; Ram, N.; Conroy, D.E. Daily physical activity and life satisfaction across adulthood. *Dev. Psychol.* **2015**, *51*, 1407–1419. [CrossRef] [PubMed]
52. Wicker, P.; Frick, B. The relationship between intensity and duration of physical activity and subjective well-being. *Eur. J. Public Health* **2015**, *25*, 868–872. [CrossRef] [PubMed]
53. Panza, G.A.; Taylor, B.A.; Thompson, P.D.; White, C.M.; Pescatello, L.S. Physical activity intensity and subjective well-being in healthy adults. *J. Health Psychol.* **2017**, *24*, 1257–1267. [CrossRef]
54. Wang, J.-C.; Yan, W. A Research on Relative Income Level and Urban Residents' Sense of Gain. *J. Cent. Univ. Financ. Econ.* **2019**, *10*, 119–128.
55. Bracke, P.; Pattyn, E.; von dem Knesebeck, O. Overeducation and depressive symptoms: Diminishing mental health returns to education. *Sociol. Health Illn.* **2013**, *35*, 1242–1259. [CrossRef]
56. Bracke, P.; van de Straat, V.; Missinne, S. Education, Mental Health, and Education–Labor Market Misfit. *J. Health Soc. Behav.* **2014**, *55*, 442–459. [CrossRef]
57. Shi, Z.-L.; Yang, Y.-Z. Are People with Higher Education More Likely to Get Depression? The effect of education on adults' depressive symptoms. *J. Beijing Norm. Univ. (Soc. Sci.)* **2020**, *2*, 148–160.
58. Pedišić, Ž.; Greblo, Z.; Phongsavan, P.; Milton, K.; Bauman, A.E. Are Total, Intensity- and Domain-Specific Physical Activity Levels Associated with Life Satisfaction among University Students? *PLoS ONE* **2015**, *10*, e0118137. [CrossRef] [PubMed]
59. Bowling, A. Associations with life satisfaction among very elderly people living in a deprived part of inner London. *Soc. Sci. Med.* **1990**, *31*, 1003–1011. [CrossRef] [PubMed]
60. LaFontaine, T.P.; DiLorenzo, T.M.; Frensch, P.A.; Stucky-Ropp, R.C.; Bargman, E.P.; McDonald, D.G. Aerobic Exercise and Mood. *Sports Med.* **1992**, *13*, 160–170. [CrossRef]
61. Petruzzello, S.J.; Landers, D.M.; Hatfield, B.D.; Kubitz, K.A.; Salazar, W. A Meta-Analysis on the Anxiety-Reducing Effects of Acute and Chronic Exercise. *Sports Med.* **1991**, *11*, 143–182. [CrossRef]
62. Wang, J.-W. Analysis of the impact of square dance on the physical and mental health of middle-aged and elderly people. *New West* **2013**, *12*. [CrossRef]

behavioral sciences

MDPI

Article

Clear Yet Crossed: Athletes' Retrospective Reports of Coach Violence

Sima Zach [1,*], Shlomit Guy [2], Rinat Ben-Yechezkel [1] and Liza Grosman-Rimon [1]

[1] Levinsky-Wingate Academic College, Wingate Institute, Tel Aviv 6937808, Israel; rinrin1973@gmail.com (R.B.-Y.); l.grosman.rimon@gmail.com (L.G.-R.)
[2] School of Physical Education, The Kaye College of Education, Beersheba 8414201, Israel; guyshlomit1@googlemail.com
* Correspondence: simaz@l-w.ac.il

Abstract: Aims: This study aimed at examining coach-athlete violence based on the retrospective reports of adults who had been athletes as children and adolescents; predict variables that contribute to the existence of such violence; describe difficulties that the participants encountered as young athletes following such violence; and reveal the outcomes of such violence on their emotions and behaviors, in the past and present. Methodology: The applied mixed methods comprised quantitative self-reporting questionnaires and qualitative interviews. The former included 440 participants (mean age 27.6) who had trained for at least one year in a sports union youth department; the latter included 14 participants (aged 23–37). These competitive athletes came from eight branches of sports. The interviews were analyzed based on the Narrative Approach. Results: According to the quantitative study, all participants had experienced coach violence at least once during their career, mainly psychological violence and neglect, followed by physical violence. Sexual violence was least reported. The age of their retirement from sports and the number of coaches that they had had were significant predictors of violence. Thematic analysis of the qualitative interviews resulted in six types of coach-athlete violence: (1) psychological violence; (2) verbal violence; (3) starvation and food fattening; (4) non-proportional punishing; (5) physical violence; and (6) sexual violence. Conclusions: It is vital that coach-athlete violence is addressed in public discourse, that the topic of young athletes' safety is introduced into coaching education, and that a position holder is nominated to be in charge of such safety in all sports organizations.

Keywords: coach-athlete violence; psychological violence; physical violence; verbal violence; starvation and food fattening; non-proportional punishing

1. Introduction

Physical activity is known to have a beneficial impact on people's physical and emotional health and wellbeing [1,2]. However, it can also have negative outcomes, such as physical injuries, especially in athletes who train at high levels and frequencies [3]. An additional yet much less researched negative impact of physical training relates to athletes who are subjected to maltreatment and even violence [4,5]. Such verbal or physical abuse may include a range of aggressive behaviors directed towards athletes by their peers, parents, coaches, and other professional staff members [6]. Moreover, interpersonal violence against young athletes has been associated with mental health problems and reduced quality of life in adulthood [7].

Not surprisingly, this phenomenon is often kept under wraps. For example, young athletes' eagerness to be on an elite team and to compete at international levels may overcome their desire to speak out about what they have endured; others may fear that they will either not be believed or that they will be discriminated against for reporting such behaviors. Over the years, little improvement can be seen in child protection within sports, despite attempts to increase public attention, create relevant policies, and enforce immediate implementation of such acts and guidelines [7]. Moreover, sports organizations may even perpetuate the abuse of young athletes by sweeping such occurrences under the rug, conducting slow and private investigations, silencing victims, persuading athletes not to submit a report, and more [8]. Despite its detrimental outcomes, this phenomenon is greatly under-studied [9].

The term violence refers to a large range of behaviors that may differ greatly from one another, for example, in why it emerges, how it is expressed, and what its outcomes are Matthews and Channon [10]. Many definitions have been given to this concept, referring to violence as an attack or use of force that results in physical or psychological damage to those who are attacked, for example Audi [11], or a violation of people's human rights or basic needs [12]. Matthews and Channon [10] distinguish between direct and indirect interpersonal violence, whereby the former relates to attempts to physically harm someone else's body, while the latter relates to attempts to harm someone else's property and assets. Such violence is intentional, intended, and expressive [13]. Direct violence can also be psychological rather than physical, causing severe emotional harm and distress [14]. In cases of physical violence, psychological harm is also inevitable. In 1991, Bourdieu [15] coined the term symbolic violence to describe a variety of situations in which people are excluded, treated in a derisive manner, or receive unequal treatment that leads to direct or indirect harm.

Studies on violence in sports tend to focus on a number of different themes, such as fan violence, that may occur before, during, and after sports events [16]; different types of violence in different types of sports [17]; and violence between rivals between and during competitions [18]. Yet one type of violence in sports that is much less addressed in the literature relates to violence exhibited towards athletes by coaches and other staff members, especially towards younger athletes [7]. One reason for this under-researched phenomenon is the difficulty to determine what is considered violent behavior in the coach-athlete relationship [19].

There is no dispute that coaches are required to help athletes achieve optimal performance. To do so, they must use a range of mental and physical methods, such as raising their voice or applying physical pressure. When used to a reasonable degree, such methods are perceived as legitimate and even necessary tools. For example, Jacobs et al. [20] found that coaches and team managers positively perceived a range of behaviors as an acceptable means for motivating and encouraging athletes—actions that may be perceived by others as less than desirable. A similar approach was seen in Stirling and Kerr [21], where one athlete who was interviewed said, "A tree is measured by its fruits, and if they reached their achievements in this way, there must be something right about it". In other words, even athletes themselves may perceive such abuse as a necessary part of their training. This was also seen in Gervis et al. [22], who found that young athletes were more accepting of coaches' violent behaviors towards children at high levels of sport. Yet, in contrast to this forgiving approach, other studies found that athletes reported emotional abuse that left them scarred even years after retiring. Kerr et al. [23], for example, interviewed eight female athletes from Canadian national sports teams of various disciplines, including Olympic athletes. In retrospect, the interviewees stated that the period in which they were athletes was the worst time of their lives. Even years after retiring, they still needed psychological therapy to help them deal with the emotional abuse that they had experienced.

A dearth of literature on coach violence in sports can be seen, with similarities and differences between countries and cultures. For example, when presenting athletes and coaches in the UK with a series of vignettes that depicted a coach's emotionally abusive behavior towards a 14-year-old athlete, Gervis, Rhind, and Luzar [22] found that perceived competitive levels and athletic performance were negatively associated with perceived abusive coach behaviors. In other words, the higher the perceived athletic performance, the lower the perceived abuse. Additionally, McDonald and Kawai [24] examined perceptions of punishing coach behaviors among students from ten universities in Japan; these researchers found that participants normalized acts of coach violence and accepted them as necessary forms of discipline, often even interpreting such acts as indicative of coach care and kindness.

In the USA, Zogg, et al. [25] explored interpersonal violence in sports and perceived coaching styles among more than 4000 college athletes. The researchers found that almost 10% of the respondents reported having experienced at least one type of interpersonal violence during their college sports careers, even in the weeks immediately leading up to the study. Participants who reported having been exposed to interpersonal violence also reported worse psycho-social outcomes, including increased burnout, an expressed desire to quit their sport, and even decreased emotional well-being, especially among participants who identified as female and with non-heterosexual orientations.

In Portugal, Marracho et al. [26] asked young athletes about their experience or exposure to undesirable coach behaviors. As victims, no participants reported having experienced mistreatment behaviors in their athlete-coach relationship; yet as observers, many reported having witness various forms of abuse, including verbal and emotional abuse, as well as a lack of attention and support. Finally, in Sweden, Johansson and Lundqvist [27] explored sexual harassment and abuse, as well as coach–athlete relationships. The participants included more than 450 current and former sports-club athletes, of whom 5.5% reported some form of sexual harassment and abuse by their coach—mainly inappropriate, unpleasant, or offensive physical contact. No differences in coach harassment and abuse were seen between genders, sport performance levels, or individual/team sports. Moreover, 13–39% of the participants reported having experienced dependency, substantial coach influence over their personal-life, non-instructional physical contact, sexualized comments and jokes, and flirting. Such findings from different countries and regions suggest that coach behaviors and coach-athlete relationships are culturally rooted and may require major reconsideration of the role of sports in education. Comparative studies between countries could be especially beneficial in future research to further understand the culturally rooted issue of coach abuse.

Despite the relatively small degree of sports violence that has been reported [9], these can be categorized by a number of themes, such as research goals, gender differences, or types of violence. Psychological violence may include the restricting of movements, belittling, scapegoating, threatening, intimidating, discriminating, or ridiculing [28]; verbal violence may include profanities and humiliation [29–31], starvation or fattening [32–34], non-proportional punishing [30], and bullying, ignoring, or even expelling [35]; physical violence may include kicking, hitting, and beatings [9]; and finally, sexual violence may also occur against young athletes [36].

A human rights report that was recently published in Japan revealed vast violence by coaches towards athletes [37]. In Canada, this issue was placed on the public agenda following a series of revelations about the abuse of athletes between 1994 and 2005 (e.g., [23,37]). Recent years have seen an increase in awareness of the scope of the problem and its consequences [38]. In turn, increased efforts can be seen to gather global data as a means for equipping all parties involved in children and youth sports with relevant knowledge [5,39]. Moreover, acquiring such important data could enable the defining of rules, regulations, and codes of conduct, as well as the setting of ethical standards as a means for ensuring the physical and mental health and wellbeing of athletes.

Initially, the agenda for child protection in sports was driven by sexual abuse scandals [40], yet today it also addresses physical violence, psychological abuse, and even verbal hostility. While in the 1990s, few sports organizations acknowledged or addressed child abuse and protection (mainly in the UK, Canada, and Australia), an increase has been seen over the past decades in the international interest in this issue [40]; moreover, greater attempts have been made to describe the scope, characteristics, nature, and implications of this undesirable and harmful phenomenon [21].

In line with this literature review, this study presents four research objectives. First, based on the quantitative methodology approach, adults (aged 18+ years) who had been athletes as children and adolescents were asked to retrospectively report the types and frequencies of violence to which they were subjected by their coaches. Following their input, the research then attempted to differentiate between types of violence by their reported frequencies, while predicting which variables contribute to their perceived explanations for such violence. Next, based on the qualitative methodology approach, participants were asked to verbally describe the types of violence and difficulties that they had experienced as young athletes when faced with violence by their coaches. Following their input, the research then attempted to reveal how athletes perceive the consequences of such violence on their emotions, behaviors, and decisions, as both adolescents and as young adults.

2. Materials and Methods

The current study uses a Mixed Methods Phenomenological Research (MMPR) approach, specifically an exploratory sequential design. This means it starts with quantitative and continues with qualitative data to make the quantitative assessment more precise [41]. The reason for using MMPR is that phenomenological and quantitative methods can work well together under one main framework. Even though they have different beliefs about reality and knowledge, they share similar values and methods that make combining them possible [42].

Phenomenology, often considered a human science approach, shares scientific nature with deductive approaches, justifying the adoption of an MMPR approach. The flexibility of phenomenological methods, rooted in understanding subjective experiences, complements the strengths of quantitative methods. By incorporating multiple methods within a single study, researchers can enhance validity, minimize bias, and capitalize on the strengths of each method. The integration of quantitative methods can provide orientation, identify relevant phenomena, and test theories developed through phenomenological inquiry. Overall, the philosophical rationale for MMPR is grounded in the idea that combining phenomenological and quantitative methods under a single paradigm can yield a comprehensive and nuanced understanding of research phenomena [43]. Each section is presented separately in the paper.

2.1. Part 1—Quantitative Design

2.1.1. Participants

The study included 440 participants (173 (39%) females), aged 27.6 (SD $\pm$ 8.48), who had trained for at least one full year in the youth department of a sports union in Israel. The participants' average number of training years was 11.47 (SD $\pm$ 5.91) and their average age of retirement was 20.66 years (SD $\pm$ 7.61). They had an average of 5.3 coaches throughout their athletic career before the age of 18 (SD $\pm$ 4.37). Of the 440 participants, 164 had competed on an international level, 197 on a national level, and 64 on a country regional level, while 15 had not been competitive athletes. Among them, 204 (46.5%) had taken part in individual sports and 235 (53.5%) had taken part in team sports, as follows: 255 (60%) participated in ball games, 45 (10.6%) in martial arts, 56 (13.2%) in aquatic sports, 32 (7.5%) in track and field, and 37 (8.5%) in movement and dance. Finally, while most participants (302) had specialized in only one field of sport, 138 of the respondents had participated in more than one sport. Finally, 201 participants (46.1%) reported that their current field of occupation is related to sport, while 116 (26.6%) reported that it is not. The remaining 119 (27.3%) participants were still students at the time of the study, and as such did not yet have a clear field of occupation.

2.1.2. Questionnaire

The aim of the questionnaire was to discover general trends of violence against boys and girls in child and youth sports departments. The questionnaire was developed and validated by Parent et al. [44]. In Parent et al. [44], exploratory structural equation modeling (ESEM) was used to identify latent factors that underly the various versions of the VTAQ. Their results showed that the VTAQ-Athlete includes nine items with three factors: psychological, physical, and sexual; The VTAQ-Coach includes 36 items with three factors: psychological/neglect, physical, and sexual, and the VTAQ-Parent includes 25 items with two factors: psychological/neglect and physical. We have translated it from French to Hebrew and back to French, using the back-translation approach (e.g., [45,46]).

While the original questionnaire included three sections (violence by friends, by coaches, and by parents), the current study only utilized the section on violence against athletes by their coaches. The questionnaire included 34 items that the participants were asked to rate on a Likert-like scale from 1 (never) to 4 (Very often more than 10 times), such as "Did the coach shake, push, grab, or throw you?" or "Did the coach throw an object at you?".

2.1.3. Procedure

The study was approved by the Institutional Review Board at the authors' affiliated academic institution Kaye College for Education. To recruit participants, the questionnaire was sent to all sport unions and federations across Israel via e-mail, asking them to kindly forward it to their past and current athletes who are currently aged 18+ years. The same request was also sent to the Israeli Olympic Committee. In addition, the snowball method was applied via the authors' personal social media pages.

The interviews, which were conducted via the Zoom platform, lasted 50–120 min and, with the participants' approval, were recorded and transcribed. Upon completing the online questionnaire, the interviewees had stated that they would be willing to further discuss the issue of coach violence with the researchers. Our contact details (names, telephone numbers, and e-mail addresses) were included on the form. As with the questionnaire, complete confidentiality was ensured to all interviewees.

Analysis of the qualitative data was conducted by the first two authors and then reviewed by the additional two authors. The achieved input was analyzed and coded according to anticipated potential categories, based on the theoretical framework of the study, namely the types of violence. In other words, the data from the interviews underwent stages of categorization, including the describing, comparing, and relating of data to existing knowledge, as suggested by Attride-Stirling [47] and Bazeley [48]. Finally, trustworthiness was established using investigator triangulation [49], i.e., the participation of multiple researchers in the data interpretation process [50], as a means for enhancing clarification and accuracy.

For legal purposes, we chose to only include athletes over the age of 18; had we been exposed to violence against younger athletes, we would have had to report this to the police, according to the Child Protection Law that was enacted in Israel in 1995, and as such, would not have been able to maintain complete confidentiality for the respondents.

2.1.4. Statistical Analysis

All data were analyzed using the SPSS software, version 18.0 (SPSS Inc., Chicago, IL, USA). Continuous variables are presented as mean $\pm$ SD, while categorical variables are presented as frequencies and percentages. Linear univariable analyses were performed to identify possible socio-demographic factors that are associated with coach violence scores. Multivariable linear regressions were performed forcing all covariates (socio-psychological and demographic variables) with a statistical significance of <0.175 into the model. Backward variable elimination was used to develop the regression model. Variables with a significance level of <0.1 were retained in the final model. The questions in the Violence Toward Athletes Questionnaire—VTAQ were divided into the following three categories: Psychological violence, physical violence, and sexual violence. The percentage of the scores for each category was calculated by dividing the reported score by the maximal score for the categories and then multiplying this number by 100. One-way analysis was performed to compare psychological, physical, and sexual violence with Bonferroni corrections. A p-value of <0.05 was considered significant.

2.2. Part 2—Qualitative Design

2.2.1. Participants

This part of the research included 14 adults (9 females and 5 males), aged 23–37. They had all been competitive athletes for 10–15 years from the following branches of sports: surfing (1), gymnastics (2), judo (1), swimming (3), soccer (2), basketball (2), team handball (1), and tennis (2). While two had reached international competition levels, all others had stayed at the regional or national levels.

2.2.2. Procedure

The interviews were conducted via Zoom and lasted 48–120 min. These interviews were initiated by the participants, who, after completing the questionnaire described above, had stated that they would be willing to further discuss the issue of coach violence with the researchers. Our contact details (names, telephone numbers, and e-mail addresses) were included. As with the questionnaire, complete confidentiality was ensured to all interviewees. A narrative approach [51] was applied by listening to the participants to as great an extent as possible while asking very few questions. The initial question of each interview was always: Tell me your story.

2.2.3. Data Analysis and Trustworthiness

With the participants' permission, the interviews were recorded and transcribed. Data analysis was then performed by the two first authors of this article and reviewed by the additional two authors. The input achieved was analyzed and coded according to anticipated potential categories based on the theoretical framework of the study, namely types of violence. The choice of three classifications suited the nature of the material, as reflected through the participants' verbal expressions that were uttered during their interviews [52]. In other words, the data received from the athletes' interviews underwent phases of categorization that included the describing, comparing, and relating of the data to existing knowledge, as suggested by Attride-Stirling [49] and Bazeley [48]. Finally, trustworthiness was established using investigator triangulation [49], i.e., the use of multiple researchers in interpreting the data [50] for clarification and accuracy.

3. Results

3.1. Part 1—Quantitative Design

The purpose of the qualitative section of the study was to examine how adults retrospectively perceive the extent of coach violence towards them as child or adolescent athletes. Table 1 presents the distribution of the questionnaire answers.

All participants experienced violence from their coach at least once during their career. Regarding physical violence, about 15% of the participants reported that their coach had shaken, pushed, or grabbed them; 12% reported that their coach had directly thrown an object at them; and 22% reported that they had been hit by an object that was not aimed directly towards them. In addition, about 28% reported that the coach had forced them or asked them to do extra high-intensity and excessive training until they were physically exhausted; 23% reported that they had been forced or asked to exercise while injured, despite having a medical opinion to the contrary; about 20% reported that they were forced or asked to perform movements or technical actions that were too difficult in relation to their abilities (physical or psychological) that could have or that actually had negative consequences on their health and safety. Psychological violence was more prevalent, with approximately 30% reporting that they had been yelled at, insulted, humiliated, and mocked; about half reported that they had been excessively criticized, expelled or suspended, ignored, or treated with indifference. Reports concerning sexual violence, however, were negligible.

Table 1. Distribution of the Questionnaire Answers in Percentages (n = 440).

	Items	1 Never	2 Rarely (1–2 Times)	3 Some-Times (3–10 Times)	4 Very Often (>10 Times)
1	Shook, pushed, grabbed, or threw you	84.5	11.2	2.3	2
2	Threw an object directly at you	88.2	8.1	3.0	0.7
3	Hit you with the hand (for example, slaps)	92.0	4.1	3.0	0.9
4	Punched or kicked you	97.0	1.1	1.6	0.3
5	Hit you with an object (for example, sports equipment)	91.1	6.9	1.1	0.9
6	Tried to strangle you	98.0	0.4	1.4	0.2
7	Hit or threw objects that were not aimed directly at you (e.g., water bottles, pens)	78.0	12.0	8.0	2.0
8	Forced you/instructed you to injure an opposing player	90.5	6.4	2.0	1.1
9	Forced you/instructed you to humiliate or mock an opponent	92.0	6.1	1.4	0.5
10	Forced you/instructed you to threaten or hurt an opponent	92.0	5.0	2.3	0.7
11	Allowed you to injure an opposing player (with a punch, sports equipment, etc.) in a competition, without intervening	93.6	5.2	1.2	/
12	Allowed you to humiliate or mock an opponent in a competition, without interfering	90.7	6.1	2.3	0.9
13	Allowed you to threaten or hurt an opponent in a competition without intervening	91.8	4.5	3.0	0.7
14	Threatened to leave/abandon you	88.9	5.5	4.3	1.3
15	Threatened to harm you	91.4	3.6	4.3	0.7
16	Threatened to harm someone or something you love	95.2	3.4	1.4	/
17	Yelled at you and insulted you, humiliated you, and mocked you	59.5	23.0	11.4	6.1
18	Criticized you excessively (e.g., about your performance or your attitude)	50.2	23.6	18.9	7.3
19	Expelled or suspended you	72.5	20.9	4.6	2.0
20	Locked you in a closed room or tried to limit your freedom of movement (e.g., locking you in the locker room, tying you up)	97.7	1.1	1.1	/
21	Asked you to limit or reduce your social connections (with friends, romantic partners, or family member) to enable you to invest more of yourself in your sports	77.0	15.9	5.9	1.1
22	Ignored you or treated you with indifference (e.g., refused to talk to you, ignored your existence)	66.6	20.5	9.1	3.9
23	Forced you/instructed you to do extra high-intensity and excessive training until you were exhausted	72.5	15.2	8.9	3.4
24	Forced you/instructed you to exercise while injured despite having a medical opinion to the contrary	77.0	13.0	6.6	3.4
25	Forced you/instructed you to perform movements or technical actions that are more difficult than you are capable of (physically or psychologically) that had or could have had negative consequences on your health and safety	78.2	16.4	3.4	2.0
26	Asked you to use prohibited substances to reach the desired weight for the sport (fasting, vomiting, pills)	96.8	1.6	1.1	0.5
27	Asked you to use prohibited substances to improve performance (steroids, hormones)	97.1	1.1	0.2	/

Table 1. *Cont.*

	Items	1 Never	2 Rarely (1–2 Times)	3 Some-Times (3–10 Times)	4 Very Often (>10 Times)
28	Knew that you had used prohibited substances to reach the desired weight for the industry	98.2	0.5	1.1	0.2
29	Knew that you had used prohibited substances to improve performance	98.6	0.5	0.9	/
30	Asked you to stop going to school or suspend your studies in order to devote yourself to sports	88.2	7.7	2.0	2.0
31	Made rude, insulting comments that made you uncomfortable about your sex life, your private life, or your physical appearance (for example, comments about you or your partner's intimate body parts)	87.3	8.6	2.7	1.4
32	Behaved sexually in a way that made you feel uncomfortable (for example, rubbing you, staring at you, undressing you with their eyes, whistling at you, and massaging you)	88.2	8.4	1.7	1.7
33	Watched you or force you to perform a sexual act (touching yourself, themselves, or others)	94.3	3.9	1.4	0.5
34	Photographed you while you were having sexual activity (touching yourself, themselves, or others)	97.7	1.4	0.7	0.2

The ratio of the questionnaire's three types of violence were then calculated: psychological violence and neglect was most prevalent, followed by physical violence; sexual violence was the least reported factor (18.10 ± 4.22; 7.9 ± 2.02; 0.69 ± 0.17, respectively). One way ANOVA shows a significant difference between these three factors ($F_{(1,439)}$ = 8453.002, $p < 0.001$), as seen in Figure 1.

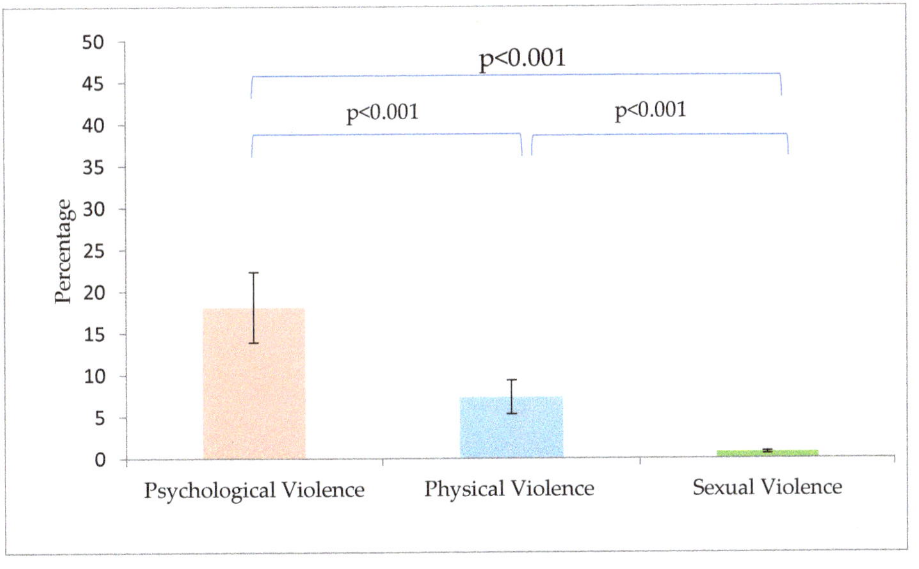

Figure 1. Differences Between the Questionnaire's Factor Scores.

When multivariable linear regressions were performed for all variables (age, gender, sport branch, individual/team sport, age of retirement from sports, number of training years, professional achievements, number of coaches, and place of residents), only two variables were significant predictors of violence: age of retirement and number of coaches, as seen in Table 2.

Table 2. Predictor of VTAQ Score Using Linear Regression Analysis.

Variable	Standardized β (CI)	t	p
Age	−0.05 (−0.15–0.04)	−1.08	0.27
Gender	0.08 (−0.25–3.22)	1.67	0.94
Sport type	−0.13 (−0.75–0.56)	−0.27	0.78
Individual/team	0.23 (−1.30–2.16)	0.48	0.62
Age of retirement	0.12 (0.01–0.257)	2.15	0.032 *
Retirement: yes/no	−0.06 (−2.97–0.59)	−1.30	0.19
Achievements	−0.01 (−1.16–0.92)	−0.22	0.81
Years of practice	0.09 (−0.003–0.29)	1.926	0.055
Number of coaches	0.14 (0.108–0.496)	3.056	0.002 *
Occupation	0.031 (−0.787–1.575)	0.655	0.513
Residence	−0.012(−1.717–1.342)	−0.241	0.810
Zone	0.029 (−0.386–0.716)	0.0589	0.0556

* = $p < 0.5$.

3.2. Part 2—Qualitative Design

After assessing the frequency of violent occurrences in the first part of the study, we were interested in understanding the types of violence and difficulties experienced by young athletes in greater detail. We also sought to reveal what they felt, how they coped, and how they perceive the consequences of such violence on their emotions, behaviors, and decisions in retrospect as today's adults.

The thematic analysis that we conducted led to the emergence of six forms of coach-athlete violence. These themes are presented in the following sections together with quotes that support and expand on each of these themes: (1) psychological violence; (2) verbal violence; (3) starvation and food fattening; (4) non-proportional punishing; (5) physical violence; and (6) sexual violence. In addition to quotes that depict the violence to which the participants were subjected as young athletes, we have also added quotes that present the consequences of such violence as perceived by the participants today.

3.2.1. Theme 1: Psychological Violence

This theme included restriction of movement, patterns of belittling, denigrating, scapegoating, threatening, scaring, discriminating, ridiculing, and other nonphysical forms of hostile treatment, such as rejection, expulsion, ignoring, bullying, or hazing. The following citations indicate psychological violence.

There were things that today as a grownup, I cannot comprehend how they were allowed to exist at all. For example, once I forgot to bring my bathing suit to practice. So she [the coach] said to me, 'Okay, then swim in your underwear'. A 12-year old girl in a pool filled with people, open to the public. It doesn't make sense to swim in your underwear, not even as a six-year-old girl. She said this in anger, 'Swim in your underwear!'. There was no other option. She said, 'Swim in your underwear or go home'. So I swam in my underwear.

> But he would scream at me, terrorize me, swear at me. Later, there was a very, very strong issue of control. Who I could go out with, what I was allowed to say. It was like the 'thoughts and feelings police'. If you lost a competition but didn't really seem miserable—in his opinion—then he thought something was wrong with you. You should be sad because you lost and vice versa. If you wear certain clothes then it's not appropriate, because it attracts too much attention. He brought me into sports at the age of eight, and we finished at the age of 30. We went through three Olympic Games, crises, and breakups. She ignored me every

> time I said something that didn't meet her expectations. She actually expected us to be silent. She could ignore me for a whole week, like a punishment... So I learned to always keep my mouth shut. (Nurit)

> He would scream so much, until he lost his voice, just because he was mad at something that we had done wrong. (Shir)

> When we traveled, he kept my money. He would decide whether to give it to me or not. He used to threaten me and sometimes he even acted on his threats, and we couldn't buy anything with our own money. In addition to expressing psychological violence, the interviewees spoke of how they coped with such violence, as seen in the following quotes. (Ori)

> As a result, I lost my faith in her [the coach]. Training wasn't fun anymore. But I kept on trying not to disappoint my parents. I retired with the feeling that I had dedicated my life to sports but had nothing to show for it... This was very difficult for me to let go of. I think you can see this even now as I talk about it, I'm still very emotional. I couldn't talk about it for about a year. I wasn't ready to talk about sports at all, at all... I also had issues with food, that was a very difficult relationship, I wanted to inhale everything without stopping to breathe. My parents started to worry about me. They would say, 'You're eating like a truck'... I simply replied that now that my coach isn't there anymore, nobody can tell me what or what not to eat. I gained a lot of weight, and I was very upset that I had gained weight but then I didn't know how to lose it. I was afraid of being hungry... I retired with the feeling that I was nobody, that I was a loser, that I wasn't successful. I felt that I didn't know who I was because I hadn't succeeded. These feelings were with me all the time. Until I slowly started to recover and tried to escape from such associations as much as possible, from such people. The truth is that at first, I constantly needed feedback. Every time I did something, I needed someone to tell me if it's okay or not. I had lost my self-esteem... There was no me. There was only a robot. I had to rebuild myself, and that was very, very difficult. (Tamar)

3.2.2. Theme 2: Verbal Violence

This category of psychological violence included cursing and humiliation, as seen in the following citations.

> Screaming like crazy at a young girl for minutes on end because she made a mistake?! That's overreacting, right? And you would often hear crazy yelling. But you get used to it. You know you'll be screamed at. You just don't know when. (Tamar)

> The following citation shows the outcome of this violence:

> You say to yourself, it is what it is, there's nothing I can do about it. Is there any other way to be on the national team and achieve your dreams? What can you do? He's the coach. If you don't want to [put up with it], you can stop. But if you want to move forward and make your dreams come true, then this is the only way. (Shir)

> He knows how he behaves. It's not a secret. Everyone knows it, everyone knows that he loses control and shouts and goes on a rampage and does illogical things... But it's all part of the sport. He's the coach. He wants you to succeed, he pushes you. So where's the line? It's really problematic. (Nave)

> When I was 14, he would always laugh at me because of how I looked. He would tell me not to eat and that if I did eat, I should only eat salad. I was larger than my teammates. He used to call me: a pig, ball, fat, big butt. I couldn't stand it. I felt humiliated. It was really unpleasant for me, I dedicated my life to swimming. And I really tried to improve, I came to all the training sessions, I never caused

any problems. I always did as I was told. I even started running as well, and ate much less, but didn't lose any weight. I was hungry all the time. Eventually I dropped out of the swimming team. (Noga)

She would humiliate me by imitating me crying. She was disrespectful towards my parents. She humiliated me in front of all the younger girls. But I did nothing. I just took it and took it. I didn't enjoy the training sessions anymore. Once when a substitute coach arrived, I enjoyed myself so much that I suddenly remembered why I love gymnastics so much. (Tamar)

Whenever we saw him walking angrily down the corridor, no one wanted to even get close to him. No one wanted to accidentally see him. Think of how many hours, days, and weeks we spent with him... and when the atmosphere is so aggressive, you start to feel ill. You carried the fear with you.

He insisted that our lives be devoted to sports. No family distractions, no boyfriends, no work, no school. We had to be sport nuns... (Yael)

3.2.3. Theme 3: Starvation and Food Fattening

This theme included weight cycling practices and rapid weight loss, as seen in the following quotes.

She would weigh me four times a day. Before training, after the first training, before the second training, and after the second training. Every single time. One day, the goal was to reach 48 Kg. But if I had reached 48, she would have demanded that I reach 47. It would never end. One day, I weighed 50 kg I think at the beginning of training, so I was supposed to weigh 47 by the end. You have to understand how thin I was... But she just said: 'You don't start training until you're 47 kg, I don't care how, do whatever you want, hang me, take pills, throw up. I don't care what you do, you're not starting until you're 47 kg. I'm lucky I don't like to throw up. I said OK. She told me to start running, even though I have stress fractures. I started running, I ran for like an hour. I lost one kilo. Then I only drank water. No food. Just water. But I couldn't keep running anymore. I was on a treadmill so I started walking. I said to myself, at least I'll walk, I can't run. It wasn't like I was running with a T-shirt and leggings. You need to understand how I was dressed. I was wearing long pants, a short-sleeved shirt, a long-sleeved shirt, a lined jacket, and a coat when she came to check on me. But when she saw that I was walking and not running, she started screaming and swearing at me, like she had completely lost control. She shouted at me to start jumping next to her with the jump rope. So for the next two-and-a-half hours, I jumped rope next to her. I was not allowed to stop!!! My legs were on fire. I couldn't feel them anymore. It hurt like crazy. After that, she told the personal trainer to take me to run in the sand dunes. It was like that almost every evening. He weighed me and I was 47.7 kg. He was so kind, he just said, 'Well, without your clothes your weight is OK'.

I swear I hadn't eaten, I wasn't allowed to drink. She wouldn't let me drink. She said it makes my muscles swell and makes me heavy.

Needed to see me sweat, huge amounts of sweat. So what did I do? I wouldn't drink all day and then I would come to the room at the end of training and drink 3 L. But then I would feel really heavy, I was gaining 2–3 kg just from the water I drank, and then the next morning, she would weigh me again and ask why I had eaten the night before. She would shout at me that I'm a liar, a thief. And I would try to tell her that I've only been drinking, not eating, and then she would scream even more, saying, 'But I told you not to drink!'. How was I supposed to exist if I couldn't drink during the day, couldn't drink at lunchtime, couldn't drink in the evening, couldn't drink at night...?

> At first, I tried really hard to do what she told me to do. She was my mentor, she knows what's right... I really did what she told me, but it was just impossible to function like that. Absolutely impossible. At breakfast, she would give me one cucumber and an egg. Sometimes I had lunch, sometimes not, depending on my weight. If I was given lunch, it was a salad or even just an apple, and then in the evening... vegetables and maybe some yogurt. I was always hungry. I would think about food all the time, even while training. (Noa)

The following quotes exemplify the consequences of such violence:

> For years I suffered from eating disorders and from a distorted body image.
>
> I gained weight and then had no clue how to lose it... (Noa)

3.2.4. Theme 4: Non-Proportional Punishing

One of the themes that emerged from the qualitative study was non-proportional punishing, as seen in the following quotes.

> My friend was fooling around before the game. The coach got angry and threw him off the field. I begged him to punish him after the game. He was our leading player. But he just screamed at me too and told me to get off the field. I didn't play that day. I had been preparing for this game for months, my parents had come especially to see me play. I sat outside feeling very humiliated. (Ofek)

> In general, it's humiliating when you're a mature person and you're being yelled at in front of other people, in front of the other competitors. There were loads of comments all the time. Even about other teammates. Like the pants that she was wearing that had to many frills. He [the coach] thought they were attracting too much attention, so he said to her, 'If you want attention, win some medals. But don't wear those pants anymore'. Then one day she wore them on purpose, and he just dropped her off in the middle of nowhere while we were on the way to the airport in Berlin! She had to make her own way to the airport! (Ofek)

In response to such non-proportional punishing, two interviewees expressed the following outcomes:

> When I [later] became a coach myself, I knew how *not* to behave towards my young athletes. (Yam)

> At the time, we were very obedient. No one wanted to be punished or thrown off the team. We knew that we depended on him, and he was considered the best. (Gonen)

3.2.5. Theme 5: Physical Violence

This theme included kicking, punching, and beatings, as seen in the following quotes.

> I just didn't do the entrance of the choreography the way she wanted me to. So she gets up, tugs on my arm, and shouts, 'What did you do?!'. And then she steps on me. She knew I had a stress fracture... I'd had it for about two years, but she stood on me!... There were other little girls in the gymnasium... It was really unpleasant. Then suddenly something occurred to me, and I answered her! For the first time ever, I answered her. I was really angry and I said, 'Enough is enough!'. She was so shocked that I had even reacted. But then she looked at me and yelled, 'What did you say?!'. (Tamar)

> She took me by the hand just like that and then pushed me. She really shoved me and I fell. And then she started kicking me, and shouted, 'Get out of here!'. I was so humiliated, so, so humiliated. All the little girls were watching... I just got up, took my bag, and left.

> All the time I felt like I wasn't OK. No matter what I did. During training, the coach would swear at us, shout and humiliate us. He didn't care that I was

> in pain. For example, I had stress fractures in my legs. But he thought I was inventing my pain. He would say that I was making it up just so that I wouldn't have to make an effort. But he knew that I had a stress fracture in my leg. I told him that my leg was hurting. One day I really couldn't jump because of the pain. When I told him, he asked where the pain was. I thought he was asking because he cared. But he just started standing on my leg—really hard, again and again! He told me that I need to go beyond the pain. And I was really trying to overcome the pain and not think about it. (Ofek)

> You could have some kind of injury. A tear, a torn or stretched ligament, or something like that. You know it takes six weeks to heal, let's say, but if you have a competition or training camp coming up, then you go to compete or train even with your injury. Instead of letting it heal properly. Because you understand that if you don't, you'll be out of action for much longer than the six weeks. Because you've already missed some competitions that were the basis for further competitions. So you compete like this. (Nir)

> Once she got mad at me for being sick, I really didn't feel well. We were at a training camp and the pool was really cold, I was running a fever of 40. So she told me to get into the water to cool down. She said that I have to take part in the training. (Shahar)

In relation to physical coach-athlete violence, the following outcomes were also conveyed in the interviews:

> Unless you're dead or dying... even if you're really ill, you just stay quiet. Otherwise they'll say that you're whining. Even though it's better to miss one training session, rather than killing your body, but I'm like... I'm telling you, everyone around me, myself included, will come to train even if we're really ill. Everyone's afraid to say that they're not coming. (Ofek)

3.2.6. Theme 6: Sexual Violence

This theme included behavior of sever harassment, exploitation, and abuse as described by Fejgin and Hanegby [53].

> We were in the hot tub, like, after training we usually go into the hot tub, and he [the coach's son], held on to me and took his penis out. At first I thought it was his toe. I was an innocent 14-year-old. I didn't know what it was, I'd never seen anything like it in my life. When I eventually realized what it was, I froze, I froze in my place. I couldn't do anything, I just froze... One of the other girls said that he used to touch her, and suddenly all the girls were sitting down with us, talking about it. He'd done that to many of the girls. It was very comforting to know that we weren't alone. But we didn't do anything about it. Nothing. (Noga)

> From time to time he would touch me, more and more. It got steadily worse. It started with him touching my genitals. Then he would ask me to play something that requires concentration, and I would be really concentrating on the game with the remote control. And he would start to touch me. Then he would pull me on top of him. At first he was fully clothed, but then very gradually, very gently, he would take his pants off. He would also put cream on. The last time it happened, he took me to his room... and lay me on the bed, and started rubbing himself against me. He almost penetrated... I have a picture in my head of some I of mirror on the wall, and I can see myself crying... (Nave)

For this sixth and final theme, interviewees also spoke of the outcome of their being subjected to sexual abuse, as seen in the following quotes.

> I didn't talk to anyone [about it]. I was so ashamed. I was even ashamed to tell my parents. I was really ashamed, because somehow, I felt like I was guilty. Why?

> I felt that I was guilty, like, why had I gone into the jacuzzi alone with him? Or what did I expect wearing a bathing suit? (Yonit)

> When I talked to my teammates about it, everyone thought he had a kind of deviant profile. You know, like if someone brings something up, then everyone immediately says his name or remembers how he used to behave. They all remember this. If he had been a responsible adult, this wouldn't have happened. It wasn't really a secret though. So it should have turned on a warning light for other people in the pool. This stuff went on for about a year. (Shir)

> We always have this talk, my friends and I, about the babysitter who looks after my kids. I never let my husband take her home, I always take her home myself. Not because I think my husband will do something to her, but because I don't want there to be a situation where she may not feel comfortable, or that she might say something that happened or didn't happen. My friends and I always talk about where the line should be drawn. (Nurit)

> When you send a child to a class, you know a certain person or you think you know a certain person. But then it's someone completely different at the core. That's how it was with my coach... Today I have serious trust issues and it's clear to me that it's based on something from there. I do work on these things, but my first instinct is not to trust the person, not to believe the person who is standing in front of me... (Ori)

> I felt that I was like... I was very careful to hide everything... but I felt that... When I was there, it seemed funny and I laughed about it. But then at home, I would sit and think about these things, about how to get out of this situation... I felt like I was living a sort of double life with some kind of mask that I put on in the morning and only took off at night... There were many things that never even crossed my mind as being problematic until after I stopped training. Even then I repressed many things and I am only able to see today. I might suddenly remember a certain situation... It's really difficult for me. (Yam)

> I don't remember getting out of the car [after training]... I just remember how I would feel five seconds later, because I would just sit on the steps at the entrance to my house and cry. Eventually I would collect myself, wipe away the tears, and go into the house as if nothing had happened. Then I would take a shower, and I remember scrubbing my body really hard. I felt like I really needed to clean myself. Even later, when I started dealing with these things as a more mature person, I would scrub my skin until it hurt whenever I was in a difficult situation. (Noga)

> I was afraid to talk about it. I was afraid, I didn't know... like if I look back on it today, I don't know if I was afraid of my parents' reaction, or if I was afraid for my place, or if I was afraid that he would deny everything and I would look like a liar... I don't know what I was thinking, why I didn't contact anyone, but I really remember trying to get my family to ask me what had happened or how I felt.

4. Discussion

4.1. Part 1—Quantitative Design

The aim of the quantitative section of this study was to examine the types and frequencies of violence experienced by young athletes by their coaches, as reported retrospectively by adult athletes (18 years+), to differentiate between types of violence by their reported frequencies, and to predict which variables contribute to their perceived explanations of coach violence towards young athletes. Unlike previous reports (e.g., [23,37,38]), our findings show a relatively low frequency of violence in all three factors (psychological violence, physical violence, and sexual violence).

Specifically, sexual violence was rarely reported in this study. There may be several possible explanations for these results. First, in Israel, there are laws for preventing sexual harassment [54,55]. All places of occupation in Israel are obliged to nominate a specific person who is in charge of sexual harassment in the workplace. Sexual violence is treated as a criminal act and handled by the police. Hence, public awareness towards sexual harassment has significantly increased over the past two decades. On the other hand, the underreporting of sexual harassment is a known phenomenon [55] that might have occurred in this study. With regards to physical violence, the majority of the participants reported having never experienced any of the physical behaviors that were measured in this study. Nevertheless, a "relatively" low percentage of participants did report having experienced physical violence. The question that every coach, parent, and adult that works or lives with children and youth should ask themselves is, what is "relatively"? Is it acceptable that 20% or 15% of young athletes experience physical violence by their coaches? Should we be concerned if "only" 10% experience physical violence, or should we emphasize that 90% do not?

As for psychological violence and neglect, the results are not encouraging. It seems that almost all participants experienced psychological violence to some extent. The variety of offensive/insulting/harmful/humiliating behaviors that coaches use towards their athletes is also troublesome, as athletes spend hours, days, months, and sometimes even years in the company of their coaches [56,57]. The participants expressed having experienced endless negative emotions, such as frustration, fatigue, lack of motivation, boredom, shame, and anxiety—feelings that were probably heightened by the psychological violence that they experienced. The findings of this study should ring a warning bell for all parties involved in the education and sports training of children and adolescents.

Lastly, the regression analysis that we conducted revealed that the number of coaches and the age of retirement are the only variables that predict the athletes' having experienced violence by their coaches. In other words, the older they were when retiring from their sports, the more likely they were to experience such violence. This could be explained by the parents' decreased involvement as the age of the child increases. In other words, as children age, they become less dependent on their parents. Hence the role of peers and coaches may become more prominent, as does the training environment climate [58,59]. In addition, as young athletes age, they become more competitive and the odds of their experiencing violence increase [60,61].

These findings and interpretations are important and add to the field of literature on coach violence towards athletes. Yet several limitations should be considered. First, the input received from the interviewees was based on retrospective self-reporting that is highly dependent on memories, which tend to fluctuate over time. Nevertheless, a similar method has been used in previous studies (e.g., [21]). Second, the sample in this study was not random but rather one of convenience. Yet this limitation is overcome by the relatively large sample size that presents a variety of voices.

Following this quantitative section of the study, a qualitative research design was also applied to uncover the subjective meanings and long-term effects of the violence to which the participants were exposed as young athletes.

4.2. Part 2—Qualitative Design

By analyzing the interviews conducted in this study, we were able to address our research objectives. First, we identified six forms of coaches' violent behaviors towards athletes, in line with previous studies: (1) psychological violence [28]; (2) verbal violence [29,30]; (3) starvation [33,34]; (4) non-proportional punishing [30]; (5) physical violence [9]; and (6) sexual violence [36]. Adding important information to the literature, the study presents each form of coach-athlete violence together with detailed examples and related outcomes. These reports were provided by adults who found it difficult to recall what they had been through and put their experiences into words. Even years later, some participants were afraid to be exposed through their stories.

Stirling and Kerr [21] claimed that violence affects the psychological wellbeing, training, and performance of athletes, and as such, they may exhibit frequent mood swings, anger, low self-efficacy, low self-esteem, anxiety, and even lack of a sense of accomplishment. They may also exhibit decreased motivation, reduced enjoyment during training, impaired focus, and difficulty in acquiring skills. Some athletes spoke of friends who had retired early from sports since they could not cope with their coach's violent behavior towards them. Finally, such abuse may lead to decreased levels of performance and inability to reach their athletic potential. Indeed, during our interviews, violence was described as having a far-reaching effect, beyond the scope and time of their actual career.

While some athletes stated that their coaches' constant yelling at them actually spurred them on, making them better athletes, they would not willingly go through such abuse again. Our results strengthen those of Kavanagh et al. [62], who examined retrospective reports of retired elite athletes in England. As with this study, their participants also expressed the difficult experiences that they had undergone subject to coach-athlete abuse, as well as the coping strategies that they employed in order to persist and achieve their goals. The athletes spoke of different ways in which they dealt with isolated or ongoing incidents of abuse over the years, and how they dealt with the memories and consequences of this abuse following their retirement.

Despite the important contribution of the qualitative research presented in this article, several research limitations should be addressed concerning the qualitative study. First, as the interviews employed a retrospective study, memory-related shortcomings and emotional changes may have occurred over time—for better or for worse. However, such a methodology is greatly accepted in academic research [63]. Moreover, only 14 of the 440 participants agreed to talk about their experiences in an interview. While this may be a relatively small and non-representative sample, the stories that were conveyed by these interviewees are alarming enough to call for immediate practical implications and interventions.

5. Conclusions

When combining both parts of this study—the quantitative and the qualitative—the findings indicate that athlete-coach abuse is alive and kicking. As such, it is imperative to increase public awareness on this matter, introduce the topic of young athletes' safety into coaching education, and nominate position holders to be in charge of such safety within sports organizations. The novelty of this study's results is primarily expressed through exploration of the lingering and ongoing impact of coaches' violence and abuse against athletes. Furthermore, the employed methodology, which integrated both quantitative and qualitative research, enabled the participants to sound their voice and put a so-called face to the numbers. This research approach is relatively rare in studies on violence in sports. As such, the study's significance lies in its ability to humanize the individuals behind these incidents, particularly children.

Author Contributions: Conceptualization, S.Z. and S.G.; Methodology, S.Z., R.B.-Y. and L.G.-R.; Software, L.G.-R.; Validation, S.G.; Formal analysis, S.Z., S.G. and L.G.-R.; Data curation, S.Z., S.G. and R.B.-Y.; Writing—original draft, S.Z.; Writing—review and editing, S.Z. and S.G.; Visualization, L.G.-R. All authors have read and agreed to the published version of the manuscript.

Funding: This research received no external funding.

Institutional Review Board Statement: The Kaye College of Education approved the current study on 15 February 2021.

Informed Consent Statement: Informed consent was obtained from all subjects involved in the study.

Data Availability Statement: Data is unavailable due to privacy and ethical restrictions.

Conflicts of Interest: The authors declare no conflicts of interest.

References

1. Buecker, S.; Simacek, T.; Ingwersen, B.; Terwiel, S.; Simonsmeier, B.A. Physical activity and subjective well-being in healthy individuals: A meta-analytic review. *Health Psychol. Rev.* **2021**, *15*, 574–592. [CrossRef]
2. Giles, S.; Fletcher, D.; Arnold, R.; Ashfield, A.; Harrison, J. Measuring well-being in sport performers: Where are we now and how do we progress? *Sports Med.* **2020**, *50*, 1255–1270. [CrossRef]
3. Simpson, R.J.; Campbell, J.P.; Gleeson, M.; Krüger, K.; Nieman, D.C.; Pyne, D.B.; Turner, J.E.; Walsh, N.P. Can exercise affect immune function to increase susceptibility to infection? *Exerc. Immunol. Rev.* **2020**, *26*, 8–22.
4. Brackenridge, C.; Fasting, K.; Kirby, S.; Leahy, T. *Protecting Children from Violence in Sport; A Review from Industrialized Countries*; UNICEF Innocenti Research Centre: Firenze, Italy, 2010.
5. Mountjoy, M.; Brackenridge, C.; Arrington, M.; Blauwet, C.; Carska-Sheppard, A.; Fasting, K.; Kirby, S.; Leahy, T.; Marks, S.; Martin, K.; et al. International Olympic Committee consensus statement: Harassment and abuse (non-accidental violence) in sport. *Br. J. Sports Med.* **2016**, *50*, 1019–1029. [CrossRef]
6. Kerr, G.; Kidd, B.; Donnelly, P. One step forward, two steps back: The struggle for child protection in canadian sport. *Soc. Sci.* **2020**, *9*, 68. [CrossRef]
7. Vertommen, T.; Kampen, J.; Schipper-van Veldhoven, N.; Uzieblo, K.; Van Den Eede, F. Severe interpersonal violence against children in sport: Associated mental health problems and quality of life in adulthood. *Child Abus. Negl.* **2018**, *76*, 459–468. [CrossRef]
8. Nite, C.; Nauright, J. Examining institutional work that perpetuates abuse in sport organizations. *Sport Manag. Rev.* **2020**, *23*, 117–129. [CrossRef]
9. Parent, S.; Fortier, K. Prevalence of interpersonal violence against athletes in the sport context. *Curr. Opin. Psychol.* **2017**, *16*, 165–169. [CrossRef]
10. Matthews, C.R.; Channon, A. Understanding sports violence: Revisiting foundational explorations. *Sport Soc.* **2017**, *20*, 751–767. [CrossRef]
11. Audi, R. Intentionalistic explanations of action. *Metaphilosophy* **1971**, *2*, 241–250. [CrossRef]
12. Salmi, J. *Violence and Democratic Society*; Zed Books: London, UK, 1993.
13. Dunning, E. Violence and violence-control in long-term perspective: 'Testing' Elias in relation to war, genocide, crime, punishment and sport. In *Violence in Europe*; Springer: Berlin/Heidelberg, Germany, 2008; pp. 227–249.
14. Imbusch, P. The concept of violence. In *International Handbook of Violence Research*; Springer: Berlin/Heidelberg, Germany, 2003; pp. 13–39.
15. Bourdieu, P. *Language and Symbolic Power*; Harvard University Press: Cambridge, MA, USA, 1991.
16. Ostrowsky, M.K. Sports fans, alcohol use, and violent behavior: A sociological review. *Trauma Violence Abus.* **2018**, *19*, 406–419. [CrossRef] [PubMed]
17. Mutz, M. Athletic participation and the approval and use of violence: A comparison of adolescent males in different sports disciplines. *Eur. J. Sport Soc.* **2012**, *9*, 177–201. [CrossRef]
18. Spaaij, R.; Schaillée, H. Unsanctioned aggression and violence in amateur sport: A multidisciplinary synthesis. *Aggress. Violent Behav.* **2019**, *44*, 36–46. [CrossRef]
19. Guy, S.; Zach, S. The person who loves me the most is also the person who hurts me the most: Power relations between a single coach and an athlete from the athletes' point of view. *Spirit Sport (Ruach Ha'Sport)* **2023**, *9*, 83–110.
20. Jacobs, F.; Smits, F.; Knoppers, A. 'You don't realize what you see!': The institutional context of emotional abuse in elite youth sport. *Sport Soc.* **2017**, *20*, 126–143. [CrossRef]
21. Stirling, A.E.; Kerr, G. The perceived effects of elite athletes' experiences of emotional abuse in the coach-athlete relationship. *Int. J. Sport Exerc. Psychol.* **2013**, *11*, 87–100. [CrossRef]
22. Gervis, M.; Rhind, D.; Luzar, A. Perceptions of emotional abuse in the coach–athlete relationship in youth sport: The influence of competitive level and outcome. *Int. J. Sports Sci. Coach.* **2016**, *11*, 772–779. [CrossRef]
23. Kerr, G.; Willson, E.; Stirling, A. "It Was the Worst Time in My Life": The effects of emotionally abusive coaching on female Canadian national team athletes. *Women Sport Phys. Act. J.* **2020**, *28*, 81–89. [CrossRef]
24. McDonald, B.; Kawai, K. Punishing coaching: Bukatsudō and the normalisation of coach violence. *Jpn. Forum* **2017**, *29*, 196–217. [CrossRef]
25. Zogg, C.K.; Runquist, E.B., 3rd; Amick, M.; Gilmer, G.; Milroy, J.J.; Wyrick, D.L.; Grimm, K.; Tuakli-Wosornu, Y.A. Experiences of interpersonal violence in sport and perceived coaching style among college athletes. *JAMA Netw. Open* **2024**, *7*, e2350248. [CrossRef]
26. Marracho, P.; Coelho, E.M.R.T.D.C.; Pereira, A.; Nery, M. Mistreatment behaviours in the Athlete-coach relationship. *Retos* **2023**, *2023*, 790–7989. [CrossRef]
27. Johansson, S.; Lundqvist, C. Sexual harassment and abuse in coach–athlete relationships in Sweden. *Eur. J. Sport Soc.* **2017**, *14*, 117–137. [CrossRef]
28. WHO. *Report of the Consultation on Child Abuse Prevention (No. WHO/HSC/PVI/99.1)*; WHO: Geneva, Switzerland, 1999.
29. Elliott, S.; Drummond, M. The (limited) impact of sport policy on parental behaviour in youth sport: A qualitative inquiry in junior Australian football. *Int. J. Sport Policy Politics* **2015**, *7*, 519–530. [CrossRef]

30. LoGuercio, M. Exploring Lived Experience of Abusive Behavior among Youth Hockey Coaches. *J. Sports Phys. Educ. Stud.* **2022**, *2*, 1–12. [CrossRef]
31. Raakman, E.; Dorsch, K.; Rhind, D. The development of a typology of abusive coaching behaviours within youth sport. *Int. J. Sports Sci. Coach.* **2010**, *5*, 503–515. [CrossRef]
32. Atkinson, M. Masculinity on the menu: Body Slimming and self-starvation as physical culture. In *Challenging Myths of Masculinity*; Routledge: London, UK, 2016; pp. 81–102.
33. Miles-Chan, J.L.; Isacco, L. Weight cycling practices in sport: A risk factor for later obesity? *Obes. Rev.* **2021**, *22*, e13188. [CrossRef] [PubMed]
34. Pélissier, L.; Ennequin, G.; Bagot, S.; Pereira, B.; Lachèze, T.; Duclos, M.; Thivel, D.; Miles-Chan, J.; Isacco, L. Lightest weight-class athletes are at higher risk of weight regain: Results from the French-Rapid Weight Loss Questionnaire. *Physician Sportsmed.* **2022**, *51*, 144–152. [CrossRef] [PubMed]
35. Jeckell, A.S.; Copenhaver, E.A.; Diamond, A.B. Hazing and bullying in athletic culture. In *Mental Health in the Athlete*; Springer: Berlin/Heidelberg, Germany, 2020; pp. 165–179.
36. Gaedicke, S.; Schäfer, A.; Hoffmann, B.; Ohlert, J.; Allroggen, M.; Hartmann-Tews, I.; Rulofs, B. Sexual violence and the coach–athlete relationship: A scoping review from sport sociological and sport psychological perspectives. *Front. Sports Act. Living* **2021**, *3*, 643–707. [CrossRef]
37. Human Rights Watch. I Was Hit So Many Times, I Can't Count. 2020. Available online: https://www.hrw.org/report/2020/07/20/i-was-hitso-many-times-i-cant-count/abuse-child-athletes-japan (accessed on 18 August 2022).
38. Stoltenborgh, M.; Bakermans-Kranenburg, M.J.; Alink, L.R.A.; Ijzendoorn, M.H. The prevalence of child maltreatment across the globe: Review of a series of meta-analyses. *Child Abus. Rev.* **2015**, *24*, 37–50. [CrossRef]
39. Lang, M.; Hartill, M. *Safeguarding, Child Protection and Abuse in Sport: International Perspectives in Research, Policy and Practice*; Routledge: London, UK, 2014.
40. Brackenridge, C.H.; Rhind, D. Child protection in sport: Reflections on thirty years of science and activism. *Soc. Sci.* **2014**, *3*, 326–340. [CrossRef]
41. Creswell, J.W. *Qualitative Inquiry and Research Design: Choosing among Five Approaches*; Sage: Thousand Oaks, CA, USA, 2007.
42. Mayoh, J.; Onwuegbuzie, A.J. Toward a conceptualization of mixed methods phenomenological research. *J. Mix. Methods Res.* **2015**, *9*, 91–107. [CrossRef]
43. Onwuegbuzie, A.J.; Johnson, R.B.; Collins, K.M. Call for mixed analysis: A philosophical framework for combining qualitative and quantitative approaches. *Int. J. Mult. Res. Approaches* **2009**, *3*, 114–139. [CrossRef]
44. Parent, S.; Fortier, K.; Vaillancourt-Morel, M.P.; Lessard, G.; Goulet, C.; Demers, G.; Paradis, H.; Hartill, M. Development and initial factor validation of the Violence Toward Athletes Questionnaire (VTAQ) in a sample of young athletes. *Loisir et Société/Soc. Leis.* **2019**, *42*, 471–486. [CrossRef]
45. Brislin, R.W. Back-translation for cross-cultural research. *J. Cross-Cult. Psychol.* **1970**, *1*, 185–216. [CrossRef]
46. Klotz, A.C.; Swider, B.W.; Kwon, S.H. Back-translation practices in organizational research: Avoiding loss in translation. *J. Appl. Psychol.* **2023**, *108*, 699–727. [CrossRef] [PubMed]
47. Attride-Stirling, J. Thematic networks: An analytic tool for qualitative research. *Qual. Res.* **2001**, *1*, 385–405. [CrossRef]
48. Bazeley, P. Analysing qualitative data: More than 'identifying themes'. *Malays. J. Qual. Res.* **2009**, *2*, 6–22.
49. Anney, V.N. Ensuring the quality of the findings of qualitative research: Looking at trustworthiness criteria. *J. Emerg. Trends Educ. Res. Policy Stud.* **2014**, *5*, 272–281.
50. Cho, J.; Trent, A. Validity in qualitative research revisited. *Qual. Res.* **2006**, *6*, 319–340. [CrossRef]
51. Spector-Mersel, G. Narrative research: Time for a paradigm. *Narrat. Inq.* **2010**, *20*, 204–224. [CrossRef]
52. Charmaz, K. Premises, principles, and practices in qualitative research: Revisiting the foundations. *Qual. Health Res.* **2004**, *14*, 976–993. [CrossRef] [PubMed]
53. Fejgin, N.; Hanegby, R. Gender and cultural bias in perceptions of sexual harassment in sport. *Int. Rev. Sociol. Sport* **2001**, *36*, 459–478. [CrossRef]
54. The Law for Preventing Sexual Harassment. 1998. Available online: https://www.nevo.co.il/law_html/law00/72507.htm (accessed on 9 January 2023).
55. State Comptroller Report. (2018–2019). Applying the Law. Available online: https://www.mevaker.gov.il/sites/DigitalLibrary/Pages/Reports/3285-2.aspx?AspxAutoDetectCookieSupport=1 (accessed on 9 January 2023).
56. Ericsson, K.A.; Prietula, M.J.; Cokely, E.T. The making of an expert. *Harv. Bus. Rev.* **2007**, *85*, 114. [PubMed]
57. Hassmén, P.; King, G.; Hjälm, S.; Lundkvist, E.; Gustafsson, H. Burnout symptoms and recovery processes in eight elite soccer coaches over 10 years. *Int. J. Sports Sci. Coach.* **2019**, *14*, 431–443. [CrossRef]
58. Chu, T.L.; Zhang, T. The roles of coaches, peers, and parents in athletes' basic psychological needs: A mixed-studies review. *Int. J. Sports Sci. Coach.* **2019**, *14*, 569–588. [CrossRef]
59. Vazou, S.; Ntoumanis, N.; Duda, J.L. Predicting young athletes' motivational indices as a function of their perceptions of the coach-and peer-created climate. *Psychol. Sport Exerc.* **2006**, *7*, 215–233. [CrossRef]
60. Karagün, E. Self-confidence level in professional athletes; an examination of exposure to violence, branch and socio-demographic aspects. *J. Hum. Sci.* **2014**, *11*, 744–753.

61. Parent, S.; Vaillancourt-Morel, M.P. Magnitude and risk factors for interpersonal violence experienced by Canadian teenagers in the sport context. *J. Sport Soc. Issues* **2021**, *45*, 528–544. [CrossRef]
62. Kavanagh, E.; Brown, L.; Jones, I. Elite athletes' experience of coping with emotional abuse in the coach–athlete relationship. *J. Appl. Sport Psychol.* **2017**, *29*, 402–417. [CrossRef]
63. Dai, D.Y.; Li, X. Behind an Accelerated Scientific Research Career: Dynamic Interplay of Endogenous and Exogenous Forces in Talent Development. *Educ. Sci.* **2020**, *10*, 220. [CrossRef]

behavioral sciences

MDPI

Article

Impact of the COVID-19 Pandemic on the Scientific Production of Physical Education Researchers: A Five-Year Follow-Up Study

Sarah Jane Lemos de Melo [1], Vanderlei Porto Pinto [1], Emerson Sebastião [2], Érica de Moraes Santos Corrêa [3] and Gustavo Christofoletti [1,3,*]

1 Institute of Health, Federal University of Mato Grosso do Sul (UFMS), Campo Grande 79060-900, MS, Brazil; melosarahjane@gmail.com (S.J.L.d.M.); portovanderley@gmail.com (V.P.P.)
2 Department of Health and Kinesiology, University of Illinois Urbana-Champaign, Urbana, IL 61801, USA; esebast2@illinois.edu
3 School of Medicine, Federal University of Mato Grosso do Sul (UFMS), Campo Grande 79060-900, MS, Brazil; ericamscorrea@gmail.com
* Correspondence: g.christofoletti@ufms.br

Abstract: The COVID-19 pandemic caused significant changes in society's dynamics, particularly affecting the landscape of education. Research in several areas may have been affected during periods of social restrictions. This study analyzed the curricula of 558 researchers across 27 graduate programs in physical education in Brazil to investigate the potential impact of the COVID-19 pandemic on scientific publications. Researchers' production from 2018 to 2022 underwent a comprehensive analysis, considering the total number of publications, Qualis rank, and journal impact factor. Data were analyzed using chi-squared and Kruskal-Wallis tests. Significance was set at 5%. Overall, the analyzed researchers published a total of 17,932 manuscripts from 2018 to 2022. During the COVID-19 pandemic, there was a decline of 16.4% in the number of articles published ($p = 0.001$). This decline was similar between men and women ($p = 0.603$) and was associated with a worsening in Qualis rank ($p = 0.001$). The number of studies published in journals with impact factors was also affected ($p = 0.001$). The findings suggest a potential impact of the COVID-19 pandemic on the scientific production of Brazilian researchers in the field of physical education. Funding agencies should consider the challenges associated with the COVID-19 pandemic before evaluating researchers and programs.

Keywords: COVID-19; bibliometrics; physical education and training; behavioral research

1. Introduction

At the end of 2019, the world was impacted by a new condition responsible for causing fever, dyspnea, pneumonia, and death in individuals of all ages [1]. The first cases, identified in the city of Wuhan, China, showed an alarming rate of dissemination, affecting more than 775 million people in different countries [2]. Histological analyses indicated that the disease resulted from infection with SARS-CoV-2, prompting the World Health Organization to classify it as COVID-19 (referring to the type of virus and the year of disease as identification).

The first case of COVID-19 in Brazil was reported in February 2020 [3]. Similar to other countries, this disease was highly prevalent, with more than 37 million people infected and 700 thousand deaths [2]. In Brazil, this scenario was aggravated by conflicting governmental policies that recommended the use of medications with dubious efficacy against COVID-19 and delayed vaccine acquisition [4–7].

In early 2020, the World Health Organization declared the novel coronavirus, and the associated disease, COVID-19, a global pandemic. This prompted countries, states, and municipalities to take measures to contain the spread of the virus and reduce the burden on clinics and hospitals. Mask mandates, constant hand hygiene, and shelter-in-place orders were important preventive measures for this disease [8,9]. Social isolation, although necessary to decrease the spread of COVID-19, has affected people's behavior in situations that require direct human contact [10]. For instance, physical education professionals had to adapt to the pandemic by developing online exercise programs to maintain a minimum level of physical activity for people of all ages [11–13].

In situations where social restriction and face-to-face contact were discouraged, research in physical education may have been affected. While the implementation of lockdowns has played an important role in reducing the spread of the virus, hospitalizations, and deaths caused by COVID-19, it also created challenges for conducting new studies requiring direct participant involvement, which potentially affected academic production [14].

The possible impact of the COVID-19 pandemic on scientific production is significant because universities are regularly evaluated by funding agencies based on their published manuscripts. Researchers have reported a reduction in research funding during the COVID-19 pandemic [15,16]. To secure increased financial investment and acquire additional resources, deans exert consistent pressure on researchers to increase research productivity and publish in high-impact journals.

There is growing political pressure on universities to intensify partnerships and enlarge research funding options [17]. The underlying explanation behind the "publish or perish" attitude is that programs with stronger publication records are more likely to attract additional resources. Consequently, scholars who publish infrequently or prioritize activities that do not directly result in publications may find themselves at a disadvantage when competing for academic positions (e.g., assistant professor, lecturer) [18].

In view of the aforementioned, this study investigated the potential impact of the COVID-19 pandemic on the scientific production of graduate programs in Brazil focused on the area of physical education. Confirming the hypothesis that the production of manuscripts was affected by COVID-19, funding agencies should consider the challenges posed by the COVID-19 pandemic before evaluating researchers and programs.

2. Methods

This bibliometric study targeted 558 researchers from graduate programs in physical education in Brazil. The study protocol was submitted and approved by the Internal Review Board (protocol: # 5.454.817). The study was conducted in accordance with the Guideline for Reporting Bibliometric Review of the Biomedical Literature (BIBLIO) [19].

The inclusion criteria included researchers who were faculty members of graduate programs in physical education. The exclusion criteria involved researchers who were members of programs created after 2017 because, in Brazil, a master's thesis takes up to two years to be completed and a doctorate dissertation takes up to four years; therefore, researchers of programs created after 2017 would not have their scientific production assessed before the COVID-19 pandemic. Out of the 39 graduate programs in physical education in Brazil, 27 met the eligibility criteria.

After the selection of the graduate programs, all faculty members were cataloged. The scientific production from 2018 to 2022 of the researchers was analyzed. The definition for this period was based on the COVID-19 pandemic in Brazil. Since the first case of the disease was identified in February 2020 [3], analyzing the years 2018 and 2019 would allow us to observe the scientific production before the COVID-19 pandemic. In 2020 and 2021, the disease was highly prevalent, and lockdowns and shelter-in-place (social restrictions) measures were implemented [20]. In 2022, the disease was still present, but was now mitigated by extensive vaccination of the Brazilian population [21].

Researchers' production was limited to the publication of peer-reviewed articles published in scientific journals. The other forms of scholarly work such as abstracts, event presentations, pre-prints, thesis, and dissertations were not considered in the analysis. Despite being important academic work, they are usually not evaluated by funding agencies.

The scientific production of the researchers was extracted from the Brazilian Curriculum Lattes platform (https://lattes.cnpq.br/, accessed on 1 March 2024). Briefly, the Lattes Platform is an information system maintained by the Brazilian federal government to manage information on science, technology, and innovation related to research in Brazil. This database is a digital curriculum vitae/memorial in which researchers document their scientific production [22]. By creating and submitting records to Curriculum Lattes, researchers acknowledge that this information is available to the public and authorize its use to support the evaluation of graduate programs and research. To ensure data privacy, the names of the researchers were preserved and only general information about the studies (such as year of publication and journal indexing) was extracted. In this study, the scientific production of all researchers was analyzed from 2018 to 2022 (5-year follow-up). Analyses were conducted between March and December of 2023.

The scientific production of the researchers was evaluated using the number of manuscripts published annually, irrespective of the quality of the studies. Additionally, two specific metrics known to assess the quality and representativeness of journals in the scientific community were adopted: the Qualis rank system and the Web of Science® impact factor [23,24].

Qualis is the official journal ranking system of the Brazilian government and is managed by the CAPES Foundation (Portuguese: Coordenação de Aperfeiçoamento de Pessoal de Nível Superior) [25]. This classification system assigns grades to journals based on their circulation level (i.e., local, national, or international). The current Qualis rank system categorizes journals into three main groups: "A" (this includes subcategories A1, A2, A3, and A4), "B" (this includes subcategories B1, B2, B3, and B4), and "C". Journals in the "A" category have the highest representability in the scientific community, typically featuring international circulation and indexed in important databases such as PUBMed®. Journals in the "B" category have good representability in the scientific community, generally with national circulation, and are indexed in databases such as SciELO®. Journals in the "C" category usually have a local circulation.

The impact factor of the journals was assessed using the Web of Science® Journal Citation Reports (JCR). The JCR is a comprehensive resource that provides data on academic journals in the sciences and social sciences. The journal's impact factor—one of the most well-known metrics provided by the JCR—is used to measure the importance of journals by calculating the number of times articles have been cited in recent years [26]. The higher the journal's impact factor, the better the journal's classification.

Statistical Analysis

Data were presented as absolute frequencies, means, and standard deviations. Inferential analyses were performed using non-parametric tests, as these are normally applied to ordinal and nominal data. The chi-squared test was used to analyze the variability in the total number of articles published before and during the COVID-19 pandemic. This test, along with likelihood ratio analysis, was used to assess the impact of the COVID-19 pandemic according to the region of the graduate program in Brazil, the researcher's sex, and the Qualis rank system. Additionally, the Kruskall-Wallis H test was used to analyze the impact factor of the journals in which the articles were published, with the year of publication being included as an independent variable and the impact factor as a dependent variable. For all analyses, significance was set at 5%.

3. Results

Twenty-seven graduate programs in physical education were analyzed in this study. The programs are located in different regions of Brazil: twelve are located in the Southeast, seven in the South, six in the Northeast, and two in the Midwest region of the country. There was no graduate program in physical education in the North region of Brazil that met the eligibility criteria. A total of 558 researchers were included. The majority were male (70.8%, $p = 0.001$), with a significant portion of faculty members affiliated with programs located in the Southeast region (48.9%, $p = 0.001$). Figure 1 provides detailed characteristics of the programs and researchers included in this study.

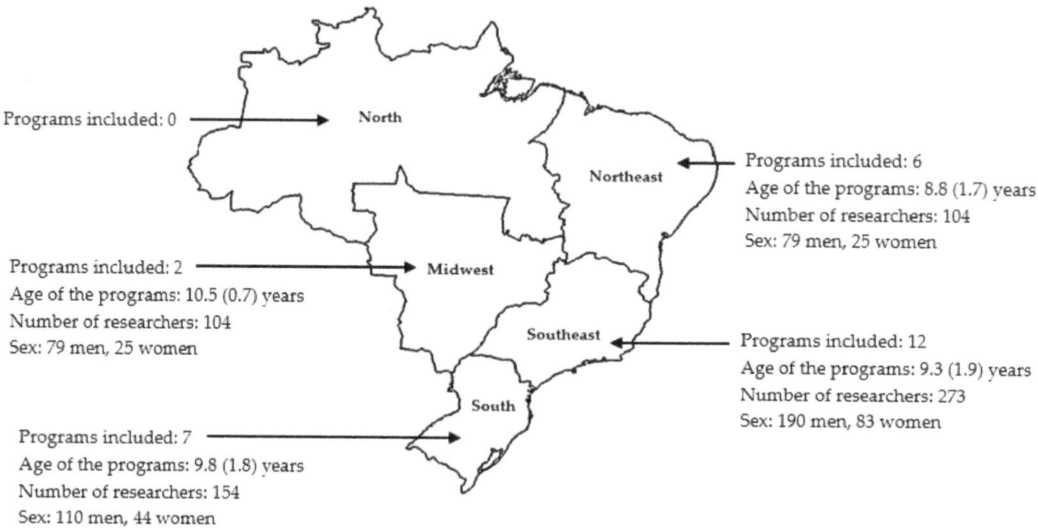

Figure 1. Characteristics of the programs and researchers in Physical Education in Brazil.

A total of 19,296 manuscripts were extracted and analyzed from the Curriculum Lattes of the researchers. Out of the 19,296 articles, 1364 were excluded due to repeated publications, which occurred when more than one researcher was involved in the same study, causing the article to be counted multiple times. Between 2018 and 2022, 17,932 studies were published. The impact of the COVID-19 pandemic on the scientific production of researchers was observed between 2021 and 2022, with a 16.4% decline in the number of articles published. This decline was observed in all regions of Brazil and was similar between men and women. Table 1 displays the number of articles published from 2018 to 2022, separated by region and sex.

Table 1. Impact of COVID-19 on the number of studies.

Variables		Year of Publication					Total	p
		2018	2019	2020	2021	2022		
Number of studies, n		3493	3311	3840	3969	3319	17,932	0.001
Number of studies by region, n	South	1169	1038	1153	1191	943	5489	0.001
	Southeast	1638	1523	1714	1747	1577	8199	
	Midwest	158	193	203	240	186	980	
	Northeast	528	557	770	791	613	3259	
Number of studies by sex, n	Male	2660	2468	2898	3008	2497	13,531	0.603
	Female	833	843	942	961	822	4401	

The COVID-19 pandemic negatively impacted the Qualis ranks of the manuscripts published. Similar to the total number of studies, the impact on the Qualis ranks occurred between 2021 and 2022, with a 14.7% decline in the publication of articles in journals categorized as "A", 21.6% as "B", and 11.1% in the "C" category. Table 2 lists the number of articles published separated by the Qualis rank system.

Table 2. Impact of COVID-19, according to the Qualis rank.

Qualis Rank	Year of Publication					Total	p
	2018	2019	2020	2021	2022		
A1	473	437	578	617	545	2650	
A2	402	390	445	483	438	2158	
A3	263	241	293	281	220	1298	
A4	292	248	297	299	230	1366	
B1	843	746	752	638	619	3598	0.001
B2	579	589	553	508	321	2550	
B3	125	147	198	206	121	797	
B4	71	89	88	70	54	372	
C	445	424	636	867	771	3143	
Total	3493	3311	3840	3969	3319	17,932	

Of the 17,932 manuscripts analyzed, 9914 (55.29%) were published in journals with an impact factor. The number of studies published in journals with impact factors was affected by COVID-19, particularly between 2021 and 2022. By contrast, the mean score of the impact factor of the journals was not affected. Figure 2 shows the number of articles published in journals with JCR impact factors and Table 3 shows the mean impact factor scores for each year.

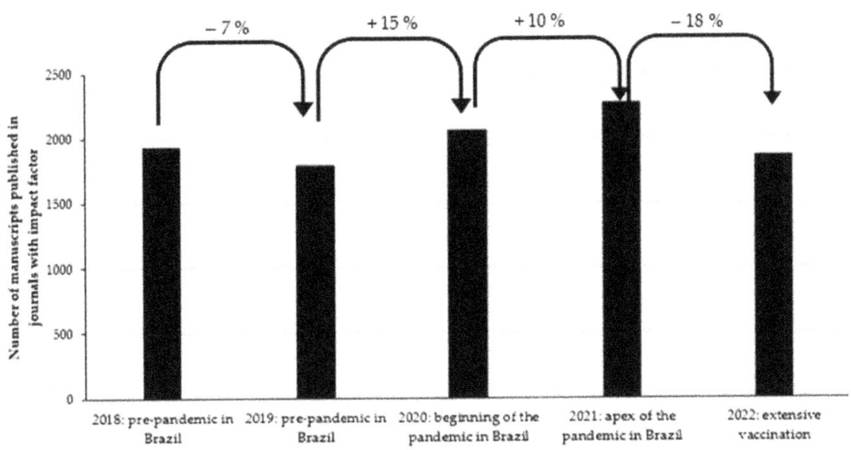

Figure 2. Impact of COVID-19 on the number of studies published in journals with impact factors.

Table 3. Impact of COVID-19, according to the Web of Science® Journal Citation Report (JCR).

	Year of Publication					p
	2018	2019	2020	2021	2022	
Mean JCR score (95% Confidence Interval)	2.501 (1.9; 3.0)	2.157 (1.8; 2.4)	3.256 (2.5; 3.9)	2.883 (2.3; 3.4)	1.932 (1.8; 2.0)	0.275

4. Discussion

This study investigated the impact of the COVID-19 pandemic on the scientific production of Brazilian researchers who are members of graduate programs in physical education. The results indicated a perceptive decline in the production of manuscripts, particularly between 2021 and 2022. The decline was similar between men and women. The Qualis rank was affected by COVID-19, resulting in a decline in publications in journals categorized as "A", "B", and "C". The quantity of articles published in journals with an impact factor was also impacted. These findings confirm our hypothesis that the scientific production and associated metrics of evaluation (i.e., quantity, journal's impact factor, and Qualis rank) would be negatively impacted by the COVID-19 pandemic. Understanding these parameters is important for analyzing the research scenario during the COVID-19 pandemic and the challenges faced by researchers and programs. This has further practical applications regarding the evaluation of researchers and graduate programs by funding agencies.

Most graduate programs in Brazil are located in the Southeast region of the country. The Southeast part of Brazil has some of the largest cities, such as São Paulo, Rio de Janeiro, and Belo Horizonte. Consequently, a significant number of researchers are in this region. This characteristic explains the data presented in Table 1, which demonstrates a higher quantity of manuscript publications in programs from this region compared to other regions.

The impact of the COVID-19 pandemic on scientific production has occurred in all regions, with a decline observed between 2021 and 2022. Considering that the first case of COVID-19 in Brazil occurred in 2020, a decline in scientific production from that year onward would be expected. However, from data collection to its publication, there is usually a time-lapse of 1–2 years [27,28]. In other words, the increase in production in 2020 and 2021 was the result of studies conducted and developed between 2018 and 2019, before the COVID-19 pandemic. Conversely, the decline in production in 2022 reflects the impact of the COVID-19 pandemic, as it encompasses articles developed between 2020 and 2021. To this end, the impact of the pandemic on the research is evident in the publications of 2022.

The number of articles published by men was greater than the number of articles published by women. These data reflect the historical profile of universities and science, which typically employ more men than women [29,30]. Considering that women represent only 29.2% of the total researchers in physical education programs in Brazil, their scientific production reaches a proportion close to this analysis (4401 articles, representing 24.5% of the production in the area). The decline in scientific production was similar between men and women. We expected to find a greater decline in the scientific production of women considering that, with the lockdown imposed during the pandemic, women were burdened with household activities and childcare in addition to their responsibilities as researchers [31]. This finding reinforces women's efforts to mitigate the impact of the COVID-19 pandemic on their scientific production, resulting in a decline similar to that observed for men.

The Qualis rank system is a method used to assess the scientific production of researchers and programs in Brazil [32]. It considers both the indexing and the Scopus quartile ranking of the journals. As these metrics are constantly changing; the Qualis rank system is, from time to time, updated by the Brazilian government. There have been many criticisms regarding Qualis as a mechanism for measuring quality. It has been argued that using a single metric to evaluate different areas of expertise tends to cause distortions in criteria [33]. In addition, journals classified in the lower categories of Qualis tend to remain in the same category because researchers do not submit their manuscripts to these journals. This prevents journals from improving their Qualis rank [34]. Despite the criticism of Qualis, we chose to use this metric because it is a federal governmental mechanism for evaluating graduate programs in Brazil.

When analyzing the Qualis rank, the total number of articles published in journals categorized as "A", "B", and "C" declined during 2021 and 2022. Considering that categories "A" and "B" denote journals of higher quality, this finding allows us to assert that not only was the quantity of manuscripts impacted by the COVID-19 pandemic, but also the quality of the studies developed.

Similar to Qualis, there are many criticisms regarding the use of impact factors to evaluate the quality of an article [35]. If a journal is evaluated based on the number of citations, there may be a bias caused by researchers and reviewers who forcibly cite and recommend their references, seeking to improve the impact factor of the journals and their chances of publication [36]. Since there is no consensus on the best form to evaluate the quality of research, we chose to include an analysis of the impact factor, along with Qualis.

Figure 2 shows that the number of articles published in journals with impact factors declined between 2021 and 2022. This finding reinforces that the impact of COVID-19 on Brazilian researchers occurred in 2022. The impact factors of the journals in which the studies were published remained consistent over the years (Table 3). This demonstrates an effort of researchers to maintain the quality of their scientific production, even though the number of articles published in journals with impact factors has declined.

For the screening of scientific production, it is possible to use the Curriculum Lattes platform or perform an active search in databases such as PubMed®, Scopus®, or EMBASE®. We opted to use Curriculum Lattes for three reasons: First, many journals are present in more than one database, which could lead to the inclusion of repetitive articles. Second, some journals do not provide an option to search for recently accepted articles; on the other hand, the Curriculum Lattes platform allows researchers to enter information about an approved article immediately after receiving an acceptance letter from the journal. Third, Curriculum Lattes is a tool that each researcher must update regularly as programs are constantly evaluated [37]. For these reasons, we chose to conduct an analysis on the researchers' Curriculum Lattes rather than on the databases.

Our findings confirm the results of previous studies on the impact of the pandemic on scientific research and clinical academic training [38–40]. According to Riccaboni and Verginer [39], the pandemic induced a sudden increase in research output related to COVID-19 and a significant drop in overall publishing rates in areas unrelated to COVID-19. Raynaud et al. [40] identified an 18% decrease in non-COVID-19 research during the pandemic. This finding is consistent with those of the present study. However, it is important to highlight that our study included only researchers working in the field of physical education, whereas Raynaud et al. [40] conducted a broader study without a focus on any specific field.

This study had some limitations. First, the exclusion of repeated manuscripts identified in Curriculum Lattes was based on the first appearance of the study in the statistical spreadsheet and did not consider the order of authorship or the research location. This might impact the number of articles developed by men or women or the region in which the study was produced. Second, it is possible that a researcher is affiliated with more than one graduate program, and their production may pertain to two distinct areas. In these cases, all the articles were counted because it was not possible to precisely identify the program to which each study belonged. Third, we standardized the use of metrics (Qualis and impact factor) of journals in 2023. It is possible that a journal had a change in Qualis or impact factor score during the 5-year timeline of this study [41]. Despite these limitations, we were able to provide valuable information on the quantity and quality of Brazilian researchers' scientific production and how it was impacted by the COVID-19 pandemic. Future studies should attempt to address the potential impact of the COVID-19 pandemic in other areas to determine if the pattern observed in physical education holds true in different fields. Since COVID-19 has waned, future studies should further investigate whether such publication metrics have returned to levels prior to the pandemic.

5. Conclusions

The COVID-19 pandemic negatively affected the scientific production of physical education researchers in Brazil. Both the quantity and quality of manuscripts were impacted with no clear distinction of such impact in the scientific production of both men and women. The results should be considered by government agencies when evaluating graduate programs in the area of physical education—although other areas have most likely been impacted as well—during the pandemic. This is important because although COVID-19 has waned, some of its consequences may still linger in different areas of society, including, but not limited to, scientific research and its protagonists: researchers and participants.

Author Contributions: Conceptualization, S.J.L.d.M., V.P.P. and G.C.; methodology, S.J.L.d.M., V.P.P., E.S. and G.C.; formal analysis, S.J.L.d.M., V.P.P., É.d.M.S.C. and G.C.; writing—original draft preparation, S.J.L.d.M., E.S., É.d.M.S.C. and G.C.; writing—review and editing, S.J.L.d.M., E.S., É.d.M.S.C. and G.C.; project administration, S.J.L.d.M. and G.C.; funding acquisition, G.C. All authors have read and agreed to the published version of the manuscript.

Funding: This study was funded by the National Council for Scientific and Technological Development (CNPq grant n. 403238/2023-4), by the Scientific Foundation of the state of Mato Grosso do Sul (FUNDECT grant n. 275/2022, SIAFEM: 32194, Process N. 71/032.871/2022), and by the Brazilian Coordination for the Improvement of Higher Education Personnel (CAPES grant number Finance Code 001).

Institutional Review Board Statement: The study was approved by the Ethics Committee of the Federal University of Mato Grosso do Sul (protocol: # 5.454.817, approval date: 7 June 2022).

Informed Consent Statement: As the data were collected from a public repository, the institutional ethics committee waived the need for written consent.

Data Availability Statement: The data presented in this study are available on request from the corresponding author.

Acknowledgments: To the graduate programs "Health and Development of the Midwest Region of Brazil (Faculty of Medicine)" and "Movement Sciences" (Institute of Health). To the Brazilian Coordination for the Improvement of Higher Education Personnel, which provided a scholarship to S.J.L.d.M. and É.d.M.S.C.

Conflicts of Interest: The authors declare no conflicts of interest.

References

1. Zhao, M.; Wang, M.; Zhang, J.; Gu, J.; Zhang, P.; Xu, Y.; Ye, J.; Wang, Z.; Ye, D.; Pan, W.; et al. Comparison of clinical characteristics and outcomes of patients with coronavirus disease 2019 at different ages. *Aging* **2020**, *12*, 10070–10086. [CrossRef]
2. World Health Organization. WHO Coronavirus (COVID-19) Dashboard. 2023. Available online: https://covid19.who.int/?mapFilter=deaths (accessed on 27 January 2024).
3. Rodriguez-Morales, A.J.; Gallego, V.; Escalera-Antezana, J.P.; Méndez, C.A.; Zambrano, L.I.; Franco-Paredes, C.; Suárez, J.A.; Rodriguez-Enciso, H.D.; Balbin-Ramon, G.J.; Savio-Larriera, E.; et al. COVID-19 in Latin America: The implications of the first confirmed case in Brazil. *Travel Med. Infect. Dis.* **2020**, *35*, 101613. [CrossRef]
4. Lotta, G.; Wenham, C.; Nunes, J.; Pimenta, D.N. Community health workers reveal COVID-19 disaster in Brazil. *Lancet* **2020**, *396*, 365–366. [CrossRef]
5. Silva, H.M. Medicines and illusions in the fight against COVID-19 in Brazil. *Ethics Med. Public Health* **2021**, *16*, 100622. [CrossRef]
6. Hallal, P.C. SOS Brazil: Science under attack. *Lancet* **2021**, *397*, 373–374. [CrossRef]
7. Gramacho, W.G.; Turgeon, M. When politics collides with public health: COVID-19 vaccine country of origin and vaccination acceptance in Brazil. *Vaccine* **2021**, *39*, 2608–2612. [CrossRef]
8. Talic, S.; Shah, S.; Wild, H.; Gasevic, D.; Maharaj, A.; Ademi, Z.; Li, X.; Xu, W.; Mesa-Eguiagaray, I.; Rostron, J.; et al. Effectiveness of public health measures in reducing the incidence of COVID-19, SARS-CoV-2 transmission, and COVID-19 mortality: Systematic review and meta-analysis. *BMJ Clin. Res. Ed.* **2021**, *375*, e068302. [CrossRef]
9. Ayenigbara, I.O.; Adeleke, O.R.; Ayenigbara, G.O.; Adegboro, J.S.; Olofintuyi, O.O. COVID-19 (SARS-CoV-2) pandemic: Fears, facts and preventive measures. *Germs* **2020**, *10*, 218–228. [CrossRef]
10. Bezerra, A.C.V.; Silva, C.E.M.D.; Soares, F.R.G.; Silva, J.A.M.D. Factors associated with people's behavior in social isolation during the COVID-19 pandemic. *Cien Saude Colet* **2020**, *25* (Suppl. S1), 2411–2421. [CrossRef]
11. Bailey, R.; Scheuer, C. The COVID-19 pandemic as a fortuitous disruptor in physical education: The case of active homework. *AIMS Public Health* **2022**, *9*, 423–439. [CrossRef]
12. Pavlovic, A.; DeFina, L.F.; Natale, B.L.; Thiele, S.E.; Walker, T.J.; Craig, D.W.; Vint, G.R.; Leonard, D.; Haskell, W.L.; Kohl, H.W. Keeping children healthy during and after COVID-19 pandemic: Meeting youth physical activity needs. *BMC Public Health* **2021**, *21*, 485. [CrossRef] [PubMed]
13. Lúcio Barbosa, N.; Burke, T.N.; Christofolleti, G.; de Alencar, G.P. Burnout syndrome, work ability, quality of life and physical activity in teachers during the COVID-19 pandemic in Campo Grande, Brazil. *Work—J. Prev. Assess. Rehabil.* **2023**, *75*, 45–53. [CrossRef]
14. Caputo, E.L.; Feter, N.; Rombaldi, A.J.; da Silva, M.C.; Reichert, F.F. What are the challenges of epidemiological research during the COVID-19 pandemic? *Motriz* **2021**, *27*, e10200200. [CrossRef]
15. Knobel, M.; Leal, F. The Tragedies of Brazilian Higher Education. *Int. Higher Educ.* **2021**, *105*, 35–36. Available online: https://ejournals.bc.edu/index.php/ihe/article/view/14397 (accessed on 15 March 2024).

16. Neves, A.A.B.; McManus, C.; de Carvalho, C.H. The Impact of Graduate Studies and Science in Brazil: An analysis in the light of the indicators. *Rev. Nupem* **2020**, *12*, 254–276. [CrossRef]
17. Muscio, A.; Quaglione, D.; Vallanti, G. Does government funding complement or substitute private research funding to universities? *Res. Policy* **2013**, *42*, 63–75. [CrossRef]
18. Rawat, S.; Meena, S. Publish or perish: Where are we heading? *J. Res. Med. Sci.* **2014**, *19*, 87–89. [PubMed]
19. Montazeri, A.; Mohammadi, S.; Hesair, P.M.; Riazi, H.; Sheikhi-Mobarakeh, Z. Preliminary guideline for reporting bibliometric reviews of the biomedical literature (BIBLIO): A minimum requirements. *Syst. Rev.* **2023**, *15*, 239. [CrossRef] [PubMed]
20. Brasil. Recommendations for the Implementation of More Restrictive Social Distancing Measures (Lockdown), in Municipalities with an Accelerated Occurrence of New Cases of COVID-19 and with Service Occupancy Rates Reaching Critical Levels. 2020. Available online: https://conselho.saude.gov.br/recomendacoes-cns/1163-recomendac-a-o-n-036-de-11-de-maio-de-2020 (accessed on 25 October 2023).
21. Castro, R. Vacinas contra a COVID-19: O fim da pandemia? *Physis Rev. Saúde Coletiva* **2021**, *31*, e310100. [CrossRef]
22. Mena-Chalco, J.P.; Junior, R.M.C. scriptLattes: An open-source knowledge extraction system from the Lattes platform. *J. Braz. Comput. Soc.* **2009**, *15*, 31–39. [CrossRef]
23. Bacal, F. Archives and the new Capes Qualis. *Arq. Bras. Cardiol.* **2009**, *92*, 395. [CrossRef]
24. Jotz, G.P.; Montefusco, A.M. International Archives of Otorhinolaryngology celebrates achievement of its first impact factor in JCR. *Int. Arch. Otorhinolaryngol.* **2023**, *27*, e547–e548. [CrossRef]
25. Marenco, A. When Institutions matter: Capes and Political science in Brazil. *Rev. Ciência Política* **2015**, *35*, 33–46. [CrossRef]
26. Moussa, S. A bibliometric investigation of the journals that were repeatedly suppressed from Clarivate's Journal Citation Reports. *Account. Res.* **2023**, *30*, 592–612. [CrossRef]
27. Camp, W.K. Why does it take so long to publish a paper in the AAPG Bulletin? *AAPG Bull.* **2024**, *108*, 225–234. [CrossRef]
28. Inman, D.J.; Wereley, N.M. How long does it take to publish a paper? *J. Intell. Mater. Syst. Struct.* **2010**, *21*, 123. [CrossRef]
29. Sanches-Oro, R.; Torres Nuez, J.; Fatahi Bandpey, M.L.; Martínez-Sanz, G. Marie Curie: How to break the glass ceiling in science and in radiology. *Radiol. Engl. Ed.* **2021**, *63*, 456–465. [CrossRef] [PubMed]
30. Segovia-Saiz, C.; Briones-Vozmediano, E.; Pastells-Peiró, R.; González-María, E.; Gea-Sánchez, M. Glass ceiling and gender inequalities in the careers of women academics in biomedical sciences. *Gac. Sanit.* **2020**, *34*, 403–410. [CrossRef]
31. Collins, C. Productivity in a pandemic. *Science* **2020**, *369*, 603. [CrossRef] [PubMed]
32. Jaffé, R. QUALIS: The journal ranking system undermining the impact of Brazilian science. *An. Acad. Bras. Ciências* **2020**, *92*, e20201116. [CrossRef] [PubMed]
33. Barata, R.B. Necessary changes in the evaluation of graduate programs in Brazil. *Interface* **2019**, *23*, e180635. [CrossRef]
34. Andriolo, A.; Souza, A.F.; Farias, A.Q.; Barbosa, A.J.; França Netto, A.S.; Hernandez, A.J.; Camargos, A.F.; Barraviera, B.; Kadunc, B.V.; Caramelli, B.; et al. Classification of journals in the QUALIS System of CAPES urgent need of changing the criteria! *Arq. Neuro-Psiquiatr.* **2010**, *68*, 327–329. [CrossRef]
35. Há, T.C.; Tan, S.B.; Soo, K.C. The Journal Impact Factor: Too Much of an Impact? *Ann. Acad. Med. Singap.* **2006**, *35*, 911–916. [CrossRef] [PubMed]
36. Peebles, E.; Scandlyn, M.; Hesp, B.R. A retrospective study investigating requests for self-citation during open peer review in a general medicine journal. *PLoS ONE* **2020**, *15*, e0237804. [CrossRef] [PubMed]
37. do Nascimento, J.L.; Nunes, E.D. Almost an autobiography: A study of social scientists in health based on the Lattes Curriculum. *Ciência Saúde Coletiva* **2014**, *19*, 1077–1084. [CrossRef]
38. Sohrabi, C.; Mathew, G.; Franchi, T.; Kerwan, A.; Griffin, M.; Soleil, C.; Del Mundo, J.; Ali, S.A.; Agha, M.; Agha, R. Impact of the coronavirus (COVID-19) pandemic on scientific research and implications for clinical academic training—A review. *Int. J. Surg.* **2021**, *86*, 57–63. [CrossRef] [PubMed]
39. Riccaboni, M.; Verginer, L. The impact of the COVID-19 pandemic on scientific research in the life sciences. *PLoS ONE* **2022**, *17*, e0263001. [CrossRef]
40. Raynaud, M.; Goutaudier, V.; Louis, K.; Al-Awadhi, S.; Dubourg, Q.; Truchot, A.; Brousse, R.; Saleh, N.; Giarraputo, A.; Debiais, C.; et al. Impact of the COVID-19 pandemic on publication dynamics and non-COVID-19 research production. *BMC Med. Res. Methodol.* **2021**, *21*, 255. [CrossRef]
41. Nascimento, O.A.S.; Filho, A.L. Scientific journals in Brazilian physical education: Publications, institutions and indexers. *Movimento* **2023**, *29*, e29048. [CrossRef]

MDPI AG
Grosspeteranlage 5
4052 Basel
Switzerland
Tel.: +41 61 683 77 34

Behavioral Sciences Editorial Office
E-mail: behavsci@mdpi.com
www.mdpi.com/journal/behavsci

www.ingramcontent.com/pod-product-compliance
Lightning Source LLC
Chambersburg PA
CBHW040746250926
51850CB00007BB/1427
* 9 7 8 3 7 2 5 8 5 4 6 9 1 *